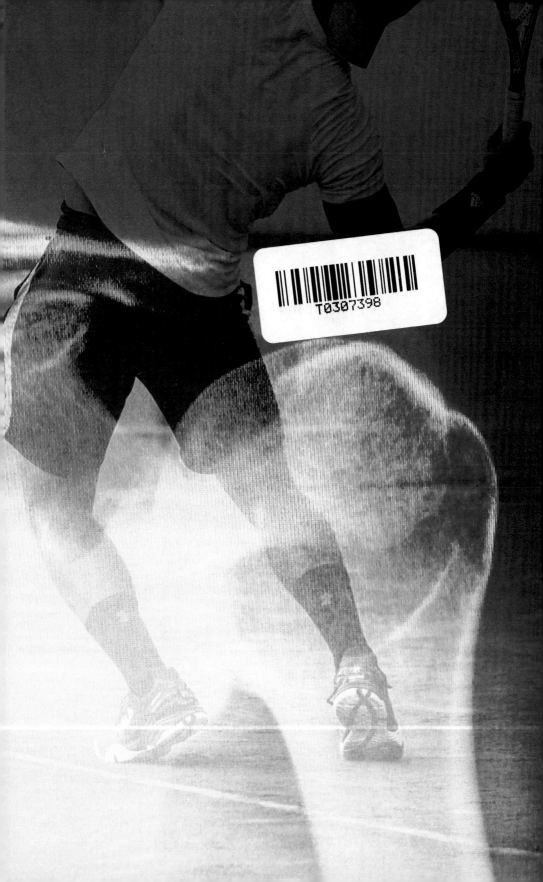

Also available at all good book stores

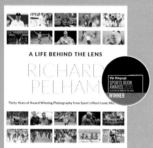

9781785315466

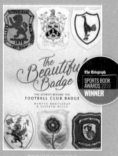

9781785313929

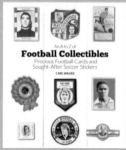

9781785315602

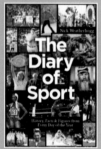

9781785316289

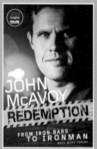

9781785316005

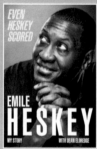

9781785315008

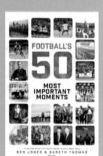

9781785316326

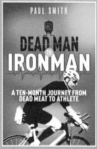

9781785316173

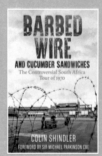

9781785316340

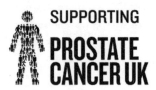

KNIFE
IN THE
FAST LANE

A Surgeon's Perspective
from the Sharp End of Sport

BILL RIBBANS

First published by Pitch Publishing, 2020

Pitch Publishing
A2 Yeoman Gate
Yeoman Way
Worthing
Sussex
BN13 3QZ
www.pitchpublishing.co.uk
info@pitchpublishing.co.uk

A CIP catalogue record is available for this book
from the British Library.

ISBN 978 1 78531 688 3

Typesetting and origination by Pitch Publishing
Printed and bound in Great Britain by TJ Books, Padstow

CONTENTS

FOREWORD – THE ATHLETE

I FIRST met Bill back in 2005 when I was being plagued by chronic ankle pain. I had not officially turned professional at this point and feared the injury would scupper my career before it had started.

Bill was a leading expert in his field of orthopaedic surgery and British Athletics asked me to seek his advice on the best course of action. After scans and assessments, a large ankle spur was found, which needed removal. I was anxious prior to the surgery; at this point I wasn't experienced in going under the knife (as I'd go on to become!), but Bill had a calm reassurance which put any fears of an unsuccessful recovery to bed. As an athlete, the urgency to get back to doing what you love is paramount. Bill has a willingness to help any athlete in the most efficient and straightforward fashion.

Sportspeople fear surgery and view it as a last resort. And while an enlightened coach will take the time to understand that surgery may be necessary, others will always believe you can push on through regardless, under the guise of 'character building'.

Bill was open to exploring alternative means of treatment before reaching for the knife, which offered a comforting balance of urgency without hastiness. There were multiple occasions on which he needed to consider countless avenues of treatment for me including injections and physiotherapy. I had two further injuries later in my career when I also finished up on his operating table.

For a professional sportsperson, developing trust and fostering an ongoing relationship with someone who fixes your body is incredibly important. I have a huge level of respect for those responsible for maintaining the inner workings of someone who relies on their body for performance. I seek advice from Bill with regards to my body even to this day.

This book is a fantastic resource for anybody, particularly athletes, who hope to gain a true understanding of what it takes to keep the body at its peak of physical fitness, and understand the methods someone like Bill uses, and meticulous duty of care he takes, in order to keep an athlete prospering. It is a must-read for those keen to understand how physical well-being is intrinsic to high-quality performance, from professional athletes to weekend joggers, and should be compulsory reading for those overseeing athletes.

I had the great honour to officially open Bill's clinic in Northampton. Considering he has worked with some of the biggest names in sport, I feel incredibly privileged that he has asked me to write this foreword. It is difficult to convey both how important a role he has played for me over the years and demonstrate on a personal level how decent and affable a human he has always been.

Greg Rutherford MBE.
Olympic, World, European and
Commonwealth long jump champion.

FOREWORD – THE COACH

MY FIRST meeting with Bill, in Northampton back in 1995, had been arranged by a good friend, Phil Pask, a part-time physio and fitness conditioner at the club. Rugby had just gone professional and we had been challenged by our great chairman, Keith Barwell, with taking the club forward into the new era.

The three of us were looking at the medical support which was going to be necessary for the emerging professional players, and the responsibility which needed to be taken by the club for their well-being. What transpired was four incredibly happy and enjoyable years, simply because everyone concerned loved rugby and the club and the challenge.

What quickly became apparent was that Bill was a sportsman as well as a surgeon and he had an understanding and appreciation of the many different aspects of a sporting environment. From the outset, his approach gave me the confidence to know that an outstanding environment was evolving.

We knocked down two changing rooms in the old wooden stand to create a medical room. Bill created a network of surgeons who would make themselves available at short notice to deal with any player emergencies. Often the player would turn up at the hospital transported in the back of Bill's car.

As a coach, I have always believed in the philosophy and approach of 'Teams within Teams', both on and off the field. The confidence I got from advice given by Bill, Phil Pask and the other medical staff took pressure away from me. It was an atmosphere created by trust and respect. They made player welfare their responsibility.

These relationships and friendships forged from our collective challenge supported an outstanding group of players, which led to

Northampton Saints' first-ever trophy – the European Cup in 2000. We had given ourselves the target of winning it in five years; it was won in four!

This book is a tremendous insight into the work and approach needed when medicine meets sport, and how interrelated those environments are if success is to be achieved.

I have been very fortunate to have had the opportunity to work with, and be advised by, people such as Bill and James Robson (my doctor with Scotland and the Lions). Without them, as a coach, I would have found it extremely difficult to have any chance of success.

Understanding players, as a coach, comes from so many different directions.

Importantly, players speak honestly in the medical room to both doctors and physios – about physical and mental well-being. Without losing confidentiality it is the advice I received from the doctors which progressively guided me on how I should adapt training and my approach to it; sometimes I cancelled it.

Having quality medical personnel alongside you creates the most valuable environment in which to perform – an honest and trusted sounding board for decisions to be made in relation to the players as a group, but more importantly as individuals.

What this book achieves so successfully is the description of the environment we both shared, of the exposure to challenge, and the need for continuous analysis, practice, repetition and review, from which comes the incredible feeling of knowing you are part of something special and learning something new and adapting every day. It is the awareness and appreciation of the differences in skills and expertise which give strength to the whole group.

Bill's experience and expertise, from being involved with so many sports at a high level, gives a breadth of knowledge and understanding that all medical and non-medical staff entering the sporting environment can benefit from. Knowing what you are coming into helps you avoid unnecessary errors and continues to enhance best practice.

Rugby is at a crossroads for player welfare, and more than ever needs clarity of thinking to ensure competitions and game management make it as safe as possible. Medical science has to be at the forefront of that thinking; lessons learnt since the days of first creating medical rooms under wooden stands have to be acknowledged and understood.

This book should be mandatory reading for all administrators who take responsibility for the direction of rugby union and the welfare of its players.

Sir Ian McGeechan OBE.
Coach to Headingley, Northampton, Wasps, Scotland
and British Lions.

INTRODUCTION

THE CONSEQUENCES of exercise are not always positive. Sport can be exhilarating to play and thrilling to spectate. However, injury and illness caused by sport remind us that it is an intrinsically precarious enterprise. Its activities can fly in the face of society's preoccupation with health and safety. A doctor's duty in sport includes trying to reduce risk. Failing this, you must strive to treat the problems with all the skills available.

I became involved in sports medicine in 1981 having enlisted as a part-time medical officer with the British Boxing Board of Control. I had no idea how my career would develop or how medicine would evolve in the following decades; sports medicine would not be recognised as a speciality for another 25 years. I chose orthopaedic surgery. Career progress was slow and uncertain. Building a career and reputation within sport depends on developing networks with fellow professionals – becoming a team-player and looking at athletes from a holistic viewpoint.

I have interwoven my own experiences of sports surgery with the broader questions that face doctors involved in sport. These doctors face difficult ethical issues: pressures from sporting establishments and changing room mutinies; confidentiality; the decision to challenge when players want untried remedies. All this while working within an increasingly litigious society.

The power of medicine and surgery to treat and return athletes to play has increased enormously. But has our increased ability really reduced injuries or are we simply returning players to face the next big hit? How far should the duty of care of doctors extend? Should we insist that sporting bodies take action to prolong careers and prevent long-term disability, as the Football Association has done recently in banning under-12s from heading while training?

INTRODUCTION

I have been blessed to have consulted with and operated on many elite sports people. They have included world champions across eight different sports and athletes with 28 medals from seven Olympiads. My clinics, though, are filled predominantly with the occasional runner and gym user.

Since training and working in London I have spent a long period practising medicine in my hometown, Northampton, where I first developed my love for all kinds of sport. It has been a privilege to look after athletes from the clubs that have been my own sporting heart for over 60 years.

This book charts the history of medical care for athletes, from the eras of football managers injecting players with monkey testicle extracts and team doctors being 'detained in hospitality'. It surveys the present scene of vast numbers of highly qualified support teams swaddling today's athletes.

There is always another side to the coin, however. Sport has become populated at its fringes with quacks and charlatans. Everybody wants a piece of the action, to bask in the reflected glory. Lack of training or science to support their offerings is no barrier; these individuals will muscle to the front of any sporting queue. Athletes are surrounded by numerous advisors but are still potential prey to unscrupulous paramedical parasites who populate the sporting shadows. Some elite athletes still want to have the afterbirth of a horse rubbed on their ankles or a witch doctor massage their thighs with leaves.

The world and his dog (especially football managers) are experts in sports medicine. I read avidly newspaper back pages and follow pronouncements on various 'new age' treatments. When media interest has evaporated, it is instructive to revisit these 'remedies' and reflect on whether the hype was justified – usually it is not.

In these pages I have chronicled some of the important welfare issues that loom large in many sports. Concussion, long-term damage to physical well-being, mental health, drug-taking and many more issues. I look at the battlegrounds where performance and welfare collide and how clinicians' roles have evolved to survive.

I have reflected on the relationship between medicine and sport. It seems a paradox at times: medicine has never been better ordered or more knowledgeable about athletes' care, but its position, function and worth must be increasingly defended against those within and without sporting organisations.

Finally, I reflect on the major changes in my profession since the early 1980s. What did we do before MRI scans? Examine patients is one answer. Did we really do charity runs to raise funds for keyhole surgery equipment? These are operations now considered to be our stock-in-trade.

If the book appears at times critical of aspects of sport, this is born of my concern for something I love. I am passionate about sport and convinced of its benefit for society. I thrill at the skills of our most talented athletes; their endeavours raise the national mood and inspire future generations. Sport encourages youngsters to spend fewer hours in front of electronic gadgets.

Mine has been a long journey but not a unique one. Many colleagues could write of similar careers. I hope this account proves of interest to sports followers, those involved in sports and health sciences, and the clinicians already involved or contemplating a career in this fascinating world.

The book is primarily about my patients, however. I learn from them every working day. I never forget that it is an honour for patients to consent and trust me to undertake surgery on them. Medicine is like sport. It is about exposure to the challenge. The need for analysis, planning, practice, repetition and review. Sporting endeavour mirrors my own ongoing professional growth: reflection, adaptation and continued learning.

Chapter 1

WEALTH, HEALTH AND SPORT

The times they are a changing
'Come gather 'round, people
Wherever you roam
And admit that the waters
Around you have grown'

Bob Dylan, 'The Times They Are A-Changin' (1964)

ON 30 July 1966 England defeated West Germany 4-2 to become football world champions. Arguably, it was the greatest sporting team triumph in English history. As a youngster, I was captivated. Scrapbooks and posters littered my bedroom. I still have a ticket from every one of the 32 games. I bought as many newspapers my pocket money would allow. I was hungry for news and comment. There was not a lot for a lad to feed on.

On the Saturday morning of the final the *Birmingham Post* found no place for the game on its front page. 'Traffic stopped by hailstones in Scotland' did make it. Page 13 had a pre-match article and team news. The *Post*'s Monday edition allowed news of the weekend's victory to creep on to page one but it was given fifth billing behind stories such as, 'Religion holds up operation'. Page 11 had a game report from the sports desk.

The *Sunday Times* featured a story on its front page but only to deal with its aftermath: 'London goes mad after World Cup victory'. Rolls Royce's jet engine order and chief superintendent MacArthur of Scotland Yard ranked higher. The match report was tucked away on page 16.

Fast forward to the 2018 World Cup. England's semi-final exit to Croatia was splashed across the front of *The Times* and covered its entire back page, and two further inside pages were devoted to the story. There was a 12-page semi-final special and a four-page wrap-around section – 'Thanks for the Memories!' What of MacArthur's Scotland Yard successors? Efforts to capture the Salisbury novichok poisoning villains were relegated to page 19.

Different times, different priorities.

Sport has preoccupied the British for centuries. For the avid follower of yesteryear, reports of sporting events came via local and national newspapers and later the radio. The first major sporting event broadcast on television was a tennis match from Wimbledon in 1937. FA Cup finals, Test matches and the Boat Race started a year later but only 20,000 television sets were in use to receive their coverage. Queen Elizabeth's coronation in 1953 is credited with the boom in TV ownership and by 1960 ten million homes had a television.

During the 1950s and early 1960s attempts were made to show football highlights on television, but it was *Match of the Day* (*MotD*) that would become the beating heart of the soccer fan. The programme was launched in August 1964 but the BBC offered highlights of one game only.

There were no slow-motion replays, no pundits. The first programme showcased Liverpool against Arsenal. It attracted an audience of just 20,000 viewers – less than half the attendance at Anfield earlier that day. By the time *MotD* celebrated its 50th birthday in 2014, seven million people were tuning in.

It's something of a cliché to talk of sport as 'big business'. The term was applied by one of the founders of the English Football League in the 19th century. In reality, many English clubs below the Premier League have a turnover lower than the Lidl supermarket around the corner. It is different in the 'promised land'. By 2017 Sky TV contracts pushed the English Premier League soccer summer transfer window spend to over £1.4bn with a net outlay of £665m. These vast sums at the top end seem as unstoppable as they are unfathomable, and affect more than just a player's bank balance.

Lottery money allocated via UK Sport comes with strings attached: medals are the currency. Underperforming sports such as handball, basketball, table tennis and wrestling found themselves jettisoned after the 2012 Olympics. Success in many sports depends as much on the quantity of money thrown at it as the skills of the athletes and coaches. This applies as much to Olympic sports as any football team.

With so much money at stake, and so much focus on performance, the health of our leading athletes has become a national obsession. Concerns fill newspapers and the thoughts of many within our country. Television bulletins, radio phone-ins and social media platforms thrum to the words of pundits. Websites such as physioroom.com provide injury tables and medical updates.

On one Monday in October 2019, over 10 per cent of *The Times* sports pages had medical themes: depression and anxiety in international cricket, the doping scandal swirling around distance running coach Alberto Salazar, and tackling and concussion debates at the Rugby World Cup. I could also read of and contemplate the dubious ethics of requesting that Caster Semenya be castrated.

The nation frets over injuries. The collective blood pressure rises as major soccer tournaments approach, as we debate the effect on our side's hopes of success. In 2006 it was Wayne Rooney's fractured metatarsal and Michael Owen's anterior cruciate ligament (ACL). In 2010 it was David Beckham's ruptured Achilles. By 2014 we were back to the ACL. This time it belonged to Theo Walcott.

The British are not alone in this. In 2018 the Egyptian population waited anxiously to hear whether Mohamed Salah would recover from the shoulder injury sustained in the Champions League Final just weeks before. At the same time, Ipanema beach regulars in Brazil waited nervously for Neymar to recover from his metatarsal fracture. Both players made it to the World Cup but did not set the tournament alight.

The earnings of footballers, golfers, tennis players, Formula 1 drivers and boxers have been at impressive levels for more than half a century. Back in 2006, the Professional Footballers' Association (PFA) estimated that the average Premier League annual salary was £676,000 – before bonuses. In 2018 Alexis Sanchez's transfer from Arsenal to Manchester United earned him a £6.7m signing-on fee and an annual salary of £20.35m. It didn't stop there. He was paid an extra £75,000 every time he played, before being bundled off to Inter Milan. Teenagers breaking into top football sides can expect to receive a weekly pay packet of 200 times the national average.

Earnings abroad can be even greater for soccer's superstars. In 2018 Cristiano Ronaldo was asking Real Madrid for a weekly salary of

£1.35m to stay with the club before accepting £26.5m a year on moving to Juventus. Messi was earning £673,000 per week at Barcelona.

Recently, other sports have raised the earning potential and profiles of their leading exponents. In 1996, the advent of professionalism in rugby union allowed players to jettison other careers. Twenty years later, Premiership rugby players were earning, on average, a shade under £100,000 a year, with the *Daily Mail* estimating that nine star players earned over £300,000 each in the 2016/17 season. Average salaries doubled in the next two seasons, with Leicester's Manu Tuilagi taking home £450,000. The latter's run of injuries only allowed him to play for his club on 36 occasions in five seasons (2013 to 2018). He cost Leicester £65,000 per game he played.

By the end of the decade, annual salaries were even higher with the £1m mark approaching. Saracens were relegated in 2020 for breaching the salary cap to keep ahead of the pack.

In cricket, the 2017 'retainer fee' for the 11 centrally contracted England players was £700,000. With considerable bonuses available for appearances and captaincy status, some salaries topped the million mark.

Riches may be accrued for the chosen few in cricket's Indian Premier League (IPL) 'auction'. Even before his 2019 man-of-the-match performances in the World Cup Final and Headingley Ashes Test match, Ben Stokes received a combined total of £3.1m for his participation in the 2017 and 2018 IPL competitions. This involved a maximum of 34 days of cricket if his side made the final each year. In 2017 he played 12 times – £590 for every ball bowled in the games in which he was involved.

The media coverage rivalled that of soccer following the heroics of Stokes, Buttler, Morgan and their mates in securing the 2019 Cricket World Cup in a nerve-shredding finale at Lord's. *The Times* produced its four-page wrap-around combined with ten pages of analysis. The victory was even dissected on its editorial page. The same paper produced a 16-page supplement the following day. In terms of column inches, cricket was beginning to rival other major sports.

Up until the early 2000s the Royal Mail depicted only the monarch and members of the royal family on its stamps – unless you were dead. Since then we have been able to lick the backs of many of our sporting heroes such as rugby and cricketing world champions and Olympians and famous footballers; even 1966 football World Cup winners Bobby Moore and Geoff Hurst were not given that privilege.

Why is this reminder of the eye-watering salaries of our star sportspeople and the media's insatiable appetite for sports stories relevant? Because the prolonged robustness of athletes affects their sporting competitiveness, the health of their finances and those of the organisations that engage and control their activities. Additionally, the improving financial position and media exposure of athletes impinges on their medical care because they have the freedom to pursue wise, and not-so-wise, clinical decisions: they are increasingly attractive prey.

For a doctor entering the world of sport, it can all be bewildering. Coming from NHS training, we are expected to 'watch the pennies' and follow evidence-based remedies. Government agencies such as the National Institute of Clinical Excellence can dictate our professional pathways. We have ingrained a 'value for money' mentality. Elite sport allows unfettered access to expensive tests and treatments. 'Just in case' or 'being seen to be doing something' (even if it involves untested remedies) frequently replace logical decision-making. It can appear as untamed as the Wild West.

Chapter 2

SPORT AND THE SURGEON

Early influences

Probably my obsession with sport began at birth.

Like many post-war families, mine was in thrall to our national game. At the end of 1954 my mother was in labour in Northampton General Hospital; my father was at a football match.

In the 1950s not all fathers were at their offspring's arrival and mine had an excuse. On this occasion he had to be elsewhere – Griffin Park in west London. Dad was working under his pen name, Flag Kick, for our local newspaper, the *Chronicle and Echo*. He was reporting on the Cobblers' (the appropriate nickname of Northampton Town FC) 3-1 thrashing of Brentford.

Flash Fowler was on the left wing that day. In 1998 he was voted by supporters the club's greatest legend and included in the club's Team of the Century. Fifty years later it was my privilege to replace Flash's hip, the appendage that had arrowed in many crosses during his 552 club games.

I reflected on the history of that damaged joint as I removed it during surgery. For me and my town this damaged bone was the equivalent of Denis Compton's shattered kneecap. The latter resides in the Lord's cricket museum. In different ways, these two wonderfully gifted sportsmen gave enormous pleasure to their communities during the austere post-war years.

From three years old I was introduced to the Cobblers from the relative comfort of the press box high up in the County Ground's old wooden stand. Visits to local cricket and rugby games followed and I played school football, cricket and athletics. I remember watching my father trudge home in his grey overcoat. It was the evening of the Munich air disaster in February 1958. He was inconsolable.

I thrilled at the achievements of Danny Blanchflower's double-winning Spurs teams. Later, Jimmy Greaves became my hero. I am still gutted that he didn't play in the 1966 World Cup Final. Father took me to Villa Park to see Argentina defeat Spain on their way to their infamous quarter-final with the hosts at Wembley. Sir Alf Ramsey described them unguardedly as animals.

In 1966 I followed my father and grandfather to Northampton Grammar School which since 1541 had educated boys of the borough and beyond. The school had a fine sporting tradition but was a rugby school. Schoolboy rugby internationals were commonplace and the school was a fertile nursery for Northampton Saints. Between the rugby pitch and athletics track I achieved regional representation and national finals. However, I was never quite good enough to reach the top of the podium.

Tyro medic

I had intended to follow my father into journalism or become a PE teacher. However, I enjoyed sport too much and considered which university degree might prolong my recreational pursuits. Architecture was one option because studies lasted seven years – but I could not draw, a slight handicap in the days before there were computers to assist.

Some of my schoolmasters had other opinions. One informed my parents that I spent too much time on sport and that there was no point in staying on for A levels, which was a red rag to this competitive bull. Psychologists refer to this as a 'spontaneous influence event' – it was burnished in my brain that I would prove my mentors wrong.

Medicine looked promising and Richard Gordon's *Doctor in the House* books had entertained me. Additionally, Francis Crick, who was the co-recipient of the 1962 Nobel prize for discovering our genetic building blocks, was born in my village and attended my own grammar school. However, A levels in history, geography and economics were not the normal route to *Dr Finlay* land. A few medical schools offered a one-year crash course in sciences and one hospital offered me a place, the Royal Free in London. It was the first place to train female British doctors. The Free medical school had opened in the 1870s but did not allow male students over the threshold until 1947.

No previous family member had stayed at school beyond the age of 15 and universities were as unfamiliar to my parents as to me. In 1973 only one in seven teenagers went into higher education and it was even rarer for those whose grandparents were bookkeepers or ran a fish and chip shop. I scrambled in by the skin of my teeth; the hospital withdrew the course the next year. The 30 students who had started were whittled down to 20 during that year.

The calibre of my contemporaries was astonishingly high. I was the only male to have come straight from school and many of the other students already had Oxbridge degrees. They included Henry Marsh, who went on to have a stellar career as a neurosurgeon and prize-winning writer with his books *Do No harm* and *Admissions: A Life in Brain Surgery*. Marsh described us as a 'slightly odd mix of students – a stockbroker, a Saudi princess, a Ford truck salesman – mixed up with other, younger students who had poor A level results'. Friends went on to professorships and even to become our country's deputy chief medical officer. Not a bad harvest for a group Marsh described as 'all desperate to be doctors and most of us felt a failure for some reason or other'. I stopped off mid-point at the Free to study exercise physiology and biomechanics. These subjects were still very much in their infancy and allowed me to extend the course to seven years.

Our mentors were an eclectic bunch. Baron Brian Mawhinney taught us medical physics but finished up in Margaret Thatcher's cabinet and later became Football League chairman. Steve Jones, the acclaimed biologist and broadcaster, taught us the rudiments of genetics. My first medical school dean was the eminent cardiologist Dame Frances Gardner. She was married to the larger-than-life surgeon George Qvist. Gardner's extra-curricular passion was gardening and before work she would often travel by milk float to her allotment. Qvist was rumoured to be one of the surgeons Richard Gordon based Sir Lancelot Spratt on in *Doctor in the House*.

In 1980 I became house physician on Dame Professor Sheila Sherlock's Hampstead liver unit. Like Gardner, Sherlock was one of the formidably talented female doctors at the Free. Despite her global academic reputation she had a soft spot for the hospital rugby team. Wherever possible she appointed the players to her staff. She rarely remembered our names but always knew our position on the pitch.

Eleven years of post-graduate training followed, of which all but 18 months were spent in London and the south-east. Working 36 hours 'on' and 12 hours 'off' and up to 126 hours per week was not conducive to a parallel sporting life or even personal life. You were timetabled from

0800–1800 hours Monday to Friday and worked countless nights and weekends. The hours were brutal, and days and nights morphed into one. At times you felt like a zombie, but the experience and training gained were phenomenal.

I escaped London twice to undertake fellowships at Harvard and Sheffield. The American year was pivotal in shaping my future career and the approach there to surgery and sports injuries was significantly different to that at home; education and research were more advanced and all-encompassing.

The consultant years

In 1991 I returned from Sheffield so completing the full circle and became a consultant back at my alma mater, the Royal Free. New appointees were encouraged to develop a pathway that interested them and avoided clashes with fellow colleagues.

I returned trained in the application of Ilizarov rings (the metal scaffolding around limbs) and established one of the first central London units offering this surgery for difficult fractures and leg lengthening. The hospital had an international reputation for HIV and bleeding disorders – principally haemophilia. These conditions often co-existed due to the importation of infected blood products. In the 1970s and 1980s, 5,000 British haemophiliacs were infected with HIV and hepatitis C. It was a scandal described as 'the worst treatment disaster in the history of the NHS' and resulted in 2,800 fatalities. It took over 30 years for the official inquiry into the disaster to start. The treatment, post-operative recovery and prognosis for HIV was not clear in the early 1990s and risks to staff were a major concern. Surgery on HIV-infected patients became the core of my PhD.

After five years sitting in central London traffic jams I made the difficult decision to displace my wife and three daughters and return to Northampton. My Hampstead colleagues asked why I wanted to leave a central London teaching hospital and a Harley Street practice to move to a market town in the East Midlands. The answer? Quality of life and a desire to return to my roots. Little moments can determine life's pathways. While contemplating whether to defy Samuel Johnson – 'When a man is tired of London, he is tired of life' – two sports-related incidents weighed heavily.

Firstly, one of my juniors asked if I would like to be involved with medical support at Saracens Rugby Club and attend matches. My reactions were visceral and surprising. I had played at Saracens for Northampton 2nd XV a decade before and would be delighted to treat any player in my clinic but couldn't contemplate sitting on a Sarries bench. Secondly, my colleague Nick Goddard took me to the Oval for a day's cricket. Nick was a fine surgeon and became involved with Surrey County Cricket Club. The quiet pride he took in helping his home county was infectious. I felt like a displaced refugee yearning for home. I found the criticism of abandoning central London a spur. I was determined to demonstrate that developing a good clinical, academic and research profile outside a medical ivory tower was possible.

In 2005 I joined the University of Northampton as visiting professor in surgical sciences. Five years later I became professor of sports medicine there and felt enormous pride working with my hometown varsity. We developed projects looking at sports injury surveillance, sports medicine ethics, the applications of cryotherapy (ultra-cold chambers) and the role of genetics in sports injuries.

As I move towards retirement, the current lack of such opportunities to pass on experience saddens me. A surgeon builds up a repertoire of operations based upon continuing education and reflection on the outcomes of their work. The latter is achieved by quietly taking pride in successes and resolving to learn from mistakes.

Surgery is awash with guiding maxims. An operation can lead doctors and patients down a slippery spiral and the words 'the patient needed every operation but the first one' are often repeated under my breath. Improving technical ability and equipment can lead to 'triumphs of technology over reason' but just because you could does not mean you should; a hard skill to acquire is the confidence not to operate on a patient, which comes with time and experience. We need to work hard to pass on that accumulated knowledge to young doctors.

In 2012 I felt that after nearly a third of a century in the NHS it was time to go. Times were changing. I was feeling like a dinosaur. When I started in medicine the NHS was 25 years old with the vigour of a young adult. Forty years later it was elderly and full of experience, but in organisational ways bloated and displaying many age-related degenerative disorders. Twenty-one years as a consultant had left me feeling powerless to implement change. I was not a politician or remotely medically clubbable and at the age of 57 I still wanted to improve as a professional. This was not possible for me within the NHS. Private practice income is comforting but was never a main driver. More important was making the right decisions at the right moment for my patients, unencumbered by bureaucracy.

I needed to be free to travel to visit colleagues, teach and attend meetings. There were research avenues I wanted to pursue. I had been asked to become Northamptonshire Cricket Club's chief medical officer and medical director for a state-of-the-art rehabilitation centre built by a local college. These were exciting and challenging opportunities. The NHS would not have allowed me the freedom to pursue them.

Northampton town – *sports town?*

Northampton ranks as the 73rd-largest English residence but could be argued to rank in the top five when it comes to sport. With London, Greater Manchester, Bristol and Leicester it hosts first-class cricket, Premiership rugby and soccer from one of the top four divisions of the Football League pyramid. Sporting riches indeed.

As a Northamptonian I possess that emotional incumbency that bonds you to the trials and tribulations of each sport. It's a lifelong tribal attachment that permits a share in their moods, the joyful feelings of rare successes, the heartache of each on-field and, more commonly, off-field, disaster.

Wherever I lived, it was news of the Cobblers I looked for first on Saturdays. It was where my grandfather stood me on the terraces and my father scribed in the press box. The year 1966 was our *annus mirabilis* – we reached the equivalent of the Premiership from four divisions down. Joe Mercer, Manchester City and later England manager, was so impressed that he said, 'The miracle of 1966 was not England winning the World Cup, but Northampton reaching division one.' Northampton rose from the Fourth Division to the First Division and back to the Fourth, all in the 1960s. We were the first club to achieve this dubious distinction. I have every programme from the 1965/66 season displayed at home – even the St Mirren pre-season friendly.

Fifty years later, the Cobblers were in financial difficulties with police trying to find the £10.25m lent by the local council to finance ground rebuilding. The half-finished stand stood as a monument to idiocy and greed, the club faced a winding-up order and the staff were not being paid. In the middle of all this, amazingly, the players took the Second Division title.

Half a mile away, Northampton Saints were becoming a major force in English rugby. However, they nearly sank like other great clubs such as Coventry, Moseley, Blackheath and Rosslyn Park. As English rugby union became organised into leagues the Saints were at a low ebb. In 1987 the Courage leagues were organised and clubs were placed into a tier depending upon recent results. Saints were in Division Two and should have been relegated to Division Three at the end of that year. Fortunately, the Rugby Football Union (RFU) decided not to demote anybody.

Action was required; revolution was in the air. At an acrimonious and emotional club AGM in 1988 a group of visionaries, known locally as the gang of seven, deposed the incumbents. The Saints then rose like the phoenix from the ashes and 12 years later were European champions with a side, stadium and fan base that was the envy of most.

Conversely, Northants cricket team have always been more Cinderella than Rockefella and won no titles until 1976. The club have never won the County Championship and their five white-ball (one-day) victories are spread over 40 years. However, they have produced a sprinkling of Test players, the greatest including Colin Milburn, Graeme Swann and Monty Panesar. All have been loved for their personalities as well as their skills.

Devoid of Test ground status Northants have no significant local revenues or a war chest and survive on England and Wales Cricket Board (ECB) handouts. By 2015 the club needed emergency financial help and were considering a fire sale of assets. The local council helped with a £250,000 loan. 'Put it this way, we're counting every loo roll,' explained Gavin Warren, the Northamptonshire chairman in 2016.

Sporting Northamptonians have certainly had to roll with the punches over the years. Despite the crises, the town is attuned to high-level sport. Many of its inhabitants follow its teams. For me, it has been a fascinating place for an orthopaedic sports surgeon to work.

Chapter 3

THE CALL OF THE CHANGING ROOM

*'I don't miss playing football, but I do miss
going into the dressing room every day
and having a laugh.'*

**Alan Hansen, ex-Liverpool and Scotland
soccer player, television pundit**

The Sanctum Sanctorum

The changing room is a special place. Before a game everything seems possible. Whether you are an elite athlete or Sunday morning footballer, you are with your mates and all is well with the world. Together any obstacle can be defeated.

Close to kick-off, time-honoured routines driven by superstition and custom are observed: choice of changing peg, order of kit-donning, and the strategic application of embrocation or Vaseline. Individuals morph into 'The Team' glued together by final talks, battle exhortations and warm-up routines that can border on primeval. After the battle, the team returns to its lair licking its wounds in defeat or exhilarated by victory. It can be a place of great succour but equally harsh or comical. There is no hiding place.

Even in individual sports or dance companies, the changing room harbours special affections. In 2018, the ailing Andy Murray admitted, 'I love being around the locker room, chatting with players and everything.' The interactions are the stuff of a psychologist's dreams. The positive energy that radiates from a successful changing room allows the group to reach beyond the sum of its parts.

Powerful role models set the tone. Exemplifiers of professionalism and determination raise standards and their colleagues observe what is required to reach the summit. Within rugby union, the Jonny Wilkinson work ethic was almost maniacal, and in the 1980s, decathlete Daley Thompson's mantra was to train twice on Christmas Day, calculating that his rivals might exercise only once. Conversely, athletes can exert negative influences through attitude and behavioural problems – both on and off the field; poor values exhibited by influential characters can undo the hard work done on the training paddock and contribute to team implosion. This can affect communal attitudes to injury and rehabilitation as much as training and performance.

This concept of mass influence in the workplace is credited to the work of industrial psychologist Otto Köhler in the 1920s. It applies equally to the changing room. Under positive influences, weaker members aspire to match the leaders, so long as the talent and achievement gap is not too wide. However, too easily the reverse occurs. In 2018, the leadership group concept was brought into unwelcome spotlight by the Australian cricket team when their sandpapering of the ball in front of television cameras in Cape Town dismayed the sporting world. The instigator was the vice-captain, egging on his captain and an inexperienced, impressionable colleague.

An independent inquiry concluded that players were encouraged to 'play the mongrel' and that they operated in a disconnected 'gilded bubble'. Wider responsibility was placed on Cricket Australia (CA) itself. CA was accused of 'bully tactics or worse' and viewed as 'arrogant and controlling'. This appears to have affected senior players' behaviour. In a desire to 'fit in and be valued', the younger player lost his moral compass.

Across the Tasman Sea a more positive experience was developed. The All Blacks had dominated world rugby for 34 years but had failed to win the World Cup since the inaugural 1987 competition. To help regain that title they introduced a self-policing changing room strategy entitled 'no dickheads', which is credited to the team's mental skills coach Gilbert Enoka. Individuals who put themselves above the team or who exuded a sense of entitlement were excluded. The Kiwis became world champions in 2011 and 2015.

One of my most cherished experiences as a team doctor is to be invited into the changing room – the *sanctum sanctorum*. The changing room is a living organism. Its tissues and organs are the players, the team captain its beating heart. Ideas and views develop via communication. It is an evolving and ever-changing creature with component parts exiting and arriving. However much a team may have internal issues, players will usually present a common front and support a wounded team-mate.

The changing room is not just an entity around game-time but exists during daily training. With tensions less coiled, discussions are far-ranging and friendships forged. The loss of involvement with the changing room entity contributes to higher depression and suicide rates in retired sportsmen than in the normal population. It expands to fill hotels and training facilities. It is why major sports lavish millions on the development of suitable locations for training, relaxing and planning. The medical room acts as an extension of the changing room and injured players being treated receive unannounced visits from inquisitive colleagues.

During the game the team bench, pavilion balcony or theatre wings become the scene of observation and analysis as the spectacle unfolds. Frequently I find myself seconds behind the action – looking to see who is slow up from a tackle, monitoring players carrying injuries and looking out for those seen limping from the last line-out. You must remain icy cool – even when you are positioned close to the action. That is what is expected; a player needs to hear only positive comments from the medical staff. Athletes who have been repeatedly skinned by their opposite number or carted repeatedly to the boundary know they have made mistakes and do not need reminding. Behaving like a fan of the team you're working for or letting loose at the opposition does not help your reputation. Recently, a rugby doctor allegedly abused an opposition player and landed in hot water with the authorities.

'Now is the time to say goodbye, now is the time to yield a sigh'

'Goodbye-ee'. Popular song by Peter Cook and Dudley Moore (1965)

My own goodbye to the changing room came in Cape Town on the morning of the British Lions versus Springboks first Test at Newlands in 1997. I was playing in a veterans' rugby match against Hamilton, the oldest club in South Africa. Their ground is situated at Sea Point, where the Atlantic Ocean lies in front and Table Mountain behind. Now it is also next to the Green Point stadium, which was built for the 2010 FIFA World Cup. Our captain was Graham Price, the Welsh and Lions prop. Our team manager, Willie John McBride, the greatest Lion of all, gave an unforgettable pep talk before we trotted out.

Rather inadvisably we sported red Lions shirts and followed local touring rules, including no kicking to touch. But within minutes we pleaded for the ball to be allowed beyond the whitewash to enable us to breathe again and recover from the hits. Exhausted at the end, I sat and admired the view. It was time to retire. I was 42. I was christened William John and hoped that one Willie John felt that this Willie John had not made a fool of himself.

'Let's get ready to rumble!'

Pre-game-time is busy for the doctor. The medical bags must be stocked, and away from home a reconnaissance of the medical room and equipment is mandatory. You must locate the emergency medical equipment such as spinal boards, splints and defibrillator; there must be introductions to the opposition's medics and the waiting ambulance team. You must confirm exit points for the emergency removal of stricken players, and directions and contact numbers for local hospitals.

In contact sports I will find a corner of the medical room and lay out dressing packs, local anaesthetic, needles, syringes, sutures and instruments. Head injury assessment forms (HIAs) will be at hand. Rugby union 'blood bin' regulations allow 15 minutes for assessment and wound stitching, gluing or 'butterfly stripping', so there's no time to waste in finding equipment at the bottom of my case with a player prostate and a pressure swab over his forehead. For head lacerations, a potential concussion must be considered and HIAs undertaken when necessary. These tasks require organisation and rehearsal. Once your severed scrum-half is sutured and back on the pitch, cleaning up and restocking begins.

I was once asked to cover a regional cup final at an unfamiliar neutral ground. The home medical team were not present and there was a reluctance to accommodate my request for entry to the locked clinical room. Politely I informed the hosts that the game could not start until medical facilities were accessible.

On another occasion I dealt with three English scalp lacerations in the first half of an international against France at Twickenham. Players are impatient to be back on the park and the noise from 80,000 spectators outside feels as though it is coming under every door and through every window, yet you must concentrate on your needlework, determined that the first contact with another blue shirt doesn't undo your best darning.

Half-time intervals can be feverish and when coaches earn their stripes with analysis and subtle tactical variations; in my experience the hair dryer brigade is a minority. Master strategists like ex-British Lions coach Ian McGeechan speak clearly and precisely while retaining that passion in their voice. Usually the treatment room is adjacent to the changing room and players flow in and out for injury assessments, re-taping and massages for stiffening segments. Coaches put their heads round the door. How much has a player 'left in the tank'?

Medical rooms can also appear in unexpected places. In 1994, Northampton Town FC moved from the County Ground to Sixfields, but there was an oversight: nobody remembered that a medical room was needed and Dennis Casey, our lead physiotherapist, only found out a week before the first game that none existed. A large walk-in storeroom was designated. It was intimate but still accommodated two examination couches. However, some managers used it as their chill-out space at half-time meaning that coaches, players, physios and medics participated in 'excuse-me dances'. Such were the joys of lower league football. Twenty years later a more suitable area was allocated.

The physiotherapist Mark Buckingham attended two Olympic Games at which the warm-up tracks next to the main stadium were his daily base. From there he provided treatments for competing athletes. He saw only one session during either Olympiad – the final-day relays. Glamorous our life is not.

The result of a match flavours the end-of-game scene. Defeat is frequently accompanied by restrained speech. Poor performances, narrow losses and controversial decisions may increase the volubility; exhausted players slump into their seats. Coaches and senior pros are encouraging and try to lift spirits. Conversely, smiles and congratulations greet a win. Rehydration, energy products and ice baths may follow, whatever the result.

The day's injuries file into the medical room after the game where a phalanx of clinicians awaits. An ailment triage follows. Aching limbs are dragged to the massage table and swollen knees to the physio examination couch. Cuts and concussion victims go to the medics. Plans are formulated. A scan? A Monday review? Coaches want updating. With a player's permission, timelines for recovery are communicated. The drug-testing team may appear with clipboards, specimen bottles and randomly selected victims' names for screening. The post-game assessment process can go on long after the ground has emptied of fans.

Big sporting events are tending to start later and later to accommodate media requirements, and the clinical staff's days can extend beyond the witching hour. Post-game engagements mean that weary bodies do not return to their accommodation until long after the final whistle. Physiotherapists need to be flexible. Phil Pask, the England rugby physio, has frequently used his bedroom during away tours as a treatment room into the early hours of the morning. Similarly, on one Saturday evening I was asked to examine a player during an Ashes series. I met the injured player at the hotel bar. The only place of privacy to examine and give confidential advice was the player's bedroom.

> *'Cricket – a game which the English, not being a spiritual people, have invented in order to give themselves some conception of eternity.'*
>
> **Lord Mancroft, British politician. From**
> ***Bees in Some Bonnets* (1979)**

The cricket changing room and its extensions – balcony, dugout, analysis room, medical room and hotels – has a feeling distinct from other sports. Four nights in a hotel in Chester-le-Street, the furthest outpost of English cricket, helps cement bonds and friendships as well as the occasional tensions and hangovers, especially if the weather intervenes. Four- and five-day games ensure players spend long spells confined together. Players rest, practise in the nets, speak to colleagues, coaches and friends. They play cards or darts, rehydrate, watch television, have physiotherapy or massage treatment, and watch the game in which they are active contestants. The red-ball format means players must be at the ground early. It involves a different circadian rhythm of exercise expenditure to that of football and rugby players, who are more used to later kick-offs.

Cricket contains individual duels within a team game. A bowler may regard an incoming batsman as his 'bunny'. Each opposition member's strengths and weaknesses are analysed. Plans are sketched on changing room boards and enacted with specific field placings and bowling changes. Players may stop for lunch or tea during a match-winning century or bowling spell. They can be stranded in the nervous nineties attempting to win or save a match at 6pm and face a night's fractured sleep before they can resume combat. This leaves more than enough time for various mental demons to appear.

Cricket teas for village teams are the stuff of folklore but their professional counterparts keep up the standards. Edgbaston has a conveyor belt of culinary delights during T20 finals day. However, Lord's takes the biscuit with its legendary lunches. With only 40 minutes before the bell tolls for the afternoon session, meals are meted out with military precision. For purely medical research I sampled the nutritional benefits of the offerings at 'Headquarters'.

The players' dining room at Lord's is intimate, with decor not out of place from the 1950s. We had tomato soup and lasagne; apple crumble and lashings of custard followed. I wondered about a post-prandial snooze; the well-upholstered blue seating encircling the visitors' changing room was inviting. Scampering a swift single could not have been further from my mind. Northants were skittled out for 71 in the afternoon. Despite the result, digesting lunch on the players' away-team balcony was a treasured moment.

Cricket allows for time to assess and treat injuries in a less frenzied atmosphere than large-ball games. First-morning soft tissue strains may be rehabilitated before day four. In soccer and rugby the player would miss the entire game. Inclement weather involves teams spending time watching rain reduce their run chase to ruins. Players may spend the whole day padded up while their mates spank the opposition seamers to all corners and then, after a protracted vigil, enter the arena and receive an unplayable first ball. They return to the balcony with unseemly haste. Unsurprisingly, gloves may fly, bats connect with locker doors and red mists descend.

In most team games, sides generally vacate and return to changing rooms together. In cricket, this is not always the case. A batsman returns either alone or with his accomplice. Back slaps follow a dazzling century or hoisting the opposition quickie to the boundary in pursuit of victory. Alternatively, dismissal following an ill-judged single or flail outside off-stump may be greeted with silence.

As Northamptonshire's chief medical officer, I juggle normal clinics and operating while following a game's proceedings. The BBC Sport website is invaluable for game progress reports. During home games I try to visit the ground daily for injury assessments. Requests for finger X-rays or stitches are common. For away games, I maintain contact by text or phone.

Time at the ground is important for assessing collective and individual physical and psychological well-being. Sitting on the balcony and in the changing room talking to players about the game and 'life' is not wasted time. It builds relationships and helps us understand stresses – both sporting and extraneous. A good coach knows which players to put an arm around and which to beast. A sports doctor needs to know how a player will react physically and mentally to injury and setbacks.

Knowing people over years helps predict player reactions and plan management on an individualised basis. It helps us identify the more introspective and hypochondriacal from those who play through thick and thin. It provides a strong advertisement for continuity of care from medical teams embedded over long periods of time. Additionally, time on the balcony allows us to build relationships with the coaches. Their insight has helped me appreciate better the game's subtleties. With players' permission, joint, informed decisions can be made about progress, return to play and workload management.

In 2013 Northamptonshire reached their second T20 finals day. Confidence was high but we were still the outsiders. We were playing Essex in the semi-final. I sat in the small dugout at Edgbaston in front of the Priory Stand, with the coaches and support team. My wife and father were also at the ground and I texted to confirm they had found their seats. That's when the security team pounced. I had forgotten the mobile phone ban in the players' area and might have been contacting the subcontinent with the next bowling change, to secure untold riches for illegal betting rings. My more mundane domestic explanation seemed rather weak. I was let off with a warning.

After a straightforward victory, we retreated to the changing room for the obligatory victory song, 'The Fields Are Green'. We were to make our first appearance in the final. Celebration time, I thought, but Cameron White, our impressive Australian Test batsman, quickly grounded everybody.

'You have won nothing yet,' he said. 'Return to the hotel and prepare for the last challenge against Surrey.'

Effective and statesmanlike, it did the trick: Northants subsequently claimed their first title for 21 years and only their fourth ever. This feat was repeated three years later and on both occasions the changing room celebrations included not only players but families, friends and staff. It was raucous and spontaneous, and a privilege to be there.

On several occasions I have been invited into the England cricket dressing room. The first time was at Old Trafford one day before a Test. Players were coming to and from nets practices. I was discussing recent surgery and rehabilitation with the medical team when our confidential discussions in one corner were interrupted. One player wanted news of his mate and had emerged from the showers naked. He stood amid us drying his genitalia. It was my first meeting with that individual and thankfully my last. Happier memories include being welcomed into the dressing room during the nail-biting Edgbaston Test of the 2005 Ashes. You felt honoured to be close to the characters and a sporting occasion remembered for its tension, skill and moments of sporting camaraderie.

> *'There may be trouble ahead*
> *But while there's moonlight and music and love*
> *and romance*
> *Let's face the music and dance'*

Irving Berlin, 'Let's Face the Music and Dance' (1936)

Professional dancers are no less than any elite athlete. Skills, strength and self-control honed by years of training place them on the highest performance pedestal.

Ballerinas may look like porcelain but their inner toughness is equal to any sportsperson. I have worked with various dance companies since the early 1990s. The ballet fraternity and their unique physical demands offer a natural counterpoise to the 100kg-plus rugby players in my clinics.

A dance company is like any major sports team. The demands are enormous. The English National Ballet (ENB) travels the length and breadth of this country and abroad. They learn, practise and execute many different dance productions annually. Several years ago I reviewed their programme for the year. The company had to master eight different and difficult productions performed in 13 different venues. Three-quarters of the dancers were from overseas, representing 19 countries.

Dance companies spend months closeted together, bonding, supporting and exchanging opinions. Friends' rehabilitation from injuries are monitored; the perceived skills of clinicians are mentally marked and disseminated for discussion. There is no hiding place in the dressing room.

For the changing or dressing room to gel, obstacles created by different cultures and languages must be overcome. The natural order of a dance company is less egalitarian than that of most sports, and ranges from lead principals to principals, character artists, first soloists, soloists, junior soloists, first artists and the corps de ballet. Everybody understands their place; it is not unlike the military. Leading lights have their own dressing room and artistic directors wield similar power to a soccer manager.

For many years the ENB had its home in Jay Mews behind the Albert Hall but in 2019 it moved to Canning Town. While performing in London dancers can retreat to their headquarters for rehearsal, relaxation and rehabilitation. On tour, hotels and less familiar theatres must suffice and travelling physiotherapists must make do and mend. Small spaces in the backs of theatres are converted into injury treatment areas. It has been my pleasure to watch the ENB perform in the Albert Hall and in widespread smaller venues, which gave me the chance to carry out pre-performance reviews of injured dancers and the opportunity to observe from the wings, which gives an entirely different perspective.

The dancers' preparation pre-appearance on stage is fascinating. Their knowledge of the production and their role within it is ingrained. Waiting for their entrance dressed as the Sugar Plum Fairy or a cygnet they talk about news or after-show plans – always with an ear on the music. At the appropriate moment they break off, park the can of Coke and metamorphose into character. Gliding on to stage, they transfix the audience then pirouette out of sight of the stalls and carry on where they left off. Remarkable, and however often I witnessed it, I never ceased to be impressed with this chameleon-like feat.

One of the boys?
"Cause I don't wanna be one of the
boys, one of your guys'
Katy Perry, 'One of the Boys' (2008)

When difficult health assessments need to be made, you need your professional face on. Objective and weighted decisions are required. It is like coaches' judgements on selection, contracts and transfers. Being too close to a player makes the job more difficult.

Doctors cannot be 'Jack the lad' on team outings one day and the harbinger of bad news the next. A doctor is never off duty in the presence of their athlete-patients. Players have memories like elephants and one shandy too many at the Christmas party can come back to haunt you. You risk diminishing your standing in the eyes of the changing room; you need to know your players but not be their drinking mates.

Things were different in the 1960s and 1970s when the Liverpool FC dressing room dictum was 'if anyone gets injured make sure it happens in the first half before the doc has a drink!' The manager at the time, Bill Shankly, believed that the Liverpool and England defender Tommy Smith was not born but quarried – such was Smith's toughness.

During one game, Smith sustained a deeply gashed leg before half-time. After assessing the wound in the medical room, the doctor requested, 'Go get Tommy a brandy, will you, and get me one as well – a large one!' The medic drank both measures for Dutch courage but had not enough stitches for such a large laceration. The sutures were spaced out while Joe Fagan, a future manager, put his soiled fingers on the knots during tying. After the procedure Smith pointed to the large gaps. The doctor asked Tommy to push the flesh together and filled the spaces with antibiotic powder. Finally, the medic handed Smith a prescription saying, 'You're bound to have a bit of poison after all that messing around.'

Lunchtime imbibing and medical duties at rugby matches were still an occasional concern in the mid-1990s. In the middle of a Northampton Saints match I was preparing to suture a player's scalp. He looked up at me and said, 'Before you stitch me, have you had a drink? The last doc who looked after me smelt like a brewery.' I confirmed that I was stone-cold sober. I'll return later to the problems of being detained in hospitality while on duty.

The changing room beast usually comes to a consensual decision on the merits or otherwise of various medics. A surgeon is only usually as good as their last operation. Years of success can count for nothing if one player does not respond well to your ministrations; the mumblings begin. For many years, I worked with a diligent and well-informed team doctor who came under the critical spotlight of outspoken members of the changing room. This was totally unjustified in my opinion but he lost the confidence of the group and his position became untenable. His final months with the team were traumatic and he needed time abroad to recover from the experience.

Where does this leave the doc sitting?
'I'm sittin' on the doc[k] of the bay, watchin'
the tide roll away'

Otis Redding, 'Sittin' On the Dock of the Bay' (1967)

A doctor's position is not sitting on the changing room bench with the guys. That is their special place. Medics must wait to be invited into the *sanctum* rather than assuming, and remember why they are there. They are not a secondary coach or best friend and need to maintain the changing room's respect by their professionalism and skills. The player is there because of their skillset and those in it expect nothing less of the doctor. Like a player, doctors may have a sell-by date, sometimes due to circumstances beyond their control.

Above all it is an honour to be a team medic. Being present in a team's changing room during or after a major triumph or alongside an individual athlete or dancer having witnessed an extraordinary performance is a privilege. Doctors should take quiet satisfaction in any part they play in enabling the outcome, but should never forget that it is all about the athlete.

Chapter 4

DO ATHLETES HELP THEMSELVES AND THEIR DOCTORS?

'And I have bought
Golden opinions from all sorts of people'
William Shakespeare, *Macbeth* **(1606)**

RECEIVING AN appointment is a relief for patients on NHS waiting lists. Advice is absorbed and usually followed. This is not necessarily the case with athletes.

Multiple opinions are often sought. Sports organisations' wealth, Lottery funding and private health insurance facilitates this. 'Have car will travel' is the modern mantra for today's sportspeople, who criss-cross countries and continents.

The athlete, team-mate, physiotherapist, manager, coach, agent, friends, family and internet all influence decision-making. A reasonable diagnosis and plan might be forthcoming at the first consultation. This does not stop a trawl through numerous other specialists. Even team doctors are not immune from irrational behaviour.

Athletes tend to choose doctors offering the quickest route back to sport and often I feel like I am caught up in the nets of a fishing boat whose occupants are casting far and wide in the hope of catching something special. Sometimes, long-term health and reinjury risks are not considered. Many athletes believe they can defy nature because of their physical prowess. However, a damaged body segment must serve its time, although clinical support helps speed recovery.

Injured players are suggestible to all types of remedies. The most persuasive voice does not always come from the team's medical team or specialists. One sport I was involved with had an affable participant who offered medical advice to team-mates and rival teams with little understanding of the underlying problems. It was not mainstream advice and usually involved taking a flight abroad. His well-meaning consultations caused headaches for clubs and their medical teams, with players wanting to undergo expensive and unverified treatment not covered by insurance.

Multiple opinions do not always help. If the opinions are the same the athlete can be reassured, but problems occur when numerous pathways are outlined. It is better to carefully select your first opinion, accept it and follow the advice in most cases. Usually this approach serves the rest of the population well, too. Injuries can have several solutions and we orthopaedic surgeons may not help if we give different advice based on our own education, training and experience. Most treatments are variations on a theme and will succeed. However, options can confuse athletes.

Years ago I saw a Middle Eastern royal family member. He liked to train with the footballers from the club he owned. But his knee ACL had ruptured and I was his third opinion; he had already sought the opinion of the Brazilian football team surgeon in Rio de Janeiro and that of another expert in Alabama. My hospital had looked after one of his relatives but I had no idea why he had flown into London to see a newly appointed consultant.

I explained my plan to His Royal Highness. It included an eight-to ten-month recovery with no absolute guarantee of a return to five-a-side. I thought I was being realistic but he looked mournful: he had been told he could be back on the park within three months. I could not match that outcome and wished him well. I presume he returned to Rio.

I also had a memorable non-consultation involving a global sporting superstar passing through Northampton for 24 hours. Multiple opinions had been sought for a problem present for 17 years but he had still amassed a career record that remains the envy of all. The X-ray diagnosis was clear and potential solutions seemed promising. I would have enjoyed meeting the patient but informed his doctor that there was little point if the caravan was about to move out of town never to return.

At other times the sportsperson does not really want to see you, but has been told to. A cricketer referred to me had chronic foot problems. I outlined a potential surgical plan but felt retirement was the best course for the foot and its owner. It was a difficult conversation and he was devastated. My advice was dismissed. 'You cannot be any good because you work in Northampton,' he claimed. His career was in the balance and he was frightened, which was absolutely understandable. He went elsewhere but unfortunately things did not work out and he finished with unforeseen complications. I was sad for the player and reflected on how my consultation could have been better.

Demons can take hold even after making the decision to undergo surgery. An international sportsman phoned me at home one night. We had never met but had a mutual friend. He was in a hospital bed scheduled for spinal surgery the next day. Was he 'doing the right thing?' Ugh! I quickly established that his prospective surgeon had an excellent reputation. Surgery was successful and he enjoyed many further seasons at the top.

On another occasion an elite sportsperson arrived with a bone injury that wasn't healing. They could compete but with pain. Rest or surgery? There was no absolute right or wrong answer but I felt surgery was in the long-term best interest. About 12 hours before surgery, a second opinion was being sought 100 miles away. Second opinions are healthy – I encourage them for difficult circumstances – but this was self-inflicted pressure without time for reflection. It is better to postpone surgery early and reflect on various opinions.

Too brave for their own good?

Athletes perform at and beyond the limits of exhaustion. They compete while injured. This is all highlighted regularly in the media. There are also athletes whose bravery goes beyond common sense.

At the 1954 Empire (now Commonwealth) Games in Vancouver Jim Peters led the marathon by 17 minutes as he entered the stadium. He was on course to break all kinds of records having previously broken the world marathon best three times. He hit the wall inside the stadium and took 11 minutes to cover 200m before being stretchered away, still minutes ahead, without breasting the tape. He never ran again and knew he was lucky to survive.

The acrobatics of Bert Trautmann, the Manchester City goalkeeper in the 1956 FA Cup Final, also remain vivid. The ex-Luftwaffe pilot and prisoner of war had sustained multiple fractures and dislocations to his neck vertebrae in a collision with the Birmingham City player Peter

Murphy. He remained on the field to defy Birmingham's late rally. In 2018 his life story was made into the film *Trautmann*.

Damaged testicles do not seem to slow up rugby players. In 2003, Northampton Saint Budge Pountney played on against London Irish, and in 2012, the Warrington Wolves rugby league player Paul Wood played 20 minutes with a ruptured testicle. Both submitted to the surgeon's scalpel subsequently.

In 2016, Nick Blackwell sustained a brain bleed while boxing Chris Eubank Junior. He was placed in an induced coma. Blackwell recovered well but struggled with premature retirement and secretly began sparring. Eight months later he suffered another head injury and required life-saving brain surgery and was in a coma for another 31 days. His sparring partner and trainer were suspended. Blackwell survived but faced a long recovery. In 2018 he reported that his recovery was ongoing and that he had been wheelchair-bound for a long time.

Andy Murray's stellar career appeared to climax in 2016. To his name he had added a second Wimbledon title, second Olympic title, an ATP World Tour final and the coveted world number one ranking. A truly *annus mirabilis*. However, the sheer physical effort required to reach such heights seemed to take its toll and his persistent hip injury deteriorated.

Murray's playing style centred around a punishing work ethic that enabled him to perform wonders on court. Such a dynamic game plan could not countenance pain and restriction from such a key joint. After false dawns and frustrating setbacks, Murray was close to admitting defeat. However, his hip resurfacing recovery exceeded many predictions, including mine.

Why do elite athletes push themselves so hard? Is it genetic or environmental? Inherited factors are the basis for a winner. Per-Olof Åstrand, a pioneer of exercise physiology, wrote, 'To be an Olympic champion, I am convinced one must choose one's parents carefully.' However, everybody can train smart and improve their physical state and exercise potential.

In 1997 Professor Tim Noakes developed his central governor theory. It proposed that sporting fatigue is governed by the brain largely independently of the body's actual biological state. It explained that the brain's domination is designed to avoid irreversible damage to our vital organs – that it maintains the body's even keel. To facilitate this, nerve messages reduce muscle fibre activity, giving the sensation of fatigue.

The theory suggests that an individual's brain knows the fatigue limit its body can tolerate. At any one time fatigue levels during exercise can be calculated by the Borg rating of perceived exertion (RPE). Before or soon after exercise starts, our brain calculates when the activity will end. It knows our body's maximum RPE and determines the exercise intensity level our body will tolerate to complete the task without biological catastrophe. Pace is set by our fitness levels and the task ahead. Push it too hard, too early, and fatigue will accelerate and the participant will be forced to slow down. Such assessments are made by the analysis of numerous input sources from our conscious and non-conscious self. These receptors monitor chemical and physical changes throughout our body. Although developed with reference to long-distance running, this theory has been developed as a potential model for disease states including chronic fatigue syndrome.

Can elite athletes, through training, understand better their own limits by approaching them repetitively? If fatigue is determined by our brains and not primarily by our muscles, how do emotions like ambition, fear, positive and negative triggers, and determination modify our fatigue limit? Does the shattering of sporting sacred cows such as the sub-four-minute mile (1954) or the sub-one-minute breaststroke swimming record (2001) reset rivals' mental barriers? Can athletes such as Jim Peters find ways of tricking their minds into permitting their bodies to push beyond safe physical limits and cause potential harm?

It is the athlete's Icarus moment: aim for the sun. Judge it right and bask in the golden warmth of success. Overcook it and crash and burn into the waiting arms of the medical staff.

Playing while injured

Playing with injuries is part of an elite athlete's life. There is hardly any time during a sporting career when an athlete does not have some niggle or other. Rafael Nadal has had so many injuries that he lives in almost constant pain. This is the critical difference between the amateur footballer, golfer or gym bunny and professional sportspeople. The former enjoy sport mostly for physical, psychological and social benefits. Risks may be involved, such as finishing in a ditch from not unclipping quickly enough from your new cycling pedals. But the overall intention of participating is to provide health pluses rather than negatives.

For the amateur, problems arise when the individual loses sight of their recreational goals. They may pursue training regimes or take excessive risks physically or pharmacologically that jeopardise health. Even at a social level they may be involved in a sport where rules and tactics change. These increase injury probability. Rugby union may have reached this crossroads.

In professional and elite sport the athlete has chosen to cross their own personal Rubicon. Although not realising it initially, the realities soon become apparent and some athletes need rescuing for their own safety. Tommy Smith at Liverpool was one such athlete. Despite another injury he turned up in the physio room before a game to get his leg strapped to try to play. Manager Bill Shankly walked in and saw him.

'I am playing. It's my leg,' Smith said.

Shankly replied, 'It's not your bloody leg. It's Liverpool FC's leg. And you're not bloody playing.'

Because of career dreams and employer aspirations, players accept the need to play while the Sunday morning park footballer turns over and goes back to sleep. Elite athletes understand that carrying on is not good for their long-term health but it secures their families' futures. At 25 years old, you will 'never be' 65 with knees needing replacing. Moreover, I am yet to find a 65-year-old requiring a new knee who regrets the sporting decisions of their youth.

Clubs may claim ownership of their players' bodies and souls during their playing careers, but they do not pick up the tab 30 years later. It is left to organisations such as the PFA. In a 2018 survey of 350 current international rugby union players, 45 per cent felt pressurised into playing or training when not fit. 'I was taping it up, having injections, playing a game with a suppository up my arse … I was clinging on to my career,' was how one ex-international described his knee injury management.

In 2014, colleagues and I, led by my PhD student Lucy Hammond, researched the problems of 'playing injured' in English professional football. Nearly half the games we studied featured players turning out while injured. Small budgets and playing squads meant such episodes occurred more frequently and for longer in the lower divisions.

The implications are clear for clinicians working further down professional soccer's food chain. They are working with restricted finances, a higher proportion of players carrying injuries, and have no opportunity to use well-resourced rehabilitation centres. There are no suitable deputies waiting to be drafted into matchday squads.

This message was driven home in 2017 by the admission from a player in a lower league team that he could only play after taking large quantities of non-steroidal anti-inflammatories (NSAIDs) and that on one occasion the gastric side-effects of the tablets had put him in bed for a week. His club were in a relegation battle and he had torn his knee cartilage. This story resonated with me as I operated on him. Despite asking about medication history, nothing was forthcoming. I read about it in a national newspaper years later.

Self-preservation

Ever-increasing demands, particularly in contact sports, have seen some athletes take matters into their own hands.

After reaching the top of the sporting tree, a cold, January Friday night fixture at Sale Sharks or Swansea City can lose some of its allure. Tactical injuries occur allowing rest and recovery. Coaches and strength and conditioning (S&C) teams carefully map out the season's peaks and troughs. Players have their own goals. Seasoned internationals get an adrenaline rush from big tests for club and country. A desire to prolong careers and enjoy such occasions is understandable.

Rugby and cricket central contracts are engineered to preserve players for such challenges. In soccer the reverse may occur when clubs are considered more important than country. Managers withdraw players from international duty on flimsy medical grounds. Players prematurely retire from patriotic call-ups to preserve club careers.

It comes down to what discomfort level, from a menu of background problems, you are prepared to play through, balanced against the contest's importance. Is the risk of aggravating the problem during a mid-table fixture worth jeopardising missing an upcoming international?

After years at the coalface it takes longer to recover and for one experienced player I noted a seasonal pattern emerging. An autumn of significant battles would be followed by downtime of a couple of games to allow the athlete to return with all guns firing for major new year showdowns. This game management contributed to the player having a stellar career.

Arthritis and the athlete

'If little labour, little are our gains;
Man's fortunes are according to his pains.'
Robert Herrick, 'No Pains, No Gains', *Hesperides* (1648)

The phrase 'no pain, no gain' is heard in every gym and on every training field throughout the land. Achievement in any walk of life is related as much to endeavour as skill. In sport, what is the cost to body and mind? Putting limbs on the line is part and parcel of success for the elite but what are the longer-term health consequences?

Northampton Saints rugby ground, Franklin's Gardens, has a bar called the Crooked Hooker. It is a ramshackle construct; all around has been redeveloped and modernised. It epitomises the past. It is where ex-players meet before and after games.

If anybody doubts the long-term risk of playing rugby they should position themselves outside the Hooker at 2.55pm on matchdays. Heroes from my youth and ex-team-mates file out as quickly as their pegs allow. A stooped spine here, a pair of bowed legs there, their mate disappearing into the distance courtesy of his second hip replacement. Saturday afternoons of their youth have taken their toll.

Evidence suggests a link between professional football and later osteoarthritis. A 1997 report found that half of players retiring early did so because of knee injuries. A 2000 study found that half of all retired players had osteoarthritis somewhere (which developed, on average, 24 years post-retirement) and 7 per cent possessed a knee replacement.

Retired cricketers are four times more likely to require a hip or knee replacement than the normal population. A 2012 study of several sports found sportsmen had double the risk of developing arthritis and requiring a joint replacement compared to the normal male population. In the study, Dutch researchers found that from 2000 to 2014 arthritis risk in sporting knees, hips, ankles and shoulders was several times greater than for the rest of us.

The force of collisions in rugby now means that arthritis risk will increase and occur earlier, and today, more than ever, my discussions with professional players over a range of sports now centre around managing early osteoarthritis.

I once saw a twenty-something rugby player with a problem knee. As a schoolboy, I had presented him with prizes at speech day. He was an outstanding athlete in several sports but chose rugby. His progress towards senior international honours was blighted by injuries and well before he was 30, and despite several surgeries, he was arthritic.

Another patient came to see me in his thirties. A former professional, he was returning for advice. I had looked after him for 15 years with various injuries and now he was facing an imminent shoulder replacement.

One of his knees was only a couple of years behind – all devastating for patients and depressing for me.

Knee cartilage injuries and cruciate ligament tears once threatened players' careers. Now, sportspeople expect surgery to restore them back to sport. This is quite reasonable. However, the knee is never the same after surgery. The loss of your car's shock absorber affects driving comfort and removing part of your knee cartilage has the same effect. Knowing you have joint arthritis and the decision-making that results are different matters. This applies to the weekend warrior as much as to the professional.

Surgeons have a duty of care to explain the short- and long-term dangers of continuing with sport. They may feel strongly and refuse to sanction continuation. In this respect, problems can arise during signing-on medicals; I discuss this in detail in Chapter 29. It is the individual's decision; mostly, all I can do is advise, support and document.

Jabbing joints and popping the painkilling pills

Ways of controlling painful, inflamed joints and soft tissues have improved greatly.

Steroid injections for professional athletes were commonplace in the past but we are more careful now. Steroids are excellent at reducing inflammation and, used correctly, are an important part of a doctor's arsenal. They are not designed for application to joints shortly before a match, race or performance to get an athlete on the park. The opposite is required: rest.

Stories abounded in the 1960s, 1970s and 1980s of players receiving numerous injections to numb pain before games. One such player was Kevin Beattie of Ipswich and England. Bobby Robson, his Ipswich and later England manager, described him as the most gifted English player he had seen but even in his mid-twenties he was reported to have two knee steroid injections before a game and one at half-time. By 1981 his senior career was over. He was 27 years old. He had had five operations in four years.

Roy McFarland was a wonderful centre-back for Derby County and England and was selected by Sky Sports' expert judging panel for its best all-time England XI. He had many injuries. His autobiography recalls receiving a cortisone jab into a thigh injury in the dugout by the side of the pitch during a European Cup match against Real Madrid. Not the most sterile environment. This problem was not confined to football.

Ferdie Pacheco was Muhammad Ali's personal physician and known as 'The Fight Doctor'. He was a familiar figure and close to the corner of The Greatest. His 2017 obituary recounted how, pre-fight, he injected Ali's hands with cortisone and anaesthetic to numb the pain.

Many years ago, I met a former ballerina who had partnered the absolute best on London stages. The repetitive stresses from training and performance had started to take their toll when she was in her twenties. She had lost count of the number of steroid injections put into her foot joints and eventually her feet came to resemble those of a long-term diabetic: bones and joints simply crumbled with the injections the primary culprit.

Steroids placed directly into already damaged tendons are bad news. They weaken, impair healing and increase rupture risk. The damage they inflict can increase the complexity of any subsequent operation. Colleagues at home and abroad have told me their horror stories of the ravages of multiple steroid deposits on elite tendons. I myself have picked steroid crystals from the middle of professional sportsmens' ruptured Achilles.

I also know of an athlete who lost the chance of an Olympic gold medal and the attachment of his Achilles to his heel following a steroid injection before the competition. He never raced again. Newspapers still record sportspeople resorting to repeated steroid tendon injections. It is sad and not a great example to youngsters. There is another menace, however, which is just as big: the tablets we have at home.

In 1969 ibuprofen was introduced to the UK as an NSAID and marketed as Brufen and Neurofen. You needed a prescription for both, until 1983. As a junior doctor I remember the safety discussions when it became an over-the-counter medicine. Now it is in nearly every family's first aid box. For 'coarse' rugby players it had the dual benefits of reducing Sunday morning post-match pain, and the size of the hangover.

The range of NSAIDs has multiplied and they are now available in tablet form, as creams, injections and suppositories. Their potency ranges from aspirin and ibuprofen at the mild end to indomethacin, diclofenac and meloxicam at the other. They are not without risks – the gut-wrenching effects on one footballer have been described. An athlete suffered similar stomach problems and lost Olympic medal chances after taking pre-event NSAIDs. Such outcomes are not surprising as many cannot tolerate NSAIDs, with two-fifths of people experiencing abdominal symptoms.

Athletes are particularly susceptible to asthma. About 10 per cent of the general population have asthma but the reported figures in elite sport are 25 per cent of footballers, 30 per cent of rowers, 40 per cent of cyclists and 50 per cent of swimmers. Intense training in cold conditions or swimming pools can start an asthma attack. Beware. Up to one-fifth of asthmatics can experience airway constriction into their lungs (bronchospasm) after taking NSAIDs. Other serious side-effects of long-term NSAID ingestion can include heart, liver and kidney damage and increased bleeding risk. Evidence has been accumulating for a long time but the message is not getting through.

At the football Euros in 2008, 42 per cent of drug-tested players admitted taking NSAIDs in the previous three months. One in 15 of the players taking part received steroid injections either during or in the build-up to the tournament even though the governing body (UEFA) was already issuing warnings through its own medical committee.

During the 2010 football World Cup in South Africa, 40 per cent of players took these drugs. By 2012, FIFA's chief medical officer, Dr Jiri Dvorak, estimated that this figure had increased to one-half of players and reached levels of abuse. Football needed to wake up to the threat but did it? In the 2014 World Cup, 54 per cent of players were using NSAIDs.

Stars from many sports have admitted, either in studies or to me, to NSAID use to allow a return to sport, including athletics, football, tennis, rugby, cricket, golf and basketball. In the UK the risk of death from the stronger NSAIDs is about five to seven per one million prescriptions. In 2017, 100,000 hospital admissions and 16,000 deaths occurred annually in America as a result of NSAID-related complications. Surely the message must have hit home by now. Seemingly not: NSAID use appears to have become embedded in sporting culture with revelations from present and retired soccer players confirming the scale of the problem. One player took maximum-dosage diclofenac (Voltarol) for three years to control post-surgery pain. Such levels risk long-term health problems.

Rugby union has had significant problems with the use of painkillers and NSAIDs. In 2018 the retired Irish and British Lions rugby captain Brian O'Driscoll described to *The Times* the pre-match preparation of the use of drugs towards the end of his career. Other high-profile players, such as Paul O'Connell and Jacques Burger, have also reported their reliance on such pills to get through training and games.

Andrew Coombes, the former Welsh international, explained: 'You become your own chemist in a way,' while the Leicester Tiger, Lewis

Moody, believes he developed bowel inflammation (colitis) as a result of the 'smarties' he took during his career. What should be done about this? Everybody involved in sport needs to look at themselves, including doctors. Including me.

NSAIDs are not on the World Anti-Doping Agency (WADA) list of prohibited drugs. Carefully monitored, infrequent NSAID use is reasonable for most. However, the athlete should know the side-effects and risks of long-term usage. Doctors and physiotherapists should be aware of the potential pitfalls of NSAIDs and counsel their athletes correctly. Sport's culture needs challenging.

Athletes are tough and showing no weakness is a badge of honour. The pressures and rewards of participation at the high-end of sport are understood. However, the era of physios walking around changing rooms before kick-off waving an NSAID blister pack should be relegated to the past. O'Driscoll recalled that 'the doctor would have walked down the bus on the way to games inquiring who wanted what [in the way of painkillers] in advance [of kick-off]'. His successors in the Irish set-up claim the culture is changing. I hope so. The ethos must move away from that remembered by Andrew Coombes – of being told by his coach 'to f*** off' when his pain was too much to participate in a training session.

In July 2020 leading British female gymnasts Amy Tinkler and Becky and Ellie Downie revealed details of a culture of bullying and abuse. Their sport is notoriously hard but predominantly involves teenagers. Becky Downie recalled the reaction when she tried to raise concerns: 'I was shot down, called "mentally weak", and told the injury pain levels I was experiencing were in my head.'

The risks of playing through pain should be in the curriculum of all sports' coaching courses. An open culture within sport must be fostered to allow players the freedom to discuss issues of pain management with medical support teams. Athletes need access to alternative, safer pain-reduction strategies and clinicians should be allowed to work in an environment in which they will not face censure for saying 'enough is enough'.

'They tried to make me go to rehab but I said,
"No, no, no"'

Amy Winehouse, 'Rehab' (2008)

Rehabilitation times following injury and treatment (surgical or not) can be one of the most challenging to predict. Athletes want certainty where there is none. Coaches have set ideas on how long certain injuries take to recover – which are usually wildly inaccurate.

When dealing with elite sportspeople, surgeons must learn from a different chapter in the textbook to those devoted to the rehabilitation of most of our patients. Following surgery, many patients fall into one of two camps – those who need a proverbial boot up the backside and those who need sitting on. The former group often have a fear of undoing the surgical work, while a few have a low level of pain tolerance. Even professional athletes can fall into this group. They need to be recognised early and given the information, support and confidence to overcome their misgivings.

Most sportspeople populate the latter group, however. Rehabilitation estimates are challenges to be overcome like any competitive contest. It is where the importance of the team doctor, physio, S&C guys and coach play a most important role. Commonly agreed programmes must be set to ensure a smooth and safe recovery.

When counselling an athlete before surgery we discuss aftercare. Plans are formulated and apparently agreed? No. Athletes think this is a time to start to negotiate.

'You said it would take six weeks for my bone/ligament/tendon/ muscle to be strong enough to take impact, but could I start jogging at five?' This is why I went prematurely grey at 35.

In the last decade I looked after an international sportsman with a ruptured Achilles. All appeared well in the weeks after surgery and the athlete, physio and I had a long discussion about the need for gentle graduated activity over the next couple of months. That afternoon they returned to their base and tested to see if the leg would take hopping drills. Panic phone call. The athlete had suffered a re-partial tear, was back in the boot and set back by a month.

Several years ago I gave a lecture in Switzerland on rehabilitation following Achilles tendon ruptures. I had my own views but sought advice from around the globe in the time-honoured fashion: I Googled it. I found that protocols abound from world centres of excellence and there was no consensus on when patients could safely move to the next rehabilitation stage; time projections could vary by months.

It is for these reasons that many seasoned rehabilitation clinicians use goal-based targets rather than time-based ones. Athletes must achieve levels of ability across a range of activities before moving to the next stage. This is a more scientific approach. However, sportspeople, their clubs and the media remain wedded to time predictions. If pushed, I opt for my privately held view plus 10 per cent. It gives everybody breathing space. If the player returns earlier, the coach regards the athlete, physio and doctor as geniuses.

'This was the most unkindest cut of all'
William Shakespeare, *Julius Caesar* (1599)

One of the most difficult things for a surgeon to learn is masterly inactivity – I was taught that the hardest decision to make is to send a patient home from casualty. If in doubt, admit or pass the patient on to a more senior colleague. For a surgeon, recommending that the athlete does not have surgery can be the toughest call yet. I spend a lot of my clinic time persuading people not to have surgery. Patients find this odd, as they have attended a surgical outpatients; some team doctors ask their charges to see me when they don't want their athlete to have surgery!

For the surgeon, there is no kudos in telling a potential gold medallist that, in your opinion, a more prolonged period of rest should cure the problem. The quiet, inner satisfaction at the joy of seeing an athlete come back as good as ever following surgery is immeasurable. It is not the same feeling if you have simply told the patient to have more physiotherapy – even if that was the right decision. I know I'm getting more conservative as the years go by.

Seared into my professional memory are two household names who saw me about their injuries. On balance I felt that the best course for both was to rest and let nature take its path. Both individuals had a renowned strong work and training ethic. Both went abroad for surgery. For one, the procedure was a disaster and they were never the same again. For the other, surgery was followed by an enforced rest for an unrelated issue. I have no idea which effected the cure.

My instinct is to explore non-surgical alternatives wherever possible. But once, this came back to bite me painfully. In 2007 Northampton Saints contrived to get themselves relegated out of the rugby Premiership again. The jolt caused a lot of soul searching and reflection and the medical department did not come out unscathed. During the next pre-season the club contacted me. Was I free to attend a players' lunchtime meeting?

I was not prepared for the censure we were about to receive. Various physiotherapists, GPs and I were seated in front of the playing and coaching staff. It felt a bit like a firing squad or the Spanish Inquisition. The club's fall from grace had been analysed (scientifically or otherwise) and it had been decreed that a contributor had been injury levels and the perceived slowness of recovery. The players' specific criticism of me was that I did not operate on enough of them. I was surprised. I had undertaken dozens of operations on the first-team squad over the years. I replied that I was pleased that I did not have a reputation of being 'Butcher Bill' in the changing room and would do everything I could to help players rehabilitate without recourse to a scalpel.

Soon after, a club official informed me that future opinions would be sought from surgeons with central London clinic locations. However, would I still attend matches to transport players to casualty and avoid long wait times for them? Thus ended my 13-year hands-on medical association with the club. It hurt but I reflected that I was the same as a player having their contract terminated. Time to move on.

Surgery is not the answer for everything. It is often seen as a shortcut to fixing a problem that is steeped in training errors and sport-specific technical issues. These take longer to correct.

Hoisted by someone else's petard?

'If a man talks of his misfortunes there is something in them that is not disagreeable to him; for where there is nothing but pure misery, there never is any recourse to the mention of it.'

Samuel Johnson, quoted in *Boswell's Life of Johnson, Vol. 4: The Life* **(1780–1784)**

There are times when your best endeavours become exposed publicly in unanticipated ways. Increasingly, athletes want to share their problems with the world and their comments can be surprising.

Two well-known Lancashire-based sporting heroes went into the national newspapers on the same day. One of them, the Manchester United and England footballer Owen Hargreaves, had a chronic history of knee injuries. He revealed, 'It's massive surgery ... I couldn't really tell you what the exact problem has been. Tendons are something that a lot of people think they know about, but don't really, so a lot of the treatments I have had have been slightly experimental ... The surgery did its job … but I am still in the process of getting some injections to try to manage the pain.'

England fast bowler James Anderson was the other and said of his knee problems, 'Nobody knew what it was, so they just sprayed a bit of cortisone where the pain was. Now I'm bowling without any pain, which is quite nice …'

In both cases their doctors are being damned by something approaching faint praise. Both players indicate that even experienced clinicians appear to be in the dark medically and will try something out of left field or jab and hope. Andy Murray did the same in discussing his hip damage. 'They [the experts] have no idea really … I have seen many doctors and specialists, had lots and lots of different opinions on my hip and I don't believe they know.'

Sometimes the athlete or club official is even less subtle. A sportsman once saw me with minimal problems and equivocal MRI findings. He wanted to continue training and the player, physiotherapist and I were agreed that he would return for a review in a week. Within days, his injury became more uncomfortable and he saw another surgeon. His coach went on television.

'The advice we got was for him just to rest but he's been to see another knee specialist today and he's been operated on. We expect him to be out for between four and six weeks and that is obviously a big blow for us … We got some bad advice … I'm a little bit disappointed in the advice that we got but we have to move on and I'm sure [he] will rehab pretty quickly …'

That broadcast outburst provoked interesting and supportive comments from other patients. Unfortunately, the operation did not go smoothly and the player returned to me for further surgery after the manager had departed for pastures new.

Manu Tuilagi is a massive talent within rugby union but his physical style of play exposes him to risk. From 2011 to 2018 the popular press chronicled injuries to his knees, groin, chest wall, cheekbone, hamstrings and shoulder. At one stage, Tuilagi followed the Hargreaves and Anderson line by 'dobbing in' his doctors and physiotherapists with surprising revelations about his chest wall muscle injury woes.

'When I first went to see the specialist, he had a look at it and said there's a chance I could be back in six weeks.' He carried on with weight training.

'Eight weeks later I had another scan and it [the muscle] was completely off the bone. I don't understand why he didn't see it the first time.' He had surgery the next day.

In 2017, Manu announced that he had been to Samoa to banish knee, pectoral and groin injuries. He explained that Polynesian witch doctors 'are there for the illnesses that the hospitals can't cure. When I come back for a long period of time they'll have to sack all the physios.'

The witch doctor had identified the root of Manu's problems, he claimed.

'There were three lady spirits who had married themselves on to me for the last three years. The spirits wanted me for themselves – they wanted to punish me and injuring me was the way to do it.' The witch doctor had applied oils and massages designed to prevent the three unwanted wives from finding the Leicester Tiger. However, Manu was cautious, fearing that when the lady spirits 'read the newspaper they will know where I am again'.

Manu returned, seemingly free of the shackles applied by a trio of covert concubines and completed a run of four games. Sadly, a calf injury sidelined him again. Having recovered, he appeared to be hitting his straps but after another quartet of matches, a further chest muscle injury removed him from action against Wasps. Had the newspaper reached Samoa?

A year later he was back in international rugby but suffered fresh injuries including groin damage. Prior to his England recall he 'feared during every training session ... that his body would break down'.

Millions of people around the world have ingrained belief systems handed down through generations regarding witch doctors' healing powers. They have unshakeable faith in their faculties. However, I am not aware that the Tigers' physios were looking for new jobs, but who are we to argue?

After that, which doctors would want to be involved in sport?

Doctors and sport fall into three broad categories.

Some have no interest in physical exercise for themselves or others. Others enjoy sport as a welcome distraction and healthy pursuit but not as an additional professional responsibility. Finally, there is the total enthusiast who is immersed body and soul in it. Many medics in their youth have been more than passable athletes. Some achieved fame on the sports field and pursued successful medical careers off it. W.G. Grace in cricket during the 19th century and Roger Bannister breaking the four-minute mile in 1954 were examples.

Orthopaedic surgery has an attraction for athletes. Richard Dodds captained Great Britain to 1988 Olympics hockey gold before taking up the 'carpentry' trade. Two great rugby union full-backs, J.P.R. Williams of Wales and Jonathan Webb of England also became 'bone setters'. The Belgian Jacques Rogge was a renowned rugby player, world champion yachtsman and orthopaedic surgeon before becoming president of the International Olympic Committee (IOC).

Most others have had no discernible sporting talent. However, all wanted to put their knowledge towards the furtherment of health and success for athletes at whatever level. Giving advice and treatment and later witnessing your patient return to previous levels of exercise (and even beyond) is a source of enormous professional satisfaction.

Athletes can help doctors!

We all have our sporting heroes – usually from our youth when we were beginning to play our chosen sports. The footballer Jimmy Greaves and the athlete David Hemery rank in my highest pantheon.

Others appear later from reading or watching their exploits and learning of their back story. I would love to have met C.B. Fry, who died in 1956. He was a true British polymath. He held the world long jump record and at soccer played once for England and appeared in an FA Cup final. He played rugby for the Barbarians and cricket for England (captain on several occasions). After sport he helped India at the League of Nations but refused an invitation to become King of Albania. In the 1930s, as a private citizen, he used cricket as a reconciliation attempt with Germany but his invitation to the Nazi von Ribbentrop to play cricket in the Third Reich was turned down.

Andy Ripley is a more modern-day Corinthian who affected my life. Ripley was the England and British Lions rugby number eight and a superb athlete who ate up the turf with his gambolling stride. He was the embodiment of someone enjoying life for all that it offered. After international retirement he turned out for his old college, the London School of Economics, against my hospital team. What a privilege for the other 29 of us. Later, he appeared in the television programme *Superstars*, broke the world indoor rowing age-group record and nearly qualified for the Boat Race.

He demands the ultimate respect for his final race. In 2010, at 62, his fight against prostate cancer defeated him. For the five years following diagnosis with advanced malignancy he championed research and increased awareness. In 2016 more men died of prostate cancer than women died from breast cancer in this country.

Ripley talked about the need for PSA blood testing – the test for prostate cancer. There were difficult issues around the disease and its treatment – incontinence, shrinking testicles and penile dysfunction, areas men have tried to ignore with crossed-fingers and crossed-legs. A story Ripley told has remained with me: a friend of his at the Tideway Scullers Rowing Club had informed his team-mates that he had prostate cancer. Ripley and the others commiserated and resolved to get their PSAs checked. None did. Soon after, Ripley was also diagnosed.

I admired Ripley but never knew him – apart from vainly trying to tackle him around his legs – yet his death affected me. I resolved to follow his advice. Six weeks after his death I had my first PSA test. I had no risk factors, just a feeling. Eight years later and with a PSA track record I detected the first upturn in results. There were no signs, no symptoms, and I had a standalone normal test reading. My GP looked at that result only and told me I was a typical worrying doctor. But I looked at all my results and, hypochondriac or not, followed Ripley's path to The Royal Marsden in London. Three months later, my prostate and its contained unwelcome visitor lay on the pathologist's slab.

Declan Cahill and his wonderful surgical team at The Royal Marsden are confident that it has been caught early and erased. I hope so, naturally. However, I will be forever in the debt of Andrew George Ripley. I suspect many thousands more are as well. Even in death, his infectious love for life reached its altruistic apogee in encouraging others to try to prolong their own lives by taking simple measures to protect their health.

The surgical skill set

Where does this leave the sports surgeon? Needing thorough preparation, organisation and learning from experience. Some sportspeople can be the most inspiring people you will ever meet. Others can be the most exasperating. My duty is to consider the problem in front of me but not fail to neglect the multitude of considerations in the background. Forming strong bonds with trusted colleagues within the sports world are vital to enable the discussions of concerns that will inevitably arise. Surgeons need mileage under their professional bonnets and honesty when a problem does not fit their specific skills repertoire. I need strength to stick to my beliefs – even if they are not what the athlete wants to hear.

Chapter 5

A SURGEON FOR ALL SEASONS: THE SPORTING CALENDAR

'How many things by season seasoned are
To their right praise and true perfection!'

William Shakespeare, *The Merchant of Venice*
(1596–1598)

THE 'ENGLISH Season' is the sporting and social calendar enjoyed by nobility since the 17th century. It encompasses nine high-profile events – the Chelsea Flower Show, Glyndebourne opera, the Epsom Derby, Royal Ascot and Glorious Goodwood horse racing, Wimbledon tennis, Henley rowing regatta, Windsor polo and Cowes sailing week. These events paint a quintessential and slightly eccentric picture of England but only span late spring and summer. We have a more extensive sporting calendar, with its own rhythm, which is beloved by a wider range of sports fans.

The FA Cup third round pitches minnows against mammoths at the beginning of the year. Rugby union's Six Nations then entrances us, while March and April bring the Cheltenham Festival, Grand National, London Marathon and university boat races. The finals of various football and rugby competitions take us through to the May bank holiday, when many of us are glued to TV coverage of the World Snooker Championship Final.

Subsequent warm weather brings cricket, and various rugby teams cross the equator on tour. The Derby, Wimbledon and golf Open usher in midsummer before the Charity Shield heralds England's new football season; the Scots start their season even earlier. Into autumn runners pound the streets preparing for the Great North Run and other endurance events. Later, we welcome the southern powerhouses of rugby, and soccer's Champions League begins.

We've also interwoven iconic North American fixtures into our sporting fabric, such as February's Super Bowl Sunday and the Augusta Masters Golf in April. In July, mad men in Lycra pursue the *maillot jaune* in the Tour de France. Soon it is almost Christmas and we have the chance to relive the best action through *Sports Personality of the Year (SPOTY)*. Apologies if I have omitted your favourite sporting occasion.

Layered on top of these events are the international extravaganzas that fit into a four-year cycle.

Year 1 (e.g. 2016): Olympic Games, European Football Championships and ICC World T20 cricket competition. The European Athletics Championships and golf's Ryder Cup also take place and are repeated in year 3.

Year 2 (2017) British Lions rugby tours and Rugby League World Cup. The World Athletics Championships is held and repeated in year 4.

Year 3 (2018) FIFA World Cup, Winter Olympics and Commonwealth Games.

Year 4 (2019) Rugby Union World Cup and 50-over Cricket World Cup.

Other sports have their own yearly or biennial continental or global championships or annual world cup series that trot around the globe. It is exhausting, even for the armchair aficionado, and that is before calamities like coronavirus start interfering.

We sports surgeons keep our pulses on the ebb and flow of these endeavours, to help predict injury arrivals and aid our appreciation of elite athlete and weekend warrior timetables. To help me understand the previous, present and future challenges of patients my practice manager, Gill Hurnell, assembles an athlete's profile. Being fit for an August world championship is useless if the athlete missed the qualification time or trials two months before. I need to place the injury and athlete in the setting of their goals; a treatment or surgery may work in March but not in June if the competition is in September. The closer the problem occurs to an event the more injury management rather than eradication is the goal.

The patient will see you now, Doctor!

I spent one year working as a junior casualty doctor and many more as an on-call surgeon. Patient numbers fluctuated with the hour of the day and day of the week, although one constant was the relative quiet when football matches were on TV. Once the final whistle blew, however, fans' attention returned to their ailments and casualty units gradually filled. Lumbagos that had been grumbling for days appeared, with a request for a sick note to present on Monday morning.

In 1983, I worked in casualty at Northwick Park, the nearest hospital to Wembley. Tranquillity reigned during the FA Cup Final from 3pm to 5pm while the country marvelled at Brighton and Hove Albion's resistance to Manchester United. The noise must have been deafening at the Twin Towers but the only sound in casualty was drunk supporters' snores. They had been admitted for their own safety to sleep off hangovers, their unused cup final tickets stored securely in the hospital safe.

Patients off-piste

The piste pixie is no respecter of age or experience. Disaster can strike on the nursery slopes during that first tentative morning snowplough, or mid-afternoon after a liquid lunch high above the treeline. A favourite injury scenario involves descending backwards down a black run on the last day of the holiday. On reaching home, damaged skiers find themselves in an NHS queue longer than those of their resort's bubble lifts.

The first skiing injuries appear during Christmas week and continue arriving until after Easter. Some skiers have had surgery, suturing or scanning abroad, while others are transported straight from the airport to A&E. I also see skiers from indoor ski centres with separated thumbs or groin strains from inelegantly performed parallel turns. That appetite for a pre-holiday schuss can result in their Alpine trip being spent mostly in the piano bar – seven days in permanent après-ski mode.

There is a new skiing phenomenon – skiers who appear in the middle of our summer often after holidays in Chile or New Zealand. Their journey home is long and they are impatient to be inpatients. They dream of a rapid return to southern slopes.

New England also has a lot of snow and I experienced one snow-laden winter while at Harvard. The snow would arrive at around Thanksgiving at the end of November and last until March. There was so much of it that local golf courses doubled up as cross-country ski trails; downhill slopes further afield were a comfortable day's excursion.

I was introduced to a new winter injury: snow blower's fingers. New Englanders possess an evil machine which can despatch snow from your drive into adjacent flowerbeds within minutes – if your blower is not blocked. If it is you must remember to turn it off before inserting your fingers into its innards; in their haste people forget. The blower belches into life and hands emerge looking as though their owners are auditioning for *Edward Scissorhands*. This meant that every winter Bostonians arrived in the emergency room divorced from their digits. Often the fingers had been fished from the chute and packed in ice from the driveway, but despite heroic surgical attempts to reattach them, most fingers were consigned to the trash can.

In 2015 the *Washington Post* reported that 9,000 Americans had lost digits in domestic appliances in the previous 12 years. Over 96 per cent of those people were male. The newspaper concluded that men were more likely to be ordered out to clear the snow and suggested as an afterthought that US winter driveways had become a battleground; in 2013 three times more Americans had been injured by snow shovels than blowers.

Years ago I saw a skier who had developed foot blisters and pain due to the frightening speed at which she negotiated turns and slalom poles. We agreed that surgery was needed. I was then asked if the whole process could be filmed for BBC 2's *Ski Sunday*. No pressure, then. I complied, and, although everything went well, watching it later did not help the digestion of my Sunday roast.

Post-Yuletide exercise

The post-Christmas rush to shed the Yuletide calories is commendable even if well-meaning new year's resolutions wilt within weeks. Some people join gyms while others seek local parks and footpaths for boot camps, runs and country walks. Sharing your pain with a mate is more likely to keep you going on the fitness drive.

Advice encourages gentle progression interspersed with recovery but few take the time to follow it. Christmas could not be scheduled at a worse climatic time for our exercise rhythms. January joggers have more than their fair share of foot, ankle and shin stress fractures and as viruses abound a common mistake is trying to make up for the missing mileage too quickly. Winters are frequently raw, increasing the risk of soft tissue injury, and the danger is compounded by inadequate pre-exercise stretching and warm-ups. Short days add the potential for ankles to disappear down potholes at twilight, while the hard and frequently icy ground increases the impact on lower limbs and the risk of falling – reprieving Torvill and Dean's *Boléro* ice dance.

Our bone resilience is likely to be at its lowest in the new year. When the sun goes south in the autumn so does our capacity to use sunlight to make vitamin D, a vital element in the maintenance of healthy bones and muscles. Standing outside in your shorts on a lovely November day will have no impact on your vitamin D production and by February our vitamin levels may have fallen by a fifth. People can be deficient precisely when they decide to don their trainers and jog down the street.

A study of my surgical patients found that just one-sixth has reasonable levels of vitamin D. One in five has levels so low that they risk their bone health. Dermatologists warn us of skin cancer risks from burning but there needs to be balance. Without vitamin D and sunshine our bones risk turning to jelly, even those of athletes.

The long and winding road

> *'But still they lead me back to the long*
> *and winding road'*
>
> **The Beatles, 'The Long and Winding Road' (1970)**

Despite Pheidippides' death at the end of the first marathon in 490BC, many are addicted to running the 26 miles and 385 yards that make up a marathon. Some do not stop there with ultramarathons and Ironman triathlons also popular. Participants wear their achievements for posterity, literally: like campaign medals, logos of events are tattooed on their torsos and any other available space. However, the training for, and participation in, these events is not without hazards.

The April London Marathon and September Great North Run loom large in my clinic diary. Ballot places are treasured and runners gather sponsorship for worthy and often personal causes. Television pictures from these events are inspiring and showcase triumphs of doggedness and of spirit overcoming pain, fatigue and less than optimal genetics.

For 'London', training takes place at a time of year when throats and lungs act as an Airbnb for assorted viruses and bacteria. Hazards also abound underfoot. Tough marathon exercise schedules can be the most extreme physical activity of peoples' lives. Some runners are trying to make up for lost training or reach the starting line not fully prepared. This is where illogicality sets in.

It is not ordained that your body will respond sympathetically to the required training, and several weeks before events runners with stressed bones and sausage-shaped Achilles limp slowly into outpatients. Panic sets in and patients tell me how much sponsorship money they have raised; withdrawal is not an option, whatever the injury. Enforced rest before the big day can come as a welcome relief to battered bodies, even though the effect on runners' brain endorphins is like going 'cold turkey'.

I can only advise and spell out the risk and on London Marathon mornings I sit and hope that injured patients will make it to The Mall without irrevocable harm. The week after can be busy: new or concealed problems arrive – such as fractures to be screwed or plastered, joints to be drained and tendons to be coaxed back to normal dimensions. I absolve from blame the organisers of these events. The advice on taking part is clear. The irrationality comes from the athlete alone.

My first 'up close' experience of marathons was in 1988 at the Boston Marathon, the oldest annual marathon which was first staged in 1897. The race finished in Copley Square where an enormous marquee was erected. Rows of examination couches were assembled and space blankets and intravenous lines prepared. Medics waited for the tsunami of 30,000 runners funnelling across the finishing line. There were as many podiatrists as medics, and they were required to minister to aching and blistered feet. The elite runners were given the more salubrious surroundings of a hotel suite. I was allocated to the first 20 male and female finishers.

The men's race was won by the Kenyan Ibrahim Hussein, the women's event by the great Portuguese, Rosa Mota, whose victory was the second of three in the race and was sandwiched between successes in the Rome World Championships and Seoul Olympics.

Conditions were wet and cool and Hussein finished one second ahead of the Tanzanian Juma Ikangaa. The race was packed with great runners, including Steve Jones, whose 1985 British marathon record stood until 2018 when it was broken by Mo Farah. Hussein was as fresh as a daisy afterwards despite his superhuman efforts. Not so some of the other runners, despite their elite status. The relative lack of post-race physical discomfiture of the African top finishers was astonishing. Their rapid recovery could be credited to excellent preparation, economic mechanics, good genetics and, for many, the advantages of living and training at altitude.

For others all hell broke loose once they were in the hotel and their inability to control any muscle led to collapse and outpourings best left undescribed. Close observation, maintaining equitable body temperature and fluid replenishment were vital. When I got home that evening I resolved never to run further than a half-marathon.

It's all in the timing

Most athletes welcome the end of the season and two weeks' R&R with family and friends on a beach. This off-season for sportspeople has no parallel for the sports surgeon; usually I face the reverse. For example, Northampton Saints' victory in the 2000 European Cup at Twickenham took its toll with leading lights falling by the wayside and others just about making it to the final whistle. At that evening's celebrations I spoke to Keith Barwell, the club's owner. While he was delighted that the season was over with silverware on the mantlepiece, I explained that my season was just beginning. I was aware of what many in the squad required.

Many players limp into the off-season both metaphorically and literally. Summer breaks in football and rugby are already short enough even if players are not involved in play-offs, cup finals or summer tours. Traditionally, soccer pre-season started in early July. Now most clubs creep into flaming June. Players may get six weeks' respite if they are lucky.

Injury problems often mount during the last quarter of the season when clubs' medical teams strive valiantly to make do but not mend. If surgery is deemed inevitable, timing is everything and is governed by recovery and return-to-play estimates. If the club is mid-table the decision may be made to withdraw the player from the team to allow post-surgical rehabilitation to take place in good time for the new season.

A professional footballer saw me with a tendon injury that had been niggling all season. It was then late April and he was due to be married in the next couple of weeks – in Greece. I was adamant that his surgery could not take place before his nuptials; I want my patients as close to base as possible post-surgery. Risks such as deep vein thrombosis from air flights and swelling and wound problems from heat keep me awake at night.

His manager suggested a chauffeur drive him to Greece. But travelling 1,700 miles in four days in the back of a car carries more health risks than four hours on a budget airline. How would the patient enjoy his honeymoon in 40°C heat with a healing slash down the back of his leg? His fiancée had some say on the final decision and the club reluctantly agreed that the surgery would take place on his return, which left very little time for rehabilitation. We were lucky, though. He made a miraculous recovery and missed only a handful of games at the start of the next campaign. His team won promotion and he finished the season as top scorer.

Pre-season can be challenging, as hamstrings and calves are cranked back into gear. Injuries happen and managers lose what hair they have left when their preferred starting XI begin falling like flies in early August. Some injuries have alternative management scenarios. Managers want surety of opinion when there is no definitive black or white answer

Professional cricketers have longer off-seasons than footballers or rugby players (although some play abroad during our winter). Pitches become harder as the domestic season progresses, taking a toll on legs and backs. Symptom control and workload management strategies come into play; October is the common surgical season for the county cricketer.

Sometimes players become regular off-season customers. One ex-Test cricketer found his knee became inflamed at the first sight of an outdoor cricket net after a winter of inactivity. For several successive springs he appeared with evidence of loose debris in his swollen joint. Similarly, an international rugby player had a propensity to form loose bodies in his elbow. These nasty little pebbles caused pain and loss of joint straightening, and during several off-seasons I removed a collection of them.

School's out forever

Peaks and troughs in children's injuries occur throughout the year.

In 1988, GCSEs were introduced into the British school curriculum, including physical education, which has a practical component. Every academic year 16-year-olds appear in my clinic unable to demonstrate sufficient skill in the required sports because of injury. In addition, school sports tours have become more adventurous. The furthest my school took us was Blackpool or South Wales. Now, most of the globe has been visited by an under-16 school sports team from the Home Counties.

The first 14 years of my consultant career involved being on-call every bank holiday Monday. School holidays and half-term breaks have a feel all to themselves. I wonder if the term was coined for the damage it inflicts on many immature bones. Every open space appears to provide opportunities for kids to inflict upon themselves, siblings and friends countless concussions, sprains and strains. Between 6pm and 9pm was the worst time. Children were tired but would still perch themselves on the bough of a tree or balance precariously on their big brother's skateboard. I spent countless evenings pulling bent wrists and deformed elbows back into place. They should have been in bed long before they pitched out of the local spreading oak tree.

Work as a surgeon is never dull and changes subtly with the seasons. Injuries by their nature are unpredictable to the individual but when dealing with large groups similar patterns emerge every year. This is as true in the world of sport as it is in wider society.

Chapter 6

SHRINKING VIOLETS?

'Who are the violets now ...?'

William Shakespeare, *Richard II* (1595)

AS THE father of three daughters I have tried to be supportive and encouraging of female sports participation. The battles won by female athletes and the distances metaphorically and literally run by them have been awe-inspiring but are easily forgotten.

Britain is regarded as the motherland of many sports played worldwide. However, we have been slow to champion the female athletes among us.

'Wee, sleekit, cow'rin, tim'rous beasties'

Robert Burns, 'To a Mouse, on Turning Her Up in Her Nest with the Plough', November 1785

No females were involved in the first Olympics, in Athens in 1896, the event's instigator Baron de Coubertin declaring that women would be 'impractical, uninteresting, unaesthetic, and incorrect'. Minds changed and four years later invitations to sportswomen were sent.

A total of 19 women entered the 1900 Olympiad but it was not until the 1928 Amsterdam Games that females competed in track and field, when 11 women ran the 800m. The media reported that many collapsed at the end but footage showed that they were no more exhausted than the men after their race.

Overseas officials admonished British management for supporting female inclusion in what was described as 'not a pleasant sight' and the IOC responded by barring females from running more than 200m.

This ban remained until the 1960 Rome Olympics when the 800m was reintroduced despite concerns that it was 'too taxing for the female frame'. In Tokyo in 1964 the women's pentathlon was introduced involving five events over two days. The longest distance was 200m. In my teenage years, under-17 girls were restricted to 150 yards at our national championships.

Outside of major games females continued to push the boundaries. In 1954, 23 days after Bannister's sub-four-minute mile, the English athlete Diane Leather breached the women's five-minute barrier. Her feat was not widely acclaimed and not accredited as an official world record, merely a world best. Leather celebrated with a quiet drink with her coach and club secretary. The International Amateur Athletics Federation (IAAF) didn't recognise women's middle-distance world records until 1967.

In 1972 I watched in Munich the first-ever Olympic women's 1500m heats and, contrary to pre-Games predictions, all participants survived the ordeal. Twelve years later females achieved what many had thought impossible 20 years before and completed an Olympic marathon, the American Joan Benoit, in a magnificent time of 2.24.52, leading home Norwegian Greta Weitz and Rosa Mota. In 2003, Paula Radcliffe lowered the women's world record to 2.15.25, a time that would have left the winner of the 1952 men's Olympic marathon, Emil Zatopek, trailing by at least 2km. Rather than proving to be the famous mouse of Burns' ode, many females have proved themselves durable and powerful athletes.

It was not only in athletics where thoughts of ladies breaking into a sweat held back female sports participation, and the psychological hangovers from Victorian times of women edging shyly from bathing machines did little to increase opportunities to swim. Lady swimmers were allowed into the Olympics in 1912. However, America only permitted women to compete in any sport (including swimming) if they wore long skirts. The US was not alone in this. Australian Fanny Durack won the inaugural 100m freestyle in a woollen costume combined with a skirt, which was something of a drag, literally, and limited her leg technique. Only in 1968 could females swim more than 400m, fortunately without a full twinset and pearls in sight.

In hockey, females first appeared in the Olympics in 1980. The men had competed from 1908 yet, in my youth, girls seemed more than a match for most males.

In modern times only equestrianism permits the sexes to compete against each other on equal terms, although some events allow men and women to compete on the same team, such as ice skating, tennis mixed doubles and sailing. With some exceptions sailing was gender neutral until 1988 when the sexes were segregated. In 2016, the Nacra 17 multihull catamaran was introduced for mixed crew competition. Mixed doubles curling featured in the 2018 Winter Olympics and Tokyo 2021 will introduce the mixed triathlon relay and mixed team rifle shooting.

Female rugby started in the 19th century but early matches were met with a public outcry and rioting. The England women's rugby team played its first full international only in 1987 and by 2014 they were world champions, following a thrilling competition assiduously covered by the media. Sarah Hunter and Maggie Alphonsi were among the stars.

I was introduced to quality female rugby while living in America in the mid-1980s, when the Boston Beantown club were national titleholders. They took no prisoners. My club, Beacon Hill, shared facilities and pitches with the champion outfit. Equality was more than established and the men had to wait until the ladies had finished training and relinquished the scrummaging machine.

On one wintry Saturday afternoon our game was postponed because of snow and I went to Harvard Stadium to watch an American football game played on an underground-heated pitch. I walked through a nearby park where a large crowd was watching a rugby game – it was the Beantown ladies. No amount of snow would stop them playing. I slunk off feeling rather precious.

At the Royal Free in the early 1990s I was asked if I would help set up my hospital's ladies' rugby team. Kit sponsorship was forthcoming from a company that, appropriately, manufactured knee replacements and we arranged coaching sessions on Hampstead Heath. The squad consisted mainly of talented hockey and rowing exponents, all fit, coordinated and tactically aware. They took on the accoutrements of rugby enthusiastically; debauched annual rugby club dinners are not a male preserve.

They were also brave. Too brave. And that was their undoing. They tackled like kamikaze pilots and I winced watching. Broken noses, cut lips and knee fractures mounted up. On two Sunday evenings I opened an operating theatre to screw the players back together. Before the end of the second season the team disbanded as there were not enough fit and willing volunteers to put a XV on the park. I reflected on the errors of our collective ways. A few training sessions could not compensate for a lack of years in honing sport-specific skills; learning correct head and body tackling positions takes time.

British female rugby is well established now. The first women's World Cup was held in 1991 and not surprisingly America dominated – the same pioneers I had witnessed on tundra-resembling pitches several years before. Since then it has been all New Zealand and England.

The history of women's football has been chequered. Scottish women were reported to have played an annual competition during the 1790s and much later, during the 1914–1918 war, numerous ladies' teams emerged. Many were based in the factories where females were turning out armaments. On Boxing Day in 1920 Preston-based Dick, Kerr's Ladies FC (formed at the Dick, Kerr & Co. munitions factory in 1917) took on St Helen's at Everton's Goodison Park. A crowd of 53,000 attended; many others had to be locked out of the ground. The team's star was 6ft centre-forward Lily Parr, who scored over 900 goals in a career that lasted until 1978. This post-First World War boost for the women's game shook the men's Football Association to its dubbined boots.

In 1921 the FA banned ladies' teams from Football League grounds. It claimed their football was 'distasteful' and that the game was 'quite unsuitable for females and ought not to be encouraged'. Teams transferred to parks and rugby grounds but standards dropped and playing numbers dwindled.

The second unofficial women's World Cup Final was played between hosts Mexico and Denmark in front of 110,000 spectators in 1971. The England team for the tournament had included 13-year-old sensation Leah Caleb. The momentum in the women's game was unstoppable by then and 50 years after the FA tried to strangle female participation it lifted its ban. This came just in time. An Italian semi-professional league emerged in the 1970s and other countries followed suit. Standards have risen exponentially since then and the professional women's game in England is now well established.

The 2019 World Cup in France gave the sport another boost and prompted a huge rise in attendance for the opening six fixtures of the Women's Super League 2019/20 season, the average gate rising to 10,488 compared to the 2018/19 season's average of 873. However, while Super League games were smashing attendance records, a talented Championship player had to rely on a whip-round by her club's men's team to pay for a knee scan, and was on an NHS surgery waiting list.

Soon after, the FA announced that it would ensure that medical costs for women would be covered in the future.

Women's cricket began to emerge in 1745 when 11 'maids' from Bramley in Surrey and the famous cricketing village of Hambledon in Hampshire played against one another. By 1890 the 'Original English Lady Cricketers' were profitably touring the country until their manager (presumably male) absconded with the proceeds. The first female Test match was contested in 1934 and in 1973 the first women's World Cup was played in England, with the hosts triumphing in the final over Australia. It was another two years before the inaugural men's World Cup took place.

The quality and athleticism of female football, cricket and rugby union has risen enormously. Over the last 30 years I have looked after many players from our national teams. They display maturity and professionalism in dealing with injuries, surgery and rehabilitation, and are more likely than their male counterparts to work with me during their recovery rather than try to negotiate shortcuts.

> *'I know I have the body of a weak, feeble woman; but I have the heart and stomach of a king, and of a king of England too ...'*
>
> **Queen Elizabeth I's speech to the troops at Tilbury, August 1588**

Before Lottery funding was made available for UK Sport I felt that most elite sportswomen succeeded despite the opportunities rather than because of them. They faced many 'man-made' obstacles. The UK had no female Olympic gold medallists in athletics until 1964 and even now only nine British women have won Olympic gold in track and field. These are incredible women whose successes should be savoured.

The roll-call of female sporting superstars was small in my youth. Some loomed large, though, including Mary Rand, Ann Packer, Mary Peters, Dorothy Hyman and Lillian Board from athletics, Angela Mortimer and Christine Truman from tennis, Anita Lonsbrough in swimming, Beryl Burton from cycling and Rachel Heyhoe Flint in cricket.

These heroines won the affection of us all and are best encapsulated by Lillian Board, a true darling of the nation. At 19, Board went to the 1968 Mexico Olympics as the 400m favourite but the French athlete

Colette Besson beat her by nine one-hundredths of a second. It seemed the whole of Britain had been trying to blow Board over the line. In 1969 Board became European 800m champion and that year my family travelled to the White City Stadium to see her compete against the USA. My mother was quite overcome to stand next to her in the queue for the ladies' loo.

The next year Board died aged 22 from colorectal cancer. Her forlorn mercy dash to a Bavarian clinic during the Christmas period of 1970 was reported on TV and in the press. The country was transfixed; the outpourings of grief were almost palpable.

We also cheered on foreign leading ladies such as Fanny Blankers-Koen (FBK) and Olga Korbut. FBK was the sensation of the post-war 1948 London Olympiad, at which she won four golds on the track. The Dutchwoman was the first female to achieve this feat. She was a mother of two but threw off the shackles to achieve feats that many had thought impossible. Sexist commentary followed: she was known as the 'Flying Housewife' and her home city, Amsterdam, gave her a new bicycle 'so she need not run so much'. A 2003 biography was entitled *A Queen with Men's Legs*.

Olga Korbut was the opposite of the mature 30-year old Dutchwoman but also finished with four Olympic golds. The 17-year-old 'sparrow from Minsk' won the hearts of the world with a display of athleticism that defied her slight frame. She had a major impact on gymnastics' popularity and changed its emphasis from the balletic elegance of older competitors to the acrobatics of young pocket rockets.

I witnessed one of Korbut's performances at the 1972 Munich Games. Without a ticket for the Olympiahalle, friends and I scaled the metal exoskeleton supporting the glass dome. As the Bavarian police implored us to descend we perched precariously, mesmerised by the performances of Korbut and her Soviet colleagues in the individual apparatus finals.

'Ne'er the twain shall meet?'

Rudyard Kipling, *The Ballad of East and West* (1879)

In more recent times there have been many female elite competitors to admire and try to emulate ... Nicole Cooke, Shirley Robertson, Sarah Ayton, Sarah Webb, Victoria Pendleton, Laura Trott (Kenny), Rebecca Adlington, Katherine Grainger, Helen Glover, Heather Stanning, Nicola Adams, Beth Tweddle, Charlotte Dujardin, Jade Jones, Kelly Holmes,

Christine Ohuoruogu, Jessica Ennis, Paula Radcliffe, Dina Asher-Smith … and these are just those involved in Olympic sports.

It remains difficult to keep teenage girls involved in sport, however. Over half of 17-year-old girls have given up sport altogether and two million fewer women than men play sport regularly in the UK. The 2015 'This Girl Can' campaign aimed to encourage female participation and was supported by Sport England. It was hard-hitting, using slogans such as 'Sweating like a pig, feeling like a fox' and 'I kick balls. Deal with it'.

Historically, women were restricted by societal straightjackets and in 1905 May Sutton Bundy, the first American to win the Wimbledon women's single's title, caused a stir by rolling back her cuffs to reveal her wrists.

Progress has been swift since 1945 and has led to speculation that female sporting achievements could outstrip those of men. In general, the gender gap for sports milestones (world records and leading performances) stands in favour of men whose results are on average between 9 and 17 per cent better across a range of sports.

Experience from decades of coaching men was rapidly transferred to females once sporting suppression was lifted post-1945. This was helped by a recalibration of women's physical potential during the war years – in military and civilian activities such as the Women's Land Army. Improved nutrition and medical advances in the 1950s and 1960s helped further.

In 2008 French research charted improvements in elite sports performance over nearly a century. For many sports, men's world records were only kept from the 1920s and women's from the 1950s. Factors such as institutional drug-taking muddied the waters.

Performance for both sexes advanced across a range of sports with an initial steep improvement, particularly for females. This produced a rapid closing of the gap between the sexes, although it occurred at different times in different societies. For example, in America it took place between 1950 and 1970 and in East Germany from 1970 to 1989. China's gender gap closed in the 1990s. The gender gap then stabilised, with improvements continuing in both sexes but at an equal rate. The researchers calculated that this stabilisation period started on average across all sports in 1983 and predicted that performances will continue to improve but at an equal pace between sexes, thus maintaining the status quo. The research has not been repeated and it is not clear if the 'status quo' has continued to be maintained.

'Girls will be girls and boys will be boys ...
They're in a problem they can't solve now
Oh, don't you get yourself involved, baby.'

The Isley Brothers, 'Girls Will Be Girls, Boys
Will Be Boys' (1970)

I was on a student teaching ward round on a special care baby unit in the 1970s when the paediatrician asked several of us to examine a newborn. This we did and afterwards he asked, 'What sex is the baby?' Some replied 'male', some 'female', others simply scratched their heads. We were supposed to be intelligent undergraduates.

Welcome to the cruel world of inter-sex, or differences in sexual development (DSD), which affects about one in 5,500 people. It is far more common in athletics and concerns over sportsmen masquerading as females has existed for decades.

Stella Walsh (born Stanisława Walasiewicz) won the 100m in the 1932 Olympics. After her death in 1980 it was revealed that she had male genitalia and was inter-sex. In the 1938 European Championships the world high jump record was broken by the German athlete Dora Ratjen. Later she was arrested, sent to a sports sanatorium and charged with fraud (charges later dropped). Her name was later changed to Heinrich.

The two Russian sisters Irena and Tamara Press set 29 world athletic records between 1959 and 1966. I remember these athletes well. The media dubbed them 'The Press Brothers' amid speculation that they were either male, inter-sex, or females force-injected with male hormones.

From 1946 the IAAF required female athletes to produce medical verification that they were females. In 1966 'nude parades' were introduced for the Budapest European Athletics Championships. Each woman had to appear in front of female gynaecologists, who would determine their 'womanliness'. World record holders in three events failed to attend, including Tamara Press. Both Press sisters promptly retired. Our 1972 Munich gold medallist Lady Mary Peters described the examination as the 'most crude and degrading experience I have ever known in my life'.

Fortunately the parades didn't last and the following year the IAAF introduced buccal smears – cell samples from the inside of cheeks to determine if the donor was male or female. Sorted? No. Life is not that easy. Many people can be labelled inter-sex, DSD, or, previously, hermaphrodite. David Epstein, author of *The Sports Gene*, explained: 'Biological Sex is not binary. That means whichever line you draw between men and women it is going to be arbitrary.'

More sophisticated tests were developed and unusual results started appearing. In 1967 the Polish athlete Ewa Klobukowska was found to carry a rare abnormality of a mixture of genes – known as mosaicism – and was banned even though there was no evidence of competitive advantage. Between 1972 and 1990 an estimated 504 elite athletes were disqualified on sex-testing grounds.

In the 1976 Montreal Olympics the only female to be excused from testing was Princess Anne. It was deemed inappropriate to submit the Queen's daughter to such ignominy. Additionally, it was pointed out that HRH was competing in equestrian events where sexes took part on equal terms.

These forms of tests were stopped by the IAAF in 1991 and by the IOC in 1999. Results were simply not conclusive enough. This meant that another solution was needed. What about testosterone – its levels distinguish males from females, surely …

Testosterone levels peak in early adult life then fall from then on. Men lose 1 per cent of testosterone annually from age 40. The drop is similar for females, particularly after the menopause.

Testosterone comes from male testicles and, in lesser amounts, from woman's ovaries, and from the adrenal glands in both sexes. Normally testosterone levels are between 8.8 and 30.9 (nmol/L) in men and 0.4 and 2.0 in women. This is known as your 'T-score'. On average, men have 10–20 times more testosterone than females. However, the waters become muddied in elite sport.

In 2011, the IAAF set the upper T-score limit for females at 10, 'to protect the health of the athlete'. Above this level, athletes were diagnosed as being in a state of hyperandrogenism (high levels of male hormones in females). For those females to compete again, their high levels would need to be reduced through medical intervention.

This policy was suspended in 2014 following a successful case brought by the Indian sprinter Dutee Chand, who had T-scores over 10 (they can fluctuate so several are taken). She was dropped from the Indian 2014 Commonwealth Games team, examined by male doctors and questioned about her periods and body hair. She claimed that the Athletics Federation of India viewed cases such as hers as bringing shame upon Indian sport and took her case to the Court of Arbitration for Sport

(CAS), which ruled that the IAAF had not demonstrated that high T-scores improved performance.

Research has demonstrated that normal T-score ranges are wide with a greater overlap between sexes in elite athletes. Research in 2014 found that 16.5 per cent of male athletes had T-scores below 8.4, and 13.7 per cent of female scores were above 2.7. A study four years later reported that in certain Olympic sports a quarter of male athletes had T-scores below 10 and that 5 per cent of female scores were above 10. Could some men qualify for female events based on hormone analysis? This could be a blow for many macho men.

The IAAF needed evidence of the advantages of elevated T-scores for certain women and used 2017 research in which T-scores from the World Athletics Championships of that year were analysed. For men, T-scores were highest in sprinters and lowest in throwers, notably hammer, shot and discus participants. For females, high T-score athletes did better in the 400m, 400m hurdles, 800m, hammer and pole vault. Such advantages were not seen in male events.

The IAAF announced that for events from 400m to 1500m (including the 4x400m relays and heptathlon), females must have had T-scores below 5 for at least six months before competition. This policy was due to be implemented at the end of 2018 but Caster Semenya, the double Olympic 800m champion, said she might switch to the 5k and 10k to avoid restrictions. The South African had been the subject of much speculation since claiming the 2009 World 800m title but accusations were also made relating to the scientific robustness of the IAAF's evidence, with the 2017 researchers admitting data analysis errors.

Raised male hormones do not necessarily produce benefits in sport. Some inter-sex people have Androgen Insensitivity Syndrome (AIS), in which there is a failure to respond normally to testosterone – whatever the level. For example, Maria José Martínez-Patiño was a Spanish high hurdler in the 1980s. Initial sex tests were satisfactory, she gained her certificate of femininity and made the quarter-finals of the 1983 World Championships. Two years later, further tests showed that she carried the male (XY) chromosome pattern and she was banned. Later it was revealed that she had AIS and she was reinstated in 1988. Too late – her best years of competition were behind her. The task of establishing an individual's sensitivity to male hormones – the effect of its presence – remains difficult, even now.

The IAAF suspended the implementation of its rule changes in October 2018. The United Nations condemned the IAAF's original plan, citing possible human rights breaches. However, when Caster Semenya contested the legality of the IAAF eligibility regulations in May 2019 and brought her case to CAS, the court ruled in favour of the IAAF. While CAS had sympathy for such athletes, it argued that such measures were 'necessary, reasonable and proportionate' for 'preserving the integrity of female athletics'. In future, Semenya would be required to take testosterone-reducing drugs to compete in the 800m.

Clearly this topic is a minefield and has prominent athletes on either side of the divide. In the IAAF corner were Brits such as Paula Radcliffe, Sharron Davies and Lynsey Sharp. On Semenya's side were Billie-Jean King and the transgendered, retired elite cyclist, Philippa York (formerly Robert Millar).

The IAAF stated, 'This is about our responsibility to ensure, in simple terms, a level playing field.' However, sport has never been level, which is why 99.999 per cent of the population watch the other 0.001 per cent compete at the Olympics. The rest of us don't have the same anatomy and physiology. I am convinced that I'd have had the makings of an Olympic champion at 110m hurdles – had I been 6ft 4in with legs up to my armpits. Instead, I am 5ft 8in with legs so short that they encouraged friends to call their Shetland pony after me.

Genetics, genetics, genetics. Several hundred different gene variations have been identified to give 'chosen ones' a physical advantage. Colleagues and I have tried to piece together why some athletes are more genetically programmed to suffer injury – another key factor in athletic success. A gene called EPOR controls the number of red blood cells we have and hence our oxygen-carrying capacity, and possession of the right EPOR gene variations is described by David Epstein in *The Sports Gene* as the 'gold medal mutation'.

It will take the wisdom of Solomon to resolve this, but it seems likely that an athlete's pure T-score alone will not be the final answer. In the meantime, certain female races may be 'testosterone monitored' while other events remain a 'free for all'. Males with low T-scores can be supplemented under medical supervision, while females with a high T-score will be banned until levels drop. As Oliver Hardy said to his comedy partner Stan Laurel, 'Well, here's another nice mess you've gotten me into.'

Recently, the issue of transgendered former men competing in women's sport has become a hot topic, particularly since Canadian Rachel McKinnon won an age-group World Championships title after changing sex.

Whatever the impact of gender reassignment surgery and/or hormonal manipulation to reduce testosterone levels, the physical in-built advantages acquired during adolescence remain. Stronger muscles and bones and enhanced lung and heart capacity give extra power and endurance. Sporting organisations need to balance the individual's rights against any risks to other athletes competing against a stronger, larger or faster opponent in contact sports. We have not heard the last of this issue, but a fair conclusion must be reached; the alternatives are too harsh to contemplate for many sports.

What are the alternatives? Most seem fanciful. One could be competition in which all men compete against all women. Women would be the losers and we would usher in a new Victorian order. Alternatively, we could create numerous classifications of able-bodied competitors in the same manner as paraolympic sport. What groupings could be dreamt up? Categories based on T-scores, weight, height, your country's gross domestic product, carnivores and vegetarians, or star signs? The list is endless.

In 2019 Scottish Athletics announced its solution: a non-binary gender category which would be neither male nor female. It was an admirable fix in many ways, especially for those happy to be openly identified as such. However, there are issues with a 'third way'. If it is self-determining, might average sportsmen decide to recategorise themselves, hoping for greater glory? Would individuals who had previously kept their genetic differences a private matter want to move into such a classification? Might pressure be exerted on certain people to move into this alternative category?

In English women's cricket, players need only to self-identify as female to join a team below international level. However, in 2019 a Kent transgendered player posted a batting average of 15 in the male side and 123 for the female team. In response to the adverse media coverage, the player opted to make public her medical background and revealed that her normal T-score was 1.1 – well within the normal female range. However, there would be obvious safety issues if Jofra Archer self-identified as a female and turned out for a village ladies' 3rd XI. The ECB is seeking a solution.

In 2017 the International Cricket Council set a maximum T-score of 10 for eligibility to play in women's international games, which was endorsed by CA two years later. Sports authorities in athletics, cycling and rugby are lowering the maximum level to 5. The IOC level remains at 10. This means that, theoretically, some athletes could compete in female events in one sport and male events in others.

There are no easy solutions to these thorny issues. Every individual caught up in this physiological enigma will be different. All need our understanding.

Vive la différence

There are clear differences in anatomy, physiology, biomechanics, hormones and psychology between the sexes and these are reflected in sporting performance. They may also affect susceptibility to injury.

Testosterone is one factor, as discussed above, and most men have testosterone in spade loads. Women have less but it is still a vital component for normal metabolic activity, sexual function and exercise. Testosterone T-scores correlate with competitiveness and aggression, although these are imprecise relationships.

Many years ago I spoke with sports psychologist Bill Beswick, who had been brought into the England rugby camp by then national coach Stuart Lancaster. We were watching an England training session and talked about the differences in unifying men's and women's teams. He said that in his experience males needed to go to war before they bonded while females needed to bond before being ready to go to war. Males needed a warrior's mutual respect before becoming mates; females operated in the opposite direction.

Men and women also differ skeletally, in pelvic shape and size, and the angles formed between our arms and legs. Our fat percentages and distribution differ and males have a greater capacity to carry oxygen to exercising parts. One test of aerobic fitness, called VO2 max, is usually higher by about 10 per cent in similarly aged males and females – even allowing for differences in weight and fat percentage. Males have a greater total muscle mass than females, which is more marked in the arms than the legs. World Rugby is now considering banning transgendered players from participating in female rugby following the publication of research suggesting that other players may face an increased injury risk if they are tackled by a player who has gone through male puberty.

Many female dancers and athletes develop eating disorders, menstrual irregularities and suboptimal bone health, formerly known as the Female Triad. In my clinic, middle- and long-distance runners and triathletes, particularly, are affected.

The 1980s concept of the Female Triad has been superseded by the concept of Relative Energy Deficiency in Sport (RED-S). This recognises the inability, or unwillingness, of athletes to replenish through their diet the high energy expenditure of training and performance. This can cause damage to nearly every bodily system and remains the predominant (but not exclusive) preserve of the female athlete.

Much emphasis is placed on vitamin D status, bone biochemistry and density, and sporting organisations make recommendations regarding bone health. I was a signatory to vitamin D guidelines published by the ECB. As doctors, we need to concentrate on both the immediate problem (e.g. a broken bone) and deal with underlying causes.

Do sports injury patterns differ in females and males? Injury surveillance is a notoriously difficult area and comparing sports is challenging because of the different demands. Within the same sport, there are differences in exposure to risk based on factors such as an athlete's size. How much more likely are the tackler and tackled players in male rugby to sustain an injury than their usually lighter female counterparts? Injury rates are calculated on exposure rates – time spent training and playing the sport. This may be different for males and females, and in junior and elite sport.

We know that female horse riders are likely to suffer more from concussion and take longer to recover from them. Research also suggests that female athletes are more susceptible to knee and ankle injuries. Female soccer players have a two to three times higher risk of injury to an ACL than males relative to the same involvement in sport. Females sustain these injuries at a younger age and more often than males during games. Potential risk factors have been identified and include gender differences in sex hormones, biomechanical and anatomical variations, and muscle control mechanisms. Our research group has described genetic variations that increase the risk of female ACL rupture that are not present in males.

These risks should be known to all involved in the care of female athletes and preventative schedules enacted.

Unlike the views of the founder of the modern Olympics in 1896, we have come to appreciate and value the excellence of female sport in all its manifestations. Athletes, coaches and clinicians should appreciate the variances between the genders. These differences should be understood and embraced rather than used as an excuse to regard females within sport as inferior.

Chapter 7

THE YOUNG

Pitches, politics and participation

'The other man's grass is always greener
Some are lucky, some are not
But I'm so thankful for what I've got'

Petula Clark, 'The Other Man's Grass
(Is Always Greener)' (1967)

IN MODERN Britain, youngsters' participation in recreation and sport is widely diverse.

At one end, we have huge numbers of adolescent couch potatoes. In the middle, there is a large group that undertakes sport primarily for enjoyment, and at the other end an increasing number are involved in serious, structured sports programmes aimed at achieving elite status. Dangers abound at both ends of the spectrum.

Obstacles have been put in the way of childhood sport that did not exist in the 1950s and 1960s. We walked or cycled to school and had breaktime exercise, twice-weekly PE lessons and formal games sessions that ensured we were pushed physically as much as mentally. During holidays, weekends and after school we disappeared for hours, playing different impromptu games. Today 'stranger danger' worries and concerns about the volume of traffic have created safety fears. Most children are now ferried to school in cars or buses.

In the 2014–15 period, 20 per cent of reception class children were either overweight or obese. For year 6 (10–11 year olds) this figure was 33 per cent. In 2016, 2 per cent of the UK's under-11s cycled to school compared to 49 per cent in the Netherlands. In 2018, every primary school class had, on average, one severely obese child. Primary school sport is clearly not working and, soon, half of all children will have an unhealthy body mass index (BMI) – a measure that uses height and weight to determine healthy body size.

I live within three miles of my childhood home and it is unusual, nowadays, to see jumpers and coats piled up as makeshift goalposts in the parks in which I played. My grammar school had over 200yds of covered cycle racks. They have all been removed.

Long before my schooldays the Duke of Wellington claimed that 'the battle of Waterloo was won on the playing fields of Eton'. It was believed, then, that sport taught more than the game itself – that pupils also learnt fair play, discipline, teamwork and leadership values. Sport has become our modern but sanitised battleground, without the relative lawlessness of war. Pupils of public schools still have access to playing fields but many state-educated students do not. After the 2012 Olympics, Colin Moynihan, the former Conservative sports minister, noted that half the GB medallists were educated privately compared to just 7 per cent of British children.

The more probable reason for our success in the Napoleonic wars was our economic strength. Contrast that with 21st-century Britain in which economic realities are one of the main reasons why so much school sport has been stifled. Since the late 1970s, successive governments have sold over 10,000 school playing fields; five years after the 2012 Olympics they were being sold at the rate of one per fortnight, reducing opportunities for so many youngsters. On top of that, regulations have reduced the minimum green space schools must offer pupils for recreation.

The real tragedy, however, is that participation in school sport was improving until austerity measures were imposed, despite the sale of playing fields. In 1997 only 25 per cent of state school children received at least two hours of PE per week. By 2010 it was 95 per cent. Cuts to the School Sports Partnership (SSP) in 2020 have significantly reduced the figure. The SSP was designed to improve access to specialist sports teachers and increase the number and range of organised sports offered, but by 2013 it was estimated that the percentage of schoolchildren undertaking two hours of weekly sport had fallen to 43 per cent, demonstrating how reliant school sport was on central funding.

In March 2013 the government announced £150m would be made available annually for youngsters' sport, through the Primary PE and

Sport Premium but while very welcome, successive governments' stop-go policies have impacted greatly. Academic reorganisations have also affected sport. GCSE and A level exam dates creep towards Easter, affecting summer sport significantly, especially cricket and particularly in state schools.

That special breed of teacher who gave up their spare time to organise, train and transport school sports teams is now rare. Half a century on, I am still in touch with the three individuals from school who encouraged me in my sporting endeavours. Will my children and grandchildren maintain the same bonds? Sporting access is now increasingly dependent upon out-of-school groups, which fill the breach left by successive governments' misguided policies.

It is inspiring to see the number of parents giving up evenings and weekends at local clubs. However, these organisations still face constant challenges in funding their activities and providing coaches. The well-intentioned introduction of mandatory screening (such as the Disclosure and Barring Service) has put off some parents and helpers, who are alarmed by the pitfalls of working with youngsters.

Belatedly, government is tackling the vested interests that peddle unhealthy diets for children and is instead promoting healthy eating. But the culture that promotes sedentary post-school activities still needs reversing. Government has finally woken up to the links between poor fitness, ill health and obesity, although this seems a case of 'closing the sweet shop door after the child has bolted'. Have ministers acted because of economic pressures on our beleaguered NHS? Each taxpayer shells out an extra £409 annually to fund NHS treatment of conditions such as Type II diabetes caused by obesity. Obesity shortens life and diminishes our national productivity. The intended legacy of the 2012 Olympics, to create a fitter and slimmer generation of youngsters, remains unfulfilled.

Larger than life? Or larger-than-life needs?

'The rise of childhood obesity has placed the health of an entire generation at risk.'

Tom Vilsack, US Secretary of Agriculture (2009–2017)

Sports medicine aims to improve community health by promoting regular exercise programmes. This is infinitely more important than massaging the bodies and egos of elite athletes.

In the 1960s only 1 per cent of men and 2 per cent of women were classified as obese in the UK but overall obesity levels had risen to 15 per cent by 1993 and 27 per cent by 2018. In 1954 the average British man was 5ft 7in tall and weighed 11st 6lb and the average woman 5ft 2in and 9st 10lbs. By 2020 we were an average of two inches taller but comparatively much heavier. The average UK middle-aged male weighed 13st 5lb and female 11st 6lb. In 66 years, we have put on an average of two stone and females' average waist circumference has grown by seven inches.

A 2010 report found that we were large compared to many European countries. In France, the average male weighed 10st 9lb and had a BMI of 24, compared to the average British male BMI of 27. In Italy the average male weight was 11st 9lbs and BMI 26.

The pattern elsewhere overseas is mixed. Americans have an obesity rate of 38 per cent and, despite their associations with the outdoor active lifestyles, the obesity rate for Australia is 28 per cent and for New Zealand 31 per cent. However, the Netherlands, France and the Scandinavian countries are at least 10 per cent lower than us; Italy has an obesity rate of only 10 per cent. Over the 2016–2017 period our hospitals were filled with 617,000 obesity-related admissions – an 18 per cent increase in one year.

The causes of obesity are many and are predominantly lifestyle related. Fewer people undertake physical work, we usually rely on cars for travel and choose unhealthy diets. The obesity cost to the UK economy is £27 billion. We are all the poorer for this epidemic.

Recently an eminent paediatrician described how some parents had brought their child for investigation because of a 'failure to thrive'. They were concerned that his ribs were showing but the boy had a completely normal age-related height and weight. We are forgetting what a healthy, slim child looks like.

Minority ethnicity, geographical location and social deprivation increase obesity risk in children. In 2015 only 23 per cent of boys and 20 per cent of girls met physical activity targets for one hour of moderate exercise daily. Obese schoolchildren are twice as likely to become obese adults.

The medical consequences of this are dire and include Type II diabetes, hypertension, heart disease and certain cancers. Obesity takes up to two decades off a person's useful healthy life and reduces life expectancy by six years in females and eight years in males. The association between obesity and deficiency of vitamin D, which is so important for our bone strength, is well established. Type II diabetes is normally associated with obese adults. In 2015, 95 children were diagnosed with the condition in the UK. That figure had risen to 172 children one year later.

The COVID-19 crisis has brightened the spotlight on obesity and the importance of exercise. The death from the virus of patients with a high BMI and the need for our population to walk and cycle for personal well-being and to reduce the use of public transport have been highlighted. Even the one-time obesity 'Luddite', Boris Johnson, has changed his mind on anti-obesity measures and his government has pledged funds to facilitate safer cycling. It seems the Prime Minister did not have a conversion on the road to Damascus but after treatment for COVID-19 at St Thomas' Hospital.

What are the consequences for orthopaedic surgeons, sports physicians and therapists?

Obesity has a detrimental effect on bone health. It is believed that there is a complex relationship between fat cell stimulation and bone formation. As we age, obesity is linked with diminishing bone and muscle mass. This is known as osteosarcopenic obesity.

Obesity alters balance and movement control in children and adults and obese people are more prone to falls, trips and stumbles. Significant injury from a fall is much more likely in the obese; obese patients spend longer in hospitals and are more prone to complications following injury, including clots in the legs (deep vein thromboses) and lungs (pulmonary emboli).

Heavier youngsters in America are more likely to break limbs and then require surgery and have higher risks of leg clots and skin ulcers after injury. Studies elsewhere have confirmed that obese children are more likely to sustain fractures. Ankle sprains in high BMI children are associated with more long-term issues such as chronic pain, swelling and recurrent injuries.

Overweight children are also more likely to develop hip joint problems (slipped upper femoral epiphysis), a knock-knee condition (Blount's disease) and a hunchback posture (kyphosis).

The evidence of damage to our offspring's physical and mental well-being from excessive childhood weight is overwhelming, and it can affect the rest of their lives. Vilsack's statement was no exaggeration. As a society we need to protect our children from themselves.

To be young, gifted and 'backed'

> *'Young, gifted and black*
> *We must begin to tell our young*
> *There's a world waiting for you*
> *This is a quest that's just begun.'*

Nina Simone, 'Young, Gifted and Black' (1969)

At the other end of the scale is the 'hot-housing' of children within various sports organisations, about which I have a dilemma. I thrill at the successful end product – the majesty of Max Whitlock's gymnastic routines at Rio 2016; the dynamism and skill of an emerging football talent such as Marcus Rashford. And like most sports doctors, I was drawn to my work by my own joy in exercise participation and the pleasure of watching sports people across the globe, live or on TV.

But, once involved, my priorities changed from enjoying the opportunity to 'get closer to the action' to concern for the athletes in my care. The emergence of the next Mo Farah or Cristiano Ronaldo requires their sport to identify, coach and, ultimately, reject many hundreds of thousands of other would-be sporting greats. Youngsters participating in more than 16 hours of sport weekly carry a greater injury risk – whether this involves one or multiple sporting activities.

Academies

> *'By education most have been misled.'*

**John Dryden, Northamptonian poet and
playwright, 'The Hind and Panther' (1687)**

Most major sporting organisations worth their salt have academies in which young talent is identified, instructed and monitored. Football does it biggest and best, especially in the UK. With their seemingly bottomless pits of money and extensive scouting networks, major soccer clubs annually hoover up much of the promising young teenage talent, to the detriment of other sports at times.

In *No Hunger in Paradise* Michael Calvin assessed the development of young footballers in England. He estimated that 1.5 million youngsters were involved in organised football but that only 180 would become Premier League footballers – one in every 8,333 promising young players.

The chances diminished almost season by season. In the 2014/15 Premier League season, English players accounted for 36 per cent of total playing time. In the following season the figure fell to 31 per cent.

Is peddling the dream to youngsters and making promises to parents healthy? Are the cold statistics explained? Is everybody aware of the remoteness of success in securing a professional football contract?

The investment by children and parents in time and travel, together with the potential sacrifice of academic opportunities, are immense. Football clubs have crunched the numbers in terms of cost, time and quantity to ensure they will unearth an unpolished gem to adorn their first XI or be sold for enormous profit. You might reply that disappointment is part of growing up. That unless one tries then failure is inevitable and that somebody will succeed – why not my child?

The costs of rejection can be great. In the US in 2015, 30 per cent of young athletes were enrolled in highly specialised one-sport programmes. Research at the time found that those athletes risked 'injury and burnout' and that the degree of specialisation 'positively correlated with increased serious overuse injury risk'. Injury and burnout risk in these athletes was higher because of 'single-sport training, participation in more competition, decreased age-appropriate play, and involvement in sports that require the early development of technical skills'. Coaches could increase the risk 'by encouraging increased intensity in organized practices and competition rather than self-directed unstructured free play'.

This system of specialisation was first fostered in Eastern Europe and was believed to be the most effective way of talent identification and development. Conversely, Norway is the most successful sporting country on the planet yet has a policy of no scores kept in organised sports up to under-13s. This is designed to promote enjoyment and reduce competitiveness.

I believe that children should sample a variety of sports and participate in free and unstructured activities, allowing them to develop a range of physical skills. All children should have periodic S&C work to prepare them for whatever future sports they take up, but youngsters singled out for intense single-sport involvement need close monitoring. These kids need periods of specific work to enhance muscle control, particularly in areas of recognised weakness, to improve skill levels and, importantly, reduce injury risk.

Further benefits of exposure to different sports were emphasised in the days following the gold and bronze medals of Lizzy Yarnold and Laura Deas in the bob skeleton in the 2018 PyeongChang Winter Olympics. Both had attended the same talent-spotting event – the Girls4Gold scheme in 2008 – and Natalie Dunman, head of talent ID for UK Sport, said that youngsters such as Yarnold and Deas, with multi-sports backgrounds, were most able to learn a new sport quickly.

Since the mid-1990s, rugby union has made rapid strides in developing club academies. Youngsters are identified early and placed with coaching staff aligned to Premiership clubs. The previous system of school and representative rugby followed by club trials or joining the local junior side has been dismantled.

Rugby youngsters are given advice on how to play, train and think like a professional. When I see them because they are injured they tell me they play for an elite Premiership club. Progress into the ranks of Premiership 1st XV squads is unlikely, however, because there's so much competition. But their heads have been turned and when the probable rejection slip arrives it has consequences: youngsters feel failures; their dreams are shattered. Thirty years ago they would have been the stars of their local junior clubs because they wouldn't have been funnelled into big-club youth schemes. But now, many give up altogether having fallen out of love with their chosen sport. Involvement in extreme one-sport conditioning, injuries, the development of a limited one-sport skill set, and time away from other pursuits risks limiting their enjoyment and success in other recreational activities. The activity that consumed them at age 13 has lost its attraction five years on. Hours of training, early mornings and lost weekends, disappointing academic results, injuries, competitive failures and a desire to live a 'normal' life take their toll.

Enter stage left the sports physician or orthopaedic surgeon unprepared for the simmering underlying issues.

There are times when youngsters sustain a serious injury and are advised to refocus their dreams. My antennae must also be attuned to niggling injuries that should resolve but linger. I have to look behind the words and concentrate on the unspoken messages. These are difficult times and it helps to speak to the athlete alone without the accompanying parents or coaches. Occasionally there is a dawning realisation that the youngster wants out and is relieved that someone has taken the decision out of their hands. It legitimises their explanation to family and friends: 'I wanted to carry on, but the doctor …'

I am a great admirer of Matthew Syed's writing. Syed is an ex-table tennis champion and current sports columnist with *The Times*. He has written on the myth of talent and the power of meaningful practice to acquire the skills to become a champion, or, indeed, a leading musician, businessman or ... surgeon. His books, *Bounce*, *Black Box Thinking* and *The Greatest*, examine the requirements to reach our own pinnacles.

Syed explores the principle, popularised by Malcolm Gladwell in his 2008 book *Outliers*, that 10,000 hours of deliberate practice is the key to greatness. He asks whether early access to such quality sessions in a chosen field of life, including sport, allow a champion such as Roger Federer to emerge? The theory has been challenged but early talent recognition and engagement in relevant structured activities do appear to provide advantages, particularly in the fields of music and sport.

Gladwell also explains, however, that sufficient practice by itself is not a guarantor of success, and that the 10,000-hours-of-practice theory does not apply to sport. However, his concepts have gained popular currency and have acted as a prop to those launching youngsters into regularised sporting programmes from an early age.

Youngsters should follow their sporting ambitions, and talented and aware coaches ought to train gifted teenagers for greatness. However, from a medical viewpoint, I have concerns about the health and development of these youngsters. The improvements in sports sciences must include a capability for assessing and monitoring their danger points.

Children are not 'little adults' either psychologically or physically. Safeguarding qualifications are part of every doctor's ongoing professional education and should be mandatory for anybody involved with the development of young athletes.

Colleagues and I discuss whether certain teenage problems we see represent child safeguarding issues. They often involve recurrent or chronic injury, eating disorders and unhappy, disengaged youngsters. Concern arises when parents and/or coaches don't seem to accept the underlying causes – the punishing training and competition schedules.

We do not fully understand the long-term effects of sporting rejection on a child's development or the potential damage in areas such as education and social skills – the problems of 'putting all of one's eggs in one basket' to pursue the sporting dream.

'Owing a duty of care' and 'a duty of candour' are phrases heard frequently among clinicians. I wonder how frequently they are adhered to by major sports organisations as another annual trawl of youngsters with potential, and their parents, arrive for the first training session. Everybody needs to understand that it is a numbers game. Skill and dedication are not enough; opportunity and luck, including freedom from injury, are as important. The chances of making it are tiny and the potential physical and psychological downsides should not be ignored.

Say (Swiss) cheese!

In the early 2000s I visited the British Airways flight training centre at Heathrow as part of a Royal College of Surgeons delegation. We were meeting our aviation counterparts to discuss education and training within our respective professions. I was tremendously impressed with the equipment and ethos of the establishment.

Airlines were fostering a culture of openness and learning from mistakes. It seemed light years ahead of surgical training apprenticeship methods where mantras such as 'see one, do one, teach one' still had currency.

For pilots, a mistake was not a disciplinary offence if the individual(s) identified the issue and reported it. An open and reflective process followed to indicate if remedial training was required, which might identify a corporate issue that needed correcting. Sanctions applied only if a cover-up was attempted. Within surgery that level of transparency had not been reached; the spectre of professional proceedings or legal action hung over us.

Additionally, I was introduced to Swiss cheese, which, because of its holes, was used as a model of accident causation by the British psychologist James Reason in the early 1990s. The airlines embraced his theory early and it has since been used extensively in other sectors, including health.

Mishaps can occur because of both systems and individuals. Reason likened defences against calamities to slices of Swiss cheese stacked together. Each slice was a barrier to error. More slices, or levels of defence, reduced the opportunities for accidents. However, each slice had holes in it. These were the system's weaknesses.

If one layer of cheese was breached, the next layer should stop any further breach. In airline terms, a faulty engine should trigger an alarm on the cockpit instrument panel – the second slice. However, the holes are not static – they can enlarge, close or increase in number because of personal or system failure – and if the holes (the defects) temporarily line up, the aeroplane (or in health terms the patient) can fly through the entire cheese to disaster. Reason called it the 'trajectory of accident opportunity'.

I applied the concept when considering young athletes reaching elite status but in that case the concept applies in reverse. For each of the 882 British Olympic medallists from 1896 to 2016, multiples of that number might have triumphed but for happenstance or lack of it – if the holes had lined up they'd have sailed through to success rather than hitting the barrier of, say, injury.

With raw talent, sporty youngsters need the fates to smile favourably – supportive families, local clubs or schools that encourage the specific sport at which they excel, positive role models and outstanding coaches; freedom from injury at critical times of competition is also critical. The young athlete needs either to avoid major injuries or, at least, be fortunate enough to be treated by an experienced physiotherapist, sports doctor or surgeon at the vital time.

Factors such as Lottery funding, improved sports science and medicine, and better media exposure of varying sports have reduced the number of Swiss cheese slices and enlarged the size of the remaining holes, making it easier for the talented to fulfil their potential.

Syed explained in *Bounce* how he became our leading table tennis player. He had natural aptitude but also parents who bought a table tennis table, a competitive older brother, a gifted and enthusiastic schoolteacher and coach, and 24/7 access to facilities at the local table tennis club. This propelled him to sporting fame and produced more leading table tennis talent in his locality than almost the rest of the country put together. Large holes were created in Syed's local fromage.

An inability to tackle childhood obesity, playing field sell-offs, and reducing coaching and competition opportunities (especially in disadvantaged parts of our society) have the reverse effect. They place impenetrable slabs of good old British cheddar in the path – free from holes – that even the overweight cannot digest.

The fulfilment of sporting potential is a partnership of the individual and the system. Neither can succeed without the other. Our next gold medallist may indeed represent 'an accident of alignment'.

> *'Thank Heaven for little girls,*
> *They grow up in the most delightful way*
> *Thank Heaven for little girls.'*
>
> **Maurice Chevalier, from the film *Gigi* (1958)**

Female sport is another area of concern.

Tennis has had problems with early burnout and injury causing premature retirements of many precociously talented youngsters. Tennis academies, such as those that flourish in the Floridian sun, seemed to force the early development of their charges like flowers being prepared for the Chelsea Flower Show.

Tracey Austin was one of the first. She won the first of her two American Open singles titles in 1979 at 16. Yet before her 21st birthday she was beset by chronic injury and was finished as a major title contender. Andrea Jaeger reached the world number two slot before injury forced her retirement at 19 years old in 1985. As a result, the Women's Tennis Association bought in age eligibility rules and a 'phased in' approach to competition, which appeared to help prolong tennis careers.

However, serious injuries to young female tennis players still occur including to Britain's Laura Robson whose career has stalled. She burst on to the senior scene at 18 years old and serves as a reminder of the vulnerability of youngsters. Hopefully, the emergence at 15 of Coco Gauff in 2019 will be carefully supervised and injury-free, to allow her to fulfil her potential.

Artificial all-weather hockey surfaces started to replace grass in the 1970s. In terms of speed and skill they have transformed the game because the firm surface guarantees a truer roll of the ball. But it also takes its toll on legs and backs. In junior rugby, cricket and soccer there has been an acknowledgement that the hours and intensity of training and competition need to be controlled. However, in junior girls' hockey I have been concerned by the number of matches and practice sessions undertaken by some of my patients. Teenagers tell me of their punishing schedules – a Saturday morning school game followed by a Saturday afternoon club match, and Sunday mornings devoted to representative squad practices.

It is too much

Responsibility rests jointly with the player, parents and sports' organisations. Players fear that failure to attend a squad session will result in exclusion from future games and the chance to progress up the representative ladder; sports organisations in turn need to monitor youngsters' workloads. As the treating doctor, it is hard to be the one pulling the player and the plug on the hope of junior honours. However, long-term well-being must be the priority. Even when academy-type set-ups extend into young adult life, serious issues can continue. The Nike Oregon Project was exposed in 2019 and culminated in the ban of coach Alberto Salazar. One of his runners, Mary Cain, said, 'There is a systemic crisis in women's sport in which young girls' bodies are being ruined by an emotionally and physically abusive system.'

Teenage traumas

The increasing size of teenagers, intense one-sport training programmes and improved scientific knowledge about producing quicker, stronger and fitter young athletes have led to a rise in adolescent sporting injuries. However large and developed a 15-year-old soccer or rugby player looks they are still immature in terms of bone and muscle development. Increasingly, injuries normally associated with adult athletes are being seen in adolescents.

Certain sports have long been recognised as posing specific risks to youngsters. 'Little leaguer's elbow' causes damage to the growing plate of the elbow in young baseball pitchers and was first identified in 1960 in America. The condition requires supervision and rest to avoid long-term complications. Sports involving jumping, twisting and turning involve an increased risk of ankle ligament injuries, and I see young runners with shin splints and stress fractures of the leg, ankle and feet. Our young cricket bowlers develop stress fractures in their lower spines.

The protracted build-up to the 2012 Olympiad produced interesting referrals to my clinic. The natural national desire to shine, extra funding and the admission of several 'lesser' sports to the Games (because of our hosting status) increased the numbers of young athletes in training. After 'London' was confirmed in 2005, talent identification programmes were stepped up. Centres for individual sports were established and prepared in readiness; coaches, clinicians, physiotherapists and conditioning staff were needed. Was the depth in quality and quantity available in every category? Small clusters of injuries started appearing. Stress fractures increased, particularly from one sport, which were possibly linked to excessive conditioning work on unforgiving surfaces. I saw a grouping of Achilles ruptures in young elite gymnasts – an extraordinarily rare event.

The determination of young athletes to return to sport was epitomised by one of those gymnasts with a ruptured Achilles. Only eight weeks after my surgery, the athlete returned to asymmetric bar routines – albeit with suitable cushioning surrounds – and went on to be an Olympic and World Championship medallist. However, for 'Joe Public' the outlook is not so bright. A sizeable percentage of patients never return to the same level of sport and many do not return at all.

There has been a rise in teenage and young adult ACL ruptures in contact sports. Such injuries are bad news however old you are. If a teenager had turned up with such an injury 30 years ago every knee surgeon in the department would have discussed it. Now their arrival usually passes without comment. Surgical techniques have improved but a return to sport is not guaranteed. Damage to this key knee stabiliser can have long-term consequences for the joint and its owner. A 2017 American study reported a 57 per cent increase in ACL injuries in the 6–18-year-old age group over two decades. There have also been more ACL injuries associated with increased involvement in female soccer in America. Only 72 per cent of male and female soccer players (of all ages) returned to football after ACL surgery and only 61 per cent returned at the same level. Seven years after returning to play only 36 per cent were still playing soccer of which 9 per cent had ruptured the other knee's ACL, requiring surgery.

An earlier 2014 review highlighted the bleak picture following ACL damage when looking at 7,556 athletes. Only 81 per cent returned to any sport, 65 per cent returned to their previous level of sport and only 55 per cent returned to a competitive level of sport after the ligament was rebuilt.

Elite soccer players seem to fare better at returning to sport. The elite adult player has advantages youngsters do not have, including access to the best diagnostics, surgeons and rehabilitation. Added to this are the economic imperatives for club and player but these raise the question of whether such high returns to play are a sign of knee abuse, and whether they risk further knee injury and osteoarthritis. One study found that at around 14 years after ACL surgery the damaged knee had a three-fold increase in osteoarthritis compared to the other side – in patients of any age. Such anxieties need addressing in all patient ages and levels of sporting achievement.

One-quarter of children who undergo ACL reconstruction will re-injure the ligament, a staggeringly high rate. My Norwegian colleague Lars Engebretsen has asked whether we are 'destroying junior talent', since most of those injured are outstanding young athletes. He has confirmed that of those injured, very few will ever achieve elite status in adult sport, especially in pivoting sports, because of the injury.

In all these cases, prevention is better than cure.

Spoil sport?

How should we view sport in the young? It is a significant piece in the developing jigsaw of an adolescent's life and encourages physical and mental development. It is a useful balance to more sedentary or academic pursuits and does foster Wellington's lessons for adult life.

However, sport should be enjoyed primarily for its own sake. The identification of some aptitude for a specific pursuit rarely translates into sporting fame and riches. Parents need to question whether their personal enthusiasm for their offspring's sport is not an attempt at 'achievement by proxy' – the attainment of their own unfulfilled ambitions. We must balance the positive and negative effects of pursuing adolescent single-sport pathways.

Athletes, families and coaches must understand that enthusiasm for the sport and its training sacrifices will wane in many youngsters. Once the enjoyment ceases, it is time for the athlete to consider their options. Sadly, sustaining injury is as likely as stellar sporting achievement.

The most important aspect of adolescent sport is to develop a love of games and exercise that lasts a lifetime. Anything more should be regarded as icing on the top of a multi-tiered cake.

Chapter 8

THE YOUNG AT HEART

'For it's hard, you will find,
To be narrow of mind if you're young at heart'

Frank Sinatra, 'Young at Heart' (1963)

MY FATHER enjoyed 'shooting hoops' with friends on a Thursday evening before heading to the pub. One of his team-mates was Colin 'Ollie' Milburn, the swashbuckling Northants and England batsman.

On Dad's 40th birthday he suddenly stopped these trips to the basketball court. He wasn't injured, just taking heed of my mother's words: 'Maurice, you are far too old for that kind of thing now.' And so, without demur, Dad put his kit in the back of the cupboard, stopped his regular purchase of Elliman's Embrocation and settled down to middle age. Most people did in those times. Mother's insistence probably saved his joints, which served him well throughout the rest of his life. He grudgingly accepted life away from sport and the need for a kinder, more age-appropriate recreation to indulge the pent-up endorphins. Gardening and fishing, anybody?

Dad didn't give up on sport and put in unstinting service ferrying his kids around, standing on touchlines and providing advice. However, he shook his head in disbelief as I continued running half-marathons into my fifties. It was beyond his generation's comprehension. Views like 'growing old gracefully' and 'sport is a pastime for the young' were common among the generation born between the two world wars.

In the 1980s my bosses told me that over-35s should not be offered a knee ligament reconstruction because the knee and its owner were far too old for such a surgical insult. Nowadays, my patients look at me in incredulity when I mention such ancient myths. Patients in their sixties tell me they are elite athletes with a date with destiny in the Marrakesh Ironman in three weeks' time. 'I'm afraid you don't have,' I mumble under my breath in response. Septuagenarians also appear in my clinic with frustration seeping from every pore when they cannot maintain their marathon schedule due to calf injuries.

> *'Old age is the supreme evil, because it deprives us of*
> *all pleasures, leaving us only an appetite for them,*
> *and it brings with it all sufferings. Nevertheless, we*
> *fear death, and we desire old age.'*
>
> **Giacomo Leopardi, *Thoughts*,**
> **Translation by J.G. Nichols (2002)**

Many of my patients hope that exercise will bring the eternal elixir of life. Others hope that they are Benjamin Button, reincarnate – the F. Scott Fitzgerald character who ages in reverse. We are complicated machines with wonderful control mechanisms, but we are still machines with built-in obsolescence. Senescence is the process of ageing. Our bodily functions deteriorate progressively. Theories about ageing abound and start with our DNA. Some believe ageing occurs as a result of inherent programming. Other factors include disease, diet, smoking and exercise which cause damage that cannot be completely repaired.

As we age our response to exercise changes significantly. At 65, we have lost 30 per cent of our maximum heart rate and thus our ability to pump blood to our muscles and vital organs during exercise. Our resting heart output declines by about 1 per cent per year and our VO2 max by between 9 and 15 per cent each decade. Our lung capacity diminishes; its deterioration is accelerated by cigarette smoking.

Bone mass declines from our thirties and we need to build up our bone mass in our teens. From our mid-fifties grip strength and standing balance time correlate with life expectancy. By 65, between 8 and 27 per cent of the muscle mass of our youth has gone; testosterone levels drop relentlessly from our late thirties. By 40 years old, 40 per cent of people have some form of chronic medical condition, and the incidence of this increases by 10 per cent every decade. A total of 25 per cent of women and 20 per cent of men undertake no physical activity at all.

A lifestyle for the over-fifties should include a healthy diet, no smoking and moderate alcohol intake. The four pillars of fitness are strength, stamina, suppleness and skill. Everybody can improve their well-being with sensible, well-planned and age-appropriate exercise to boost their functional ability which will help them 'drop a decade'.

Where did this sea change in attitudes to senior sport start? Perhaps we should begin with Jim Fixx. Fixx is credited with the popularisation of jogging following his 1977 bestseller *The Complete Book of Running*, which sold over a million copies. Fixx's father died from a heart attack aged 43. Jim Fixx had many additional cardiac risk factors – a stressful job, smoking and obesity as a young adult. He preached that running improves quality and quantity of life. Despite losing 27kg his insurmountable genetics caught up with him, however, and he died from a massive coronary while out running in 1984, aged 52.

As a youngster, I 'went for a run'. Boxers did 'roadwork' to prepare for a fight. Horses jogged. William Shakespeare wrote, 'You may be jogging whiles your boots are green' in *The Taming of the Shrew*. The statement warned against being too hasty. In the same way, we should spend time bedding-in our new running shoes.

In the 1960s and 1970s the term 'jogging' was coined to describe slower, sociable running. The term was attributed to two people, New Zealander Arthur Lydiard and Bill Bowerman from the US.

Running rules, OK?

I have developed a few rules of running that I've found useful when talking to patients – particularly older ones.

#1. The big leap in training is moving from three to four sessions per week.

Runners need recovery from training and performance to avoid injury and reap the benefits of their efforts. This is particularly pertinent to 'couch to 5k' participants.

One of the hardest lessons for the weekend warrior to grasp is the beneficial effects of rest. Purposeful training four days per week means that two sessions must inevitably be back-to-back. We talk about binge-drinking and binge-eating. Binge-exercising is another example of overdoing it. Over the centuries, manual labour was part and parcel of daily fare but, in modern life, most of us have sedentary lives – for example, I struggle to hit 10,000 steps (a universally accepted target and the equivalent of about five miles) during an all-day clinic. We try to stay fit with pulses of exercise; Saturday and Sunday are our exercise times and are filled with long bike rides and country runs.

Muscles, tendons and bones need time to assimilate the impact of our exercise. Collagen is a major building block of body tissue, including tendons and ligaments, and can react positively to exercise stress. The response of type I collagen (a major player) peaks three days after intense exercise, which is probably the best time to run again, depending on how strenuous the previous exercise session was. Go back to the roads too soon and you risk damage.

Intense activity can damage muscle, particularly bouts of activity such as downhill running. The initial effect is weakening and inflammation, causing muscle soreness. With appropriate recovery muscles repair more strongly. It some circumstances, deliberate muscle-damaging workouts are used as a training tool.

Similarly, healthy bone adapts to sensible, incremental loading (this is known as Wolff's Law). The bone remodels itself and strengthens over time. If you overdo it, stress reactions and fractures occur. The reverse is true with excessive inactivity. 'If you snooze, you lose.'

Rest is vital in a training programme in all these examples. Without it, training will be inefficient, athletes will tire and injuries will develop.

Athletes must appreciate that their tissues require a planned and sophisticated maintenance programme. As youngsters, we employ the equivalent of a full, skilled and enthusiastic workforce to undertake the required tasks. Our employees are enzyme systems that control activities throughout our bodies and maintain the status quo. With suitable stimuli, our machines will purr.

Our workforce becomes lazy, inefficient and de-skilled with time, however, and we become the equivalent of the Friday afternoon car coming off the motor assembly line – prone to little errors and omissions, some exhausts starting to splutter before others. In our bodies, this variation is mostly determined by our genes, although the factors to which our genes are subjected – our lifestyle, diet and environment – make a major contribution.

#2. You can fit training for a half-marathon around your life but marathon training requires life to fit around it.

The jogging movement was given added impetus by several developments, particularly mass participation runs and adult age-group competitions.

In 1981, the London Marathon and Great North Run sparked marathon and half-marathon crazes in Britain. London was the brainchild of Chris Brasher and John Disley, who were inspired by the New York Marathon. The event enabled ordinary men and women to dream, train, and compete and by 2016 a million people had completed the London Marathon, raising over £1bn for charity. It takes place in the spring and runners build up their mileages over the winter, making it the perfect antidote to Christmas over-indulgence.

The Great North Run was the brainchild of the Olympian Brendan Foster. Every September, over 54,000 athletes run around Newcastle and South Shields in the biggest half-marathon in the world. Its timing gives focus to summer training. Although other events like the Great Manchester Run and the Great South Run attract many competitors, London and Newcastle remain the big daddies of city running.

For any jogger, enlisting for their first half- or full marathon is a major undertaking. Training plans, running partners and sponsorship forms need identifying and organising. Preparation for a 13-mile race can be undertaken sensibly and enjoyably alongside other personal, professional and other sporting commitments. However, do not follow the path of one of my patients: from zero exercise he completed a half-marathon within four months, then was so high on adrenaline that he repeated the feat the next weekend. After limping for two months he appeared at my clinic with three stress fractures in his shin. He had not built in recovery time.

Conversely, marathon training is all-encompassing and takes over your life. Families, friends and work must orbit around the central marathon planet, which the entrant briefly inhabits. It is like a military campaign. Sleep, socialising and other sporting activities are subjugated to the goal of reaching the finishing line.

Some patients extend their suffering by running challenges such as the Everest Marathon, which starts at the peak's base camp. One of my ex-GP colleagues, David Buckler, acted as the event's doctor several times and described it as like trying to run a portable intensive care unit at 17,000 feet. People react unpredictably at such rarefied heights – the fittest individuals can struggle to get enough oxygen into their screaming muscles while less fit mortals cope just fine. My respect for those who achieve these feats without injury and alarm knows no bounds.

#3. Beware trying to be first among equals.
To stay active in sport, older people in the past have traipsed around

disconsolately, miles behind the youngsters at club running sessions, or avoided the risks of contact sports such as football and rugby by giving up. This has changed, with the advent of adult age-group events. They began in the USA in the late 1960s and the World Association of Veteran Athletes was formed in 1977. Pitting oneself against similar vintages has given a new lease of life to many older enthusiasts. Veteran status commences at varying times in different sports but is commonly around 35–40 years old. It then rises in five-year bands. Worn-out tendons and joints are abused to break an age-group record and competitors seem willing to trade a lifetime of swollen Achilles, or hasten the arrival of a new knee joint, for that momentary triumph.

With age, modifications are made for weakening muscles and stiffening joints. Some sprint distances are shortened and hurdle heights lowered, despite groin muscles indicating that enough is enough. We hear inspiring tales of age-defying feats, which are newsworthy because of their rarity. The over-80 athlete completing 200m in less than 30 seconds has been very fortunate in avoiding injuries and has maintained sensible exercise programmes and lifestyle choices ... and inherited a wonderful set of genes.

One of my patients was in his fifties and had started running four years earlier. He had completed 18 marathons in that time but had painful knees. He was office-based and over time had been habitually at the front of the queue for the dessert trolley. He had osteoarthritis, but was hooked on exercise and thought that running had only beneficial effects. He was shocked and close to tears that his joints were deteriorating. Alongside the pleasure of his physical achievements he had experienced the accompanying euphoria of well-being. Exercise boosts your confidence and changes the way you are perceived by family and friends. It opens new social circles that close if injury denies you the ability to train and compete.

#4. Paste an age-adjusted performance table into your logbook.
Father Time waits for no veteran athlete but golden oldies can stay 25 years old in their heads, if not in their bodies.

Age-adjusted performance tables allow a reasonable comparison of results with those of younger athletes. A 10km run of one hour by a 60-year-old equates to a 48-minute 10km for somebody half their age. Not a bad effort. We lose 20 per cent of our endurance capacity in those 30 years, yet after age adjustment older athletes could find that they are running 'quicker' than their younger selves. From the age of 40 our speed over most middle- and long-distance events drops by 1 per cent annually. This holds true until the age of 80.

In recent years cycling has been the boom sport for silver foxes, who can compare times from younger days via such organisations as the Veterans Time Trials Association. Swimming also has various methods of performance comparison for different age groups, including the Finnish Formula, the Pitcher tables and the Alan Rowson formulae.

Frustration at deteriorating times can be replaced by pride at realising what your age-adjusted body has achieved. It boosts self-regard and, hopefully, prevents athletes embarking on unrealistic training regimes that will end in unfulfillment and injury.

#5. Everybody has only so many miles in them.

Sport can come at a cost when people have indulged in seasons of contact sport, thousands of miles of running, and carried on participating while not heeding their bodies' signals of injury and over-training.

At birth we are a brand-new machine. Prototypes piloted by our parents might provide clues as to which model we are. Sometimes we need servicing, rebuilding or replacement parts. Our machine quickly shows signs of wear if we are too heavy on the clutch, crash the gears or trash the suspension by driving off-piste. Eventually, our pistons seize up and our suspension fails. We limp along at a fraction of our previous speed in the slow lane of life's motorway.

I believe that we all have a finite number of miles on our individual clocks before the machine splutters – but careful husbandry of our engines increases longevity. Many of us never reach our limits due to minimal interest in sports. However, once you have reached your physical bank account limit, the 'bank manager in the sky' is unlikely to extend your credit. This may be why people coming to running late gain so much enjoyment and personal achievement from it; they have fewer years of abuse on the clock.

I have had knee cartilage and arthritic ankle surgery, ligaments rebuilt and screws inserted in my wrist for fractures. Dentists have implanted prosthetic teeth to replace those dislodged by over-enthusiastic rugby opponents. Hernias have been repaired several times and a hole sits in my calf muscle where it exploded during a sprint. My neck only turns in one direction because of a 'stinger' (when the neck is forcibly wrenched and the nerves of the arm are stretched or pinched), and there is a defect in my lower back which restricts sleeping positions. All these problems were directly caused or aggravated by sport. The repair bills would have funded countless holidays.

Like my patients I would not have missed one moment of my sport. In your twenties and thirties you think you are 'getting away with it' but 30-plus years on you remember exactly which tackle started each ache. Many injuries are slow burners and the body has a way of later getting revenge for all the abuse.

I have often encountered a 'grounded husband'. For many men the main competitive sports of early life have a built-in shelf life. Accepting the failure of your body leads to something akin to the five stages of grief and loss. Denial and isolation give way to anger and then bargaining. Depression for what is lost precedes acceptance. Sports-wise, men enter their wilderness years searching for an alternative adrenaline fix. I spent ten years looking, before pumping up my bike tyres.

Middle-aged men grow frustrated at the sporting impediments imposed by groaning joints. There is a childhood background of sport on which marriage and parenthood fail to apply any brakes. Initially, midweek gym sessions are merely an hors d'oeuvre to weekend team sport and the slack in domestic and parenting duties is inevitably taken up by the partner, who was often also a keen sportswoman in her youth.

By the parents' late thirties and forties the children are becoming independent and mothers consider a sporting comeback. Jogging is an option and, reluctantly, the husband provides companionship and support. Initially the male waits on the (proverbial) street corner while his partner builds her speed and stamina. Then the unthinkable occurs. The woman begins enjoying her running and, even worse, becomes decent at it. She joins the running club and finds jogging buddies.

For the male, years of kicking and being kicked on local park pitches begin to take their toll; he risks becoming 'beached'. Meanwhile, his partner has discovered the joys of major city runs at home and abroad. The male is left behind to dog walk and shepherd the teenage kids. This is not how it was planned! His partner, exiled from sport in younger adult life, is unencumbered by the years of stress and strain on her body, and is injury-free.

I hear these tales of woe from men and offer a management plan for the damaged appendage and suitable future exercise programmes. I delicately approach my running rules. The male has largely exhausted his physical bank deposits but his wife has been prudent with hers, even accumulating interest, and is enjoying the benefits of her earlier frugality.

#6. Golden oldies need to mix it up a bit.

It can be difficult to avoid putting your foot into a rabbit hole and breaking your ankle or getting your head in the way of a stray size 12 boot at the bottom of a rugby ruck. It's the price of doing sport. However, many of the chronic problems in our clinics start with faulty biomechanics and training errors rather than incidents themselves. Repetitive use of the same muscles, tendons and bones risks fatigue and the need for micro-repairs. Years of use of the same muscle groups encourages the kind of breakdown that will not respond to pitchside assistance.

For me, nothing replaces the joy of running. It is the purest of sports and requires the minimum of kit. However, there came a time when I realised that my Achilles, ankles and knees were on borrowed time. I faced hard choices but we all need to mix it up.

There are so many recreational choices now – explore them. The rules that apply to adolescent single-sport specialisation should also apply to older people. If you've not fully recovered from the previous weekend's exertions by the next Saturday, it might be time to rethink your options. Post-surgically, and having viewed images of their patched-up tendon, older runners ask the inevitable question: 'What about my running?' Running should be viewed as part of a balanced weekly programme of exercise. Share the pain and strain around your body.

I think this is why sports such as triathlon and low-impact forms of exercise have become more popular. Avoiding over-reliance on one sport reduces injury risk and helps if an injury occurs. A foot problem may ground you from running but leave you free to swim and cycle. Following injury, I try to lift an athlete's gloom by highlighting the positives of, for example, their metatarsal stress fracture taking weeks to mend. It does not mean a total embargo on exercise. Areas of weakness can be worked on. It is a matter of using your imagination.

As we become older, our body's need for self-preservation changes. Even the great Usain Bolt had to bow to the march of time. Healthy hearts and lung function are required but our emphasis must increasingly be on the retention of strength and balance. Nothing is beyond redemption.

The challenge is to reduce falls and fragility fractures in the elderly. Broken hips, wrists and vertebrae are a major challenge for our NHS. At 50 years old, 2 per cent of females will be osteoporotic, rising to 25 per cent by age 80. Fragility fractures cost the NHS £2bn annually, a figure that is rising as the population ages. Risk factors include family history, smoking, excess alcohol, steroids and a history of falls. About 76,000 people break their hips in the UK annually, of which 30 per cent recover, half are left with a disability and one-fifth die as a direct or indirect result. Preventative programmes need to start early. Youngsters should be encouraged to invest early in their bone and muscle health and, as we age, increasing emphasis should be placed on staying strong.

A word of warning: we need padding as we age. Another elderly fracture risk factor is a BMI of less than 18.5. If you fall on a banana skin at Aldi you need to bounce. The over-50s shouldn't be too hard on themselves for eating that extra chocolate Hobnob.

#7. Over 50 years of age, everybody gains a new orthopaedic problem which never goes.

Hardly anybody over 50 will escape osteoarthritis somewhere – often with no symptoms. Knee cartilages increasingly fray and those plump, water-filled spinal discs of our youth resemble dried-up prunes in later life. One-third of us dies with tears to one of the important ankle tendons that help with balance. Get used to it – splits happen!

Experience teaches doctors to identify these normal ageing phenomena in our patients and appreciate that different patients respond differently to similar-looking problems. Politicians and health managers believe that orthopaedic surgery can be reduced to that of a technician – making decisions based on algorithms and starting with X-rays. Patients, patients, patients. One man's seized hip is another's occasional groin ache, but the X-rays may look identical. I have the greatest respect for the agricultural community. The final straw for a farmer's hip is when they cannot get out of their combine harvester.

The interaction between mind and body remains the key predictor of how some cope and others don't. It is why medicine remains as much an art as a science.

#8. Your favourite Premier League footballer returned six weeks after the same injury but do not expect to follow suit.

Weekend warriors cannot understand why they do not follow the same recovery timetables as their sporting heroes. Elite athletes are usually younger and have access to daily rehabilitation staff and state-of-the-art facilities. They do not have the same concerns about work and family commitments. Professional athletes have contracts to fulfil and bonuses dependent on appearances and performance, and the returning champion is carefully monitored even after resuming play. Rehabilitation programmes are designed for the elite athlete for up to 12 months after returning to play, to minimise the risk of recurrent injuries.

The importance of stretching and pre-exercise preparation becomes ever more important as we age. In senior sport, the 'book-ends' of warming up and down can take as long as the exercise itself. Amateur athletes usually start the recovery road from injury or surgery with every good intention, but enthusiasm wanes often at about 90–95 per cent of full recovery potential. Physiotherapy has finished and further effort seems to bring little progress. Work demands get in the way and the desire to return to club games becomes too great.

Discharge from the clinic because the X-ray demonstrates your fracture has healed is just the end of the start of the process of a return to sport. There is scarring, wasting and muscle inhibition that needs reversing. The answer is intensive rehabilitation but this is not readily accessed in swamped physiotherapy NHS clinics. The outstanding results achieved by police and armed forces rehabilitation centres stand in stark contrast to the travails of many of our injured civilian population.

Sharps, sidewalks and spandex

There are a few recurring themes from my clinics, including the ravages of pointy needles in your joints, the impact of running on pavements, and the cult of middle-aged men squeezed into polyester-polyurethane co-polymer attire, otherwise known as Lycra.

Gout attacks

> *'Be temperate in wine, in eating, girls, and sloth;*
> *Or the Gout will seize you and plague you both.'*

Benjamin Franklin, American Founding Father and gout sufferer, *Poor Richard's Almanac* (1734)

What did King Henry VIII, Charles Dickens, Samuel Johnson, William Pitt, Ludwig van Beethoven, Isaac Newton and Laurence Olivier have in common? They all had gout.

Telling a patient 40 years ago that they had gout produced a reaction akin to a diagnosis of gonorrhoea. They assured me that they didn't drink. Today, gout affects one in 40 of the population, usually men. With over a million sufferers you would think doctors would have gout taped. However, it is one of the most under-diagnosed and under-treated male conditions in the country. The incidence has risen by two-thirds since 2000.

Many patients suffer for years before the penny drops. 'If it is not your big toe it cannot be gout' is the medical mantra repeated in GP practices. But gout affects many different joints, tendons and bony prominences. It is caused by needle-shaped uric acid crystals produced by purine breakdown from our own tissues and diet. Although certain foodstuffs can be implicated, it is usually our own innate inability to break urate down and excrete it quickly enough that is to blame.

It causes acute pain, redness and swelling, and is episodic. My clinching question is frequently, 'If I gave you a saw in the middle of the night during a gout attack, what would you do with it?' The universal reply? 'I would saw my foot off.' Believe me, I know. I've had it. Athletes are not immune. Gout is unpredictable, causes havoc with sport and is frequently precipitated by dehydration, often in summer.

The streets of London are paved with hard concrete not gold

*'Let me take you by the hand and lead you
through the streets of London
I'll show you something to make you
change your mind.'*

Ralph McTell, 'The Streets of London' (1969)

People from my neck of the woods visit the metropolis for work, weekend breaks and to participate in sporting events. London is a great city but Northamptonians are usually happy to get back to Euston station and start their return journey. Why? It is the toll their visit has taken on their feet.

I am told weekly about the evils of the capital. In London, people cover considerable distances on Shanks's pony. By the end of the day, bunions, hammer toes and policeman's heels are screaming for mercy. It rather contradicts the notion of the soft southerner who seems to cope admirably. I'm still to solve the mystery and want to know what goes into the concrete under the paving slabs.

Mamils

'I want to ride my bicycle
I want to ride my bike
I want to ride my bicycle
I want to ride it where I like.'

Queen, 'Bicycle Race' (1978)

Olympic and Tour de France successes have triggered an explosion in cycling in the UK. On average, 5.4 million adults cycle each week with men annually riding four times further than females. The term MAMIL – middle-aged men in Lycra – was coined for good statistical reasons: numbers of cyclists in their fourth and fifth decades outstrip all other age groups.

Motorists and pedestrians complain but fewer UK residents cycle daily than in all but two of the 27 EU countries – Malta and Cyprus. In 2016, we covered 3.5 billion miles on our bikes, which is less than a quarter of the mileage covered by our predecessors in post-war Britain.

Middle-aged men love bikes. They come with kit we can tinker with and, for many, cycling is our last refuge when all other sports have given us up. Many women feel the same. Cyclists are merely following in the great traditions of British sport. We excel at sitting-down sports like equestrian events, motor racing, rowing, sailing and canoeing. Cyclists need to eat and drink during rides to avoid 'bonking' (low blood sugar levels) and coming to a grinding halt. Wonderful.

There are medical benefits too. Cycling reduces the risk of cardiovascular and cancer-related illnesses, and mid-life cycling improves life expectancy and reduces premature death rates by two-fifths. The 2020 COVID-19 crisis and concerns over the nation's fitness, coupled with a desire to keep people off public transport (to reduce disease transmission), has made our political paymasters reconsider the benefits of two wheels.

Cycling adventures are limitless and I have succumbed myself. Following the line of ants up Mont Ventoux in Provence during a hailstorm one June, I stopped at Tommy Simpson's memorial where he laid down his bike for the last time in 1967; my daughter and I have pedalled 100 miles through London and Surrey with 25,000 others, following in the tracks of the 2012 Olympic road race.

I have joined 35,000 other cyclists on the beautiful Argus cycle tour in Cape Town. The day before, my friend, the cricketer, Allan Lamb, encouraged me to get up at 5.30am and ride with Stephen Roche, the 1987 Tour de France winner. It was a thrill of a lifetime to sit in a peloton alongside a living legend – and I don't mean 'Lamby'. There are few sports where the plodding sportsman can literally follow in the tracks of their heroes.

'He'd fly through the air with the greatest of ease
The daring young man on the flying trapeze.'

George Leybourne, 'The Flying Trapeze' (1867)

Cyclists detached from their bikes are a staple diet of fracture clinics, and broken collar bones, elbow and wrist fractures abound. Sometimes I see a broken shoulder blade. 'Clip-in calamities' occur: cyclists want to feel the power throughout all 360° of their pedal revolution so opt to progress by welding their bodies to their bikes with shoe cleats locking into the pedals. Falling off is inevitable with these cleats and a rite of passage. You forget to unclip at a junction and list like the leaning tower of Pisa in full view of nearby traffic and passers-by, finishing up on the tarmac or sprawled on a bollard or other item of street furniture.

MAMILS often challenge our clinical competencies. Many chronic overuse injuries are biomechanical and relate to the fit of the biker to the bike and vice versa. I enlist the support of our local expert 'bike fitter' in times of need. Like other sports, doctors need to understand the terminology and psyche of the serious cyclist; sportives, sprockets and seat tubes need to be assimilated into our history-taking vocabulary.

Cyclists also suffer sore necks, backs and damaged tendons, or squashed nerves and numb fingers from gripping the handlebars. Pains in the posterior are another problem. This is piriformis syndrome, also known as 'wallet syndrome', because of its location – a not inappropriate term in view of the large sums spent on cycling.

Take as much advice as possible before splashing the cash on your steed. Road test for correct frame size and set-up and consider a proper bike fit. It will pay dividends on the 'long run'.

Sport for all seasons

Participating in sport as we age enriches our lives. There is so much choice and there is an activity that suits nearly all of us. The physical and psychological rewards of sport are immense. In many ways, sport is wasted on the young: they take their health and fitness for granted.

However, be thoughtful in your choices and set goals and ambitions sensibly. Regaining fitness after periods of inactivity takes time; listen to your body, take advice early rather than soldiering on and do not be defeated by minor injuries and setbacks.

Hopefully sport can remain a part of your life for as long as you want it to.

Chapter 9

OH, THE GAMES PEOPLE PLAY!

'Oh, the games people play now
Every night and every day now'

Joe South, 'Games People Play' (1968)

IN THE late 1970s and the 1980s a group of thrill-seeking individuals gained significant notoriety and media attention. They were known as the Dangerous Sports Club (DSC) and were credited with inventing modern bungee jumping.

In 1979 the group's leader, David Kirke, bungee jumped from the Bristol suspension bridge in a top hat and tails while drinking champagne. Less than ten years later, bungee jumping was offered by Kiwis on a commercial basis. DSC's activities combined hedonism and a quest for extreme adventure. The group skied at St Moritz seated on models of grand pianos and a Louis XIV dining set. A young Nigella Lawson, a prominent member of DSC as a student, was captured on film playing croquet in a sedan chair during one of the group's tea parties at the house of the Dutch Ambassador. Tragedy struck in 2002 when two former DSC members (the group had disbanded by then) fired volunteers skywards from a large catapult. One, an Oxford undergraduate, failed to land on the safety net and died from the injuries.

Many of us would cower from similar stunts but some still attempt activities that should carry a government health warning.

Bungee jumping
Millions of people bungee jump and few under-25-year-olds return from Down Under without launching themselves into a ravine attached to an

elastic band. The safety record for bungee jumping is not unblemished and deaths have occurred. Paralysis caused by spinal injury, whiplash, sight impairment and the splitting of the brain's main artery leading to stroke are among the serious injuries previously healthy participants have suffered.

Sometimes adrenaline rushes overcome rational decision-making. In the early 1990s a twenty-something patient visited my clinic. He had suffered polio in his infancy and one of his legs did not move properly. In preparation for a bungee jump his ankles had been separately secured to the ends of the cord but during the flight the joint in his bad leg was subjected to forces not asked of it for decades. The tearing of soft tissues and bleeding into his ankle left him swollen, sore and sorry. Protracted physiotherapy restored him to former glories and he became prominent in public life in later years.

Charity parachuting

Each time I see a parachutist in my clinic I recall the various research on charity jumpers. It found that military parachutists trained for 31.5 hours on average before starting and suffered injuries in less than 1 per cent of jumps. Charity parachutists received 6.5 hours of tuition and suffered an 11 per cent injury rate. Two-thirds of their recorded injuries required hospital admission, costing the NHS between £4,000 and £5,800, which did not include the costs of an average six weeks off work. For every £1 raised for charity the NHS spent £13.75 on treatment. People should try to get as much instruction on the ground before they take to the skies and should not be surprised if their surgeon is grumpy at being called on to piece together another ankle that failed to defy Newton's law of gravity.

Tough mudders

Tough mudder, a combined mud run and obstacle course, is one of the fastest growing sports with more than three million entrants since 2010. It was started by two Englishmen living in New York and has spread across the globe. Stag and hen party-goers are among those to take part, swinging from climbing frames, suffering electric shocks and burrowing through pipes dressed as superhero characters and ballerinas, my own family included.

The craze is probably safer than charity parachute jumping and some other endurance events, but I still see many sprained ankles and swollen knees. A participant drowned in 2013 after been submerged in water for 15 minutes. In another event, competitors developed gastroenteritis caused by accidentally drinking water contaminated by livestock excrement. Participants have required treatment following electrical shocks. Entrants are advised to study in advance the obstacles they will face to ensure they can cope. Barriers such as barbed wire, ice baths and electric shocks should be avoided, and cows should be kept out of the mudbaths.

Five-a-side football

Drive around any urban area in the early evening and note the spotlights showcasing slightly rotund middle-aged men indulging in five-a-side football. Teams often comprise workmates or friends from the local boozer, whose best sporting days are behind them. Many players start five-a-side when fitness or family commitments prevent them playing eleven-a-side games at weekends.

They play after a long day at work and often without a warm-up. Pitches are smaller than those of their youth and surfaces considerably harder. Although games are shorter, the ball is in play more and ricochets around like a ball in an arcade – but the exponents are no pinball wizards.

The players are usually a stone heavier than in their pomp, which affects their stopping distance, and players frequently collide with the floor, the ball and their friends. The recent fad for encouraging 'Man versus Fat' football is designed to increase the number of fun buses participating. Grazes, cuts, and bruised legs and pride are commonplace as are torn muscles and ruptured ligaments and tendons. Employers must curse when several of the office team call in sick the next morning.

Fathers' sports day races

Yet another of the unlikely-but-true dangerous acts are fathers' (and sometimes mothers') races at school sports days.

They are usually one of the final acts of the educational year, and the weather is often hot and takes its toll on sensible reasoning. The announcement of the dads' dash is a cue for testosterone to rise and for offspring to plead with bashful dads and drag them to the start.

While nervously waiting, memories re-emerge and competitive juices boil. Some fathers note their opponents' lack of middle-aged spread and coltish demeanour. Children cheer from the sidelines and, ahead, the parallel stripes of whitewash lead to a distant land – the finishing tape. It seems such a long, long way off.

Some dads run in work trousers and shoes while others are in shorts and trainers. Some may even have trained but few stretch or warm up. In 1971 the average age of a new father was 27 and in 2004 it was 32. One in ten children are born to fathers over 40. The average age of runners in fathers' day races is rising every year.

I was cajoled into participating once, having several times done the same to my father. I'd come straight from the operating theatre, my mouth dry and my limbs like jelly. We took our marks. The man next to me adopted a crouched starting position and tried the old kidology of being last to settle. I thought, 'This really is a race!'

The starting gun sounded and we set off at varying paces. One hundred yards had never seemed so far. I could hear 'Mr Crouching Dad' breathing all the way yet astonishingly I breasted the tape inelegantly first and checked that all limbs remained attached and in working order. My emergence unscathed hasn't been the fate of others over the years; sprained ankles and torn calf muscles have not been uncommon.

One year, a patient of mine from a fathers' day race ruptured his Achilles tendon as he sprang from the start. He pitched forward, putting both arms out to save face and his face. The impact of his fall dislocated both shoulders and he made a sorry sight with both arms in a sling and his leg plastered. It was a lesson in the perils of giving in to your children and imagining never-ending youth.

However, matters are getting worse: school sports day grandparents' egg and spoon races have arrived. In my childhood, most attending grandparents looked as though they had arrived in a sedan chair. Now they are expected to risk life and limb sprinting while balancing a boiled oeuf on a plastic utensil. No health note from your GP first and all of this while being cheered on by two junior generations.

I have had that nightmare experience of watching my wife run to victory while my plans lay scrambled. I was wrestling with octogenarians and my poultry product at the rear of the field. I swear the egg had been a prototype for Barnes Wallis's bouncing bomb. At least my legs survived even if my pride did not.

Skiing

Skiing is an unusual pastime and volunteering to be tied to two planks of wood and speeding down an ice field with variable control is asking for trouble. A Ribbans unscientific rule of sports medicine is, 'Skiers are the modern equivalent of First World War pilots', whose life expectancy was several weeks. You will be shot down eventually. I have never shared a lift to the slopes with a ski instructor who has not, on finding out my profession, regaled me with a surgical shopping list containing reconstructed cruciates and clavicles – and they are supposed to be the experts.

Injuries are not exclusive to boy-racers on poorly groomed black runs. Many occur to people simply adjusting their skis, waiting for the next bubble or grappling with button lifts wedged precariously between their buttocks. Americans patrol their slopes carefully but Europeans give carte blanche to prepubescent Pierres powering their snowboards through ranks of newbie skiers. Collisions are as predictable as they are ugly.

The number of injured skiers transported down the mountain in blood wagons behind expert ski rescue teams can be huge on an icy day, and local clinics deal with 'walk-ups' and 'ski-ups' nursing sore heads, broken wrists and shattered confidences. Those with the more severe injuries are sent to regional hospitals and surgical teams experienced in ski trauma. Lesser damage is patched up efficiently and the skier despatched to the local pharmacy for slings, crutches and braces. I'm almost on Christmas card terms with some Alpine doctors, so frequent is our correspondence.

While in America I took advantage of a free ski season pass and accommodation for my family in Waterville Valley, New Hampshire. In return, I had to work in the resort's medical centre for several days. My duties extended beyond my medical training and I was expected to use the X-ray machine, which I had never done before. The forerunner of *The Idiot's Guide to Taking X-rays* was taped to the wall. The machine looked like a Second World War reject and I doubt the room had lead-lined walls. Modern health and safety executives would have had a field day. I felt like a Victorian photographer with my head under a black sheet. Surprisingly, X-rays of passable quality emerged.

I was coping until I became aware of a commotion outside the clinic door. The resort owner had been chaperoning Kennedy-clan members around the slopes when one of them came to grief. I anticipated them expecting a crack traumatologist. As soon as I spoke, the Kennedy matriarch exclaimed, 'Oh no! They've put a Limey in charge.' Despite this knock to my confidence I continued to assess the junior Kennedy. The damage was superficial and short-lived, and we all survived to ski another day.

Celebrating injuries

'Come on and celebrate, good times, tonight
(Celebrate good times, come on!)
'Cause everything's gonna be all right.'

Kool & the Gang, 'Celebration' (1980)

You or your mate score the winning goal/try/run. How do you celebrate? In recent years, many celebrations have been choreographed and practised in advance, such as Robbie Keane's somersaults and cartwheels, Peter Crouch's robot dance and Paul Gascoigne's dentist's chair antics. However, danger still lurks.

In 2016, Northamptonshire were playing Worcestershire in a T20 game and our talented young fast bowler, Olly Stone, dismissed the England player Moeen Ali. Stone leapt into the air in celebration but as he landed his knee buckled. Surgery and a long rehabilitation followed and he barely played again until 2018. Thankfully, he returned to represent his country 30 months after the incident.

Two football League Cup finals have claimed victims in similar ways. Steve Morrow scored the winner for Arsenal in 1993 and his captain, Tony Adams, lifted Morrow into the air at the end. But the game's hero fell, broke his arm and missed the rest of the season, including the FA Cup Final.

In the 2015 final Chelsea's Nemanja Matic, who was suspended and not playing, joined his team-mates at the end of the game to celebrate but in doing so injured his ankle. A year earlier, England soccer physio Gary Lewin suffered an ankle fracture-dislocation (a severe fracture) landing on a water bottle while celebrating his team's goal against Italy in the World Cup.

In 2017 American researchers chronicled 62 celebration injuries. Of those, 35 per cent involved soccer and 97 per cent were suffered by men. A quarter required surgery. Ankle and knee ligament injuries were most common but one footballer died after sustaining a spinal cord injury while celebrating. Avoidance of sliding and pile-ups is advised. In lower level football, many similar injuries may well have occurred following copycat celebrations.

What are the implications for clubs, insurance companies and players? Clubs may be forced to pay players huge salaries while they lie on the treatment table. Team performance may be affected, together with a player's career progression and transfer value, and insurance companies may have to pay big medical bills. It can all can add up to large financial losses.

Perhaps it would be better to confine oneself to more sedate actions such as Bebeto's 'baby cradling' routine displayed in the 1994 World Cup.

Pantomime villains

My favourite fracture clinic tale of woe involved a pantomime horse at Christmas.

A poor fellow came to the clinic a week after Yuletide. He had been press-ganged into spending ten consecutive performances clothed in darkness and clinging to his mate's waist with his face pressed against his friend's rear end. The temperature was equivalent to Benidorm in July. He had faith in the navigational skills and Christmas dietary palate of the sighted member of this equine double act.

One night his luck ran out. 'Dobbin' frolicked and flounced at the front of the stage and attempted too tight a 90° turn. This was not a dressage horse. The rear limbs trembled and tottered before being deposited in the orchestra pit, straddling a surprised front row of the wind section. The horse whinnied off to the wings, effectively hemi-amputated. Its separated hind legs had sustained a fractured hock. In real life, the horse might have been humanely put down. Fortunately, this ankle required only six weeks in plaster. Perhaps the moral of this tale (or tail) is when impersonating Red Rum always volunteer to be at the brains end of the operation.

Danger lurks behind every obstacle but it is preferable to suffer a sports injury than fall off the sofa as a couch potato. At times, a rapid risk assessment of your ability to survive the selected challenge will suffice. Better to bow to sense and realism and fight another day.

Chapter 10

SATURDAY ... OR ANY NIGHT ... IS ALRIGHT FOR FIGHTING!

'In the clearing stands a boxer
And a fighter by his trade
And he carries the reminders
Of ev'ry glove that laid him down
Or cut him till he cried out'

Simon and Garfunkel, 'The Boxer' (1969)

AS A youngster in the 1960s I was taken to the famous Thomas a Becket pub in London's Old Kent Road.

My father and his friend John Morris whisked me up to the first floor to one of London's spiritual homes of boxing. The boxing ring dominated the room where there were punch bags and other tools of the pugilist's trade dotted around. Boxing card posters were pasted on the walls, including those heroes of my youth – Brian London, Billy Walker, Henry Cooper. The site was Cooper's base from 1956 to 1970 and was used by many of the greats, including Muhammad Ali, Joe Frazier and Sugar Ray Leonard when they had bouts in London. The grunts, the sound of leather on flesh, and flying sweat and saliva remain vivid and started a lifelong respect for devotees of the Marquis of Queensbury rules of boxing.

Sadly, the pub is no more. In 2015 Southwark Council revoked its licence after a serious assault – perhaps appropriate given its history. Modern, air-conditioned gyms now lie behind security gates so it is nostalgic to reflect on The Greatest 'floating like a butterfly' at the pub while locals supped their beer below. The hostelry's fame was extended when David Bowie rehearsed there for his Ziggy Stardust album and 1972 tour.

John Morris was the general secretary of the British Boxing Board of Control (BBBoC) for 14 years. He was voted world commissioner of the year by both the World Boxing Association and World Boxing Council. He asked me to get involved and in 1981 I joined the BBBoC panel of ringside doctors. It was my first sortie into elite sports medicine.

When hospital duties allowed I provided medical cover for professional tournaments for the next 14 years. My last year of involvement, 1995, was a pivotal one for boxing. New health and safety recommendations had already been adopted following a bout in 1991 in which Michael Watson had suffered serious injuries while boxing Chris Eubank. That fight changed the canvas of the sport. John Morris was in the ring at the end. 'The events of that night were a catalyst for the BBBoC to strengthen further the regulations surrounding the sport. British boxing embraced independent medical expertise to provide guidance,' he told me.

My reflections date back to the period before these stricter regulations were adopted and describe a bygone age. However, the dedication of the doctors involved was never in doubt. All of them knew the potential dangers that boxers faced.

Have medical bag, will travel

In the 1980s the boxing medical panel contained an eclectic bunch of doctors including GPs, skin and gut specialists and junior doctors such as me. Every month a list of boxing cards, venues and allocated doctors arrived, with invitations to locations such as Streatham, Slough, Bethnal Green, Wembley, Park Lane and the Albert Hall.

The BBBoC appointed two doctors for each tournament. We undertook pre-fight medicals on boxers who hadn't been examined at the weigh-in, emergency equipment was checked and promoters were asked to contact the nearest neurosurgical unit to pre-warn them of potential customers. When precautions tightened an ambulance was allocated to the venue. The two medics rotated fights. One doctor was ringside while the second monitored the health of boxers involved in the previous fight and undertook running repairs.

Fight venues were of all shapes and sizes and the spectators were similarly varied. The bouts often took place at a 'gentlemen's dinner' hosted by the likes of the Anglo-American Sporting Club, the World Sporting Club or the National Sporting Club (NSC) and were held at various London venues including the Hilton Hotel, Grosvenor House in Park Lane and the Café Royal in Regent Street. In the 1960s and 1970s these dinners were organised by some of the most serious movers and shakers in boxing, such as Jarvis Astaire, Mickey Duff, Jack Solomons and Harry Levene. They attracted the glitterati of London life and beyond – greats of stage, screen and sport.

The NSC was formed in 1891 and from 1951 was based at the Café Royal. Among its founders was the Earl of Lonsdale. In 1909 his lordship and the NSC awarded the Lonsdale Belt to British professional champions at all weights. The BBBoC assumed responsibility for their award in 1929 and the tradition continues today.

The Café Royal, with its chandeliers and fine furnishings, seemed an incongruous place to witness pugilists at work. The original rules of the NSC were that guests remain quiet during the fights and respect the combatants. By the 1980s the rule was certainly in abeyance and bouts took place to a background of noise, and diners frequently had their backs to the ring, which I found ungallant. The evenings raised money for charity and were invariably black-tie occasions accompanied by a sumptuous meal. They continued until the Café Royal's closure in 2009.

One evening, I arrived at the Café Royal dressed in black tie, looking forward to supper and, hopefully, a quiet evening. As fight time arrived, I realised that this was a forlorn hope. My fellow doctor had not arrived, I had a promoter and venue manager breathing down my neck and several hundred diners waiting for the action. It was the pre-mobile phone era. Should the card be cancelled? A compromise was reached enabling intervals between bouts to be elongated. That gave me time to accompany fighters from the preceding fight to their changing rooms, satisfy myself of their well-being and return to my ringside position.

It turned out to be one of those evenings. Three of the six bouts finished with cut boxers including one in which both fighters were hurt. I undertook post-fight medical examinations and sutured cut eyebrows unaided and in poor lighting. While stitching, I became aware of a crescendo of noise and slow handclapping coming from the banqueting hall. A steward put his head round the door. 'How long?' he asked. 'The natives are getting restless.'

By the end of the evening I was getting low on suture material and my shirt was splattered in blood. I had missed dinner. I went home on the underground emotionally drained and hungry. I had to use my overcoat to hide the evidence of the evening's carnage.

The most intriguing boxing venue was York Hall, Bethnal Green, in London's East End. It opened in 1929 and was a great boxing location. Many fighters had learnt their trade in the neighbourhood and York Hall had a unique atmosphere. It had a Turkish bath in the basement and bathing for the locals above. Bathrooms were cosy and doubled up on fight nights as changing rooms. On one occasion I had to squeeze into one of the changing rooms with Gary Mason, a huge man but one of the most amiable people I have met in sport. In 1985 Mason was starting out and preparing to fight Frank 'The Tank' Robinson. He seemed to occupy the whole cubicle and my pre-bout medical examination resembled a scene from the game Twister. It lasted longer than the fight because he despatched Robinson in the first round. Mason became British heavyweight champion and retired in 1994 with only one defeat – against Lennox Lewis. Tragically, he died young in a cycling accident in 2011.

York Hall was the only boxing I ever took my wife to. Mrs Ribbans and our Swedish au pair took their seats in the fourth row. It was a typically noisy Bethnal Green evening but nearly descended into a riot; many spectators claimed the raffle had been rigged in favour of a local hoodlum. The fourth row was not far enough back to soften the full noise of punches being landed by the two combatants in the ring. The ladies, finding themselves spattered with sweat, spittle and blood, retreated to the bar and refused to return. I tried.

Our 'wages' for the night were claimed at the end of hostilities. Employees queued outside the office near the back door – programme sellers, ice-cream vendors, doctors …. The promotor's 'accountant' worked on automatic pilot – 'Name … check the money … sign here' – all without raising his eyes from the cardboard box in which brown envelopes filled with used banknotes were neatly stacked.

The Albert Hall was first used for boxing shortly after the 1918 armistice and the audience often included royalty. All the greats appeared in the famous ring and even the infamous Kray twins were on the bill in 1951. Since the millennium boxing has rarely been staged at this great auditorium. However, boxing nights of the 1980s and the 1990s were special.

Then, the historic hall was packed with roaring, expectant fans and the events were often televised. The magnificent domed ceiling, adorned with its multiple 'mushrooms' to improve sound, generated atmospheric acoustics added to by the lighting focused on the ring. The skill, stamina and courage of exponents such as Herol Bomber Graham, Michael Watson, Chris Eubank Sr, Nigel Benn, Lloyd Honeyghan and many other warriors was awe-inspiring.

Behind the scenes, facilities for the gladiators were not so salubrious, with no proper changing rooms or preparation areas. Large cloakrooms off the circular walkways had to be used by boxers and their entourages; one was my consulting room for pre-fight checks and post-match repairs. One night, an American heavyweight returned after 12 rounds with a two-inch cut above his eyebrow. It required suturing but the terrified boxer refused to have the wound stitched. 'No needles, man, no needles,' he said. Thirty-six minutes of walking on to 12-ounce leather gloves filled with menace held no fear for him but the thought of a small needle reduced our man to a quivering wreck. He returned stateside with 'butterfly' strips covering his cut.

Wembley hosted many major bouts including world championships. At the old stadium Frank Bruno beat Oliver McCall for the WBC World Heavyweight Championship in 1995. In 1963, for those with longer memories, Cooper put Muhammad Ali on the seat of his pants only for The Greatest to be saved by the bell. From 1934 most Wembley fights were inside the old Empire Pool which in 1978 was renamed Wembley Arena and then the SSE Arena in 2014. In 1977 the Wembley Conference Centre was built alongside.

I never 'doctored' bouts at Wembley Stadium itself but I am sure the open-air atmosphere must have rivalled the atmosphere of the Albert Hall. Conversely, I found the Wembley Arena and Conference Centre rather functional and lacking in atmosphere but with excellent facilities for the fighters. The Conference Centre world title fights included the infamous 1987 evening when Lloyd Honeyghan charged across the ring at the sound of the second-round bell and hit the slow-rising Johnny Bumphus before he had barely left his seat.

On another occasion I went backstage to check a vanquished overseas boxer and supervise a urine sample for drug testing. The fighter was so exhausted and dehydrated that I anticipated a long wait. We dug in for the long haul. After an hour his team were anxious to leave for their hotel. His trainer grabbed a sample bottle and disappeared into a cubicle, and a minute later offered his sample which was pale and dilute. The trainer winked and was surprised at my refusal to accept it. Another long wait ensued before I left clutching a bone fide specimen.

Frank Bruno fought the Cuban José Ribalta at the Arena in April 1992. The event was live on BBC1's *Sportsnight* and took place only seven months after the Michael Watson–Chris Eubank fight in which Watson had suffered such terrible injuries. Boxing medics always felt on trial and that night was no different for me.

Bruno was the star of British boxing. Despite it being the 36th fight of his 45-fight career, it was only his second fight in the three years since he was knocked out by Mike Tyson in Las Vegas. Ribalta had also fought Tyson, in 1986, lasting until the tenth round. Bruno was superior from the bell against Ribalta and a huge right rendered the Cuban senseless in the second round. Ribalta, complete with his sawn-off pink-striped pyjama shorts, crumpled on to the ropes and then on to the canvas. For a few concerning seconds he was unresponsive. I leapt into the ring. The papers recalled that the stricken boxer required medical attention for five minutes before he could 'remember exactly what he had come to London for'.

Eventually Ribalta responded and with assistance left for the changing room. I stayed with him all the way and, to my amazement, within five further minutes he appeared fully recovered with complete fight recall. Obsessively, I checked him several times before his departure and ensured that he would not be alone during the night. I confirmed that his entourage could identify untoward symptoms and how to contact emergency services. Ribalta went on to fight for another seven years including grappling with Larry Holmes and Vitali Klitschko, both times unsuccessfully.

Boxing – should it be banned?

I ceased acting as a ringside doctor when I moved to Northampton. People had been surprised at my involvement in boxing and, in 1994, during my time as a boxing doctor, the British Medical Association called for a ban on the sport. I have libertarian views and recoil against calls for banning anything. Boxers are fully appraised of the risks – it is like taking informed consent from my patients.

Before the mid-1990s boxing had a more prominent place than it has now on the British sporting landscape and featured regularly on terrestrial television. In the 1960s Henry Cooper became a national treasure and was the first person to win BBC TV's *SPOTY* twice. He had a large supporting heavyweight cast. Muhammad Ali was the most famous sportsman on the planet and his four interviews with Michael Parkinson (from 1971 to 1981) were the stuff of telly legend. During the 1980s and early 1990s Frank Bruno flew the flag for British heavyweights.

At lighter weights we had legendary world champions such as Chris Finnegan, Howard Winstone, Walter McGowan, Ken Buchanan and Jim Watt. Barry McGuigan's fight against Pedroza to take the world featherweight title at QPR's Loftus Road ground was among the top-ten most-watched programmes in 1985, with 20 million viewers. It was the television sporting event of that year. Like Cooper, he landed the *SPOTY* award.

The aim of boxing is to vanquish an opponent by inflicting heavy blows. However, many amateur boxing clubs have brought good to communities by providing outlets for youngsters overseen by dedicated mentors. Important values of sportsmanship, dedication to training and the acceptance of both victory and defeat with equanimity are instilled. Talented young boxers emerge who view boxing as a means of escaping their roots. Boxers deserve the quality medical care that would be denied them if the sport faded into the shadows.

The date of 21 September 1991 was a watershed day for boxing. There had been tragedies in the past, such as Johnny Owens' death in America in 1980, which reminded me sternly of my responsibilities when I started boxing medical duties a year later. Steve Watt (1986), Bradley Stone (1994) and James Murray (1995) had also died fighting.

On that autumn day, Michael Watson sustained serious brain injuries during his world title fight with Chris Eubank. I had supervised previous Watson fights and was devastated. Peter Hamlyn's neurosurgical team at the Royal London undertook multiple operations on Watson but an agonisingly long rehabilitation left him with significant disabilities. His injuries seemed different to previous incidents and the public mood appeared ready to demand even more stringent medical regulation of boxing.

Watson successfully sued the BBBoC and a £400,000 payout was agreed in 2001. The BBBoC was not insured for such eventualities and had to sell its London headquarters to cover the settlement and move to Cardiff. The new regulations had teeth. Paramedics had now to be present at fights and major tournaments needed two ambulances, otherwise the whole event was suspended. The selection of medics became more stringent and they now needed the skill to pass an airway into the lungs of an unconscious boxer. Ambulances were instructed to bypass local casualty departments and make for the nearest neurosurgery centre to ensure expert care commenced inside that critical first 'golden hour'.

These improvements do not eliminate the risk of serious complications. In 1994 Bradley Stone walked from the ring seemingly uninjured before collapsing later at his girlfriend's house and dying. However, present British medical care is at the vanguard of the sport globally. After rules were tightened, 18 years passed without a death in a British ring; stricter medical control seemed to be working. By 2018 Britain had six world champions and 1,000 registered boxers – more than in the 1950s. The sport was enjoying a renaissance. However, concerns resurfaced with the deaths of Michael Norgrove (2013), Mike Towell (2016) and Scott Westgarth (2018), who died after winning a fight in Doncaster. Four fighters died worldwide in 2019. The subject of head injuries and concussion in sport will be further explored later in this book.

The late, great Sheffield-based boxing trainer Brendan Ingle had a notice posted on his gym wall. It was for all youngsters who arrived dreaming of a better life through sport. It read, 'Boxing can seriously damage your health but teaches self-discipline and gets you fit. Smoking, drinking and drugs just damage your health.'

The final bell

A doctor's duty is to provide the best and most up-to-date healthcare for the boxer, including rigorous screening of future fighters to identify risk factors for injury. Education and advice on dangers faced should be available to all boxers. Baseline psychological testing for later comparison, regular screening during their careers and assistance beyond retirement are basic support structures. At fight time, an experienced multi-disciplinary team should be present to provide prompt and appropriate emergency care.

During my years in boxing I found boxers and their teams engaging and dedicated to their profession. Unlike many other sports, there was a keen desire to work closely with medical teams and understanding if a boxer was pronounced unfit to fight. I never felt that any manager or trainer had anything but the boxer's best interests at heart.

Chapter 11

MONKEY GLANDS, METATARSALS AND THE MEDIC MANAGER

'A plague of opinion! A man may wear it on both sides, like a leather jerkin.'

From William Shakespeare's *Troilus and Cressida* (1602)

I HAVE never met a doctor with tactical soccer nous, who knew when a Christmas tree formation (4-3-2-1) wasn't working and could quickly change it to 3-5-2 to negate the opposition's counter-attacking strength. If a doctor did know, they would never offer such advice to the manager. The same is true in other sports; hearing Sir Ian McGeechan's running analysis on elite rugby made me realise how little I knew about a game I played for 30 years. This makes the extent of football coaches' knowledge of medicine and surgery puzzling. How do they acquire it? It appears encyclopaedic and I can only assume it is achieved through correspondence courses with offshore medical schools.

Other parts of this book have identified how football managers become involved with and, occasionally, disagree with their medical teams. Managers are fawned over during press conferences and emboldened to pronounce on a range of medical issues. Nothing is sacred. From MRI interpretations to recovery schedules of star strikers, the verdicts are accepted without demur by the fourth estate.

Managers' medical advice on foot metatarsal fractures, given at press conferences, was analysed some time ago. Eight Premier League players sustained injuries and in all cases the managers' predicted return to play was six to eight weeks. The actual range was 7–34 weeks with an average of 17 weeks. Not even close.

Do clubs' medical departments supply the ammunition? The frequent misinterpretation of medical facts and wide-of-the-mark forecasts suggests that managers have often gone off-script. Are they using medical matters as a means of misinformation and mind games – a case of bluff and double bluff?

The Special One

Some high-profile coaches have become serial offenders in this and the tendency to bolt on medical masterclasses to managerial press conferences has trickled down the leagues. The self-anointed 'Special One', Jose Mourinho, operates in a league of his own in this, however, and has had a string of involvements in medical matters over the years.

For example, the *London Evening Standard* reported in March 2005 that 'Robben's rehabilitation was complicated by the resignation of the club's doctor, Neil Frazer, following a row with Jose Mourinho.' Arjen Robben had broken two bones in his foot having already missed two months of the season with a break in his other ankle. *The Independent* reported that Mourinho wanted the player fit for a Liverpool game taking place 25 days after the injury but Frazer told Mourinho that Robben would not be fit. The newspaper reported that Mourinho had then told the doctor that he was no longer wanted at the club. The player did not start another game for Chelsea that season and made only fitful appearances on the substitutes' bench. The official Chelsea line was that Frazer had left his post 'due to ill health after nearly four years with Chelsea.'

In 2006 Chelsea goalkeeper Petr Cech fractured his skull in a game at Reading. Mourinho complained that the player had to wait 30 minutes for an ambulance. A South-Central Ambulance spokesman countered that the ambulance had arrived within six minutes and that Cech reached the hospital within 26 minutes. Reading FC confirmed the timings and said that Mourinho's account contained 'very serious inaccuracies'. Even the town's MP became embroiled and was quoted saying that Mourinho had 'become an embarrassment' and had been wrong to 'take a pop' at 'hard-working' NHS staff. Mourinho claimed that 'serious questions' needed answering about the Reading FC facilities.

Twelve years later Mourinho took aim at other hard-pressed emergency services, blaming Greater Manchester Police (GMP) for the late arrival of the United bus for a fixture, a claim GMP strongly disputed.

There had been other instances before that. In 2010 Mourinho took a less-than-subtle swipe at Bryan English, who had replaced Neil Fraser as Chelsea team doctor. English has been at the vanguard of sports medicine development in the UK and had worked with Mourinho for several years at Stamford Bridge. In 2010 the Portuguese was returning to Chelsea with his new club, Inter Milan. Pre-match, Mourinho was asked if Chelsea's injured Petr Cech would play. 'Of course, I think Cech could play. I don't listen to those reports that he's out for a month or more. Dr Needles can get him healthy enough to play – and play well.'

The *Daily Mail* reflected, 'If Mourinho knows Chelsea have a method of injecting players back to fitness that is beyond the capacity of their rivals he needs to clarify this, leading to a formal investigation. Otherwise, he is casting vague and baseless aspersions to unsettle an opponent before a major game, which is a shameful tactic considering the seriousness of the issue and the professional implications.' No action was taken against Mourinho. Cech was not fit to play against Inter.

In 2014, back as Chelsea's manager, Mourinho responded to criticism of players being withdrawn from international duty. Diego Costa and Cesc Fàbregas played for Chelsea against West Bromwich Albion before being declared unfit for the Spanish squad. The genuineness of the injuries was questioned by a fellow Spanish international, Sergio Ramos. Mourinho replied, 'He is not a doctor and I am the same. I do my job the best I can, but I am not a doctor. Get a masters and become a doctor before you talk about my players' fitness.' How much reflection goes on in front of the Mourinho bathroom mirror in the mornings?

It was an incident in August 2015 that earned most publicity. Chelsea and Swansea were drawing 2-2 and the former were down to ten men. In the last minutes, Eden Hazard was tackled and left 'lying face down, rolling on to his side, holding his groin and rolling back on to his front'. The referee summoned Chelsea's medical team to assess the stricken player. When they didn't respond he summoned them again. Team doctor Eva Carneiro and the physiotherapist rushed to the player. After treatment, and according to the regulations, Hazard went to the sidelines waiting to be allowed to re-enter the field, temporarily reducing Chelsea to nine men. Words were exchanged between the manager and medic as the latter returned to her position on the bench.

In a post-match interview with Sky Sports Mourinho said, 'I was unhappy with my medical staff. They were impulsive and naive. Whether you are a kit man, doctor or secretary on the bench you have to understand the game. You have to know you have one player less and to assist a player you must be sure he has a serious problem. I was sure Eden did not have a serious problem. He had a knock. He was tired.' Dr Carneiro was removed from first-team duties and later left the club.

Mourinho's action was widely criticised by those involved in the sport and thoughtful observers beyond. Oliver Kay of *The Times* was critical of football's 'duplicitous approach to on-pitch bumps and bruises'. He asked how clinicians could have assessed Hazard's injury from 50 yards and felt that it was Hazard who, if not injured, had put his team at risk. It was time for 'managers to tell their players to save the theatrics for emergencies rather than to try and get a breather, or, in many instances, trying to get an opponent booked or sent off'. His view was that 'it is always so much easier and so much more convenient to blame the medics than to blame the game'.

Mary O'Rourke, one of our country's leading Queen's Counsellors, told the newspaper, 'They did nothing wrong because their duty was to the player as their patient. Their job is to look after the players not to run the team or be tactically aware. As soon as Eden Hazard waves his hand that he wants medical assistance, he turns himself from being a player to being a patient. All credit to the FA for recognising the need to have qualified people on the bench, but it is no good if they cannot come on and assess. If you don't go on the implications are serious.'

Ex-Chelsea player Graeme Le Saux chimed in. 'Carneiro … lost her job simply through fulfilling her professional and medical obligations,' he said, adding, 'If you want the rewards for being successful in football, you have to accept responsibilities. I don't think Mourinho has ever done that, a failure that has made life unnecessarily difficult for others.'

Carneiro took out a claim for constructive dismissal against Chelsea and a separate private action against Mourinho. In June 2016 the cases were settled with undisclosed damages awarded to the doctor. Chelsea issued a contrite statement: 'We wish to place on record that in running on to the pitch Dr Carneiro was following both the rules of the game and fulfilling her responsibility to the players as a doctor, putting their safety first.'

This didn't stop Mourinho and his medical meddling continued when he was appointed Manchester United manager in 2016. Three months after starting he was reported to be 'unhappy with Manchester

United's medical department and wants the club to undertake a review because of the number of injuries …'. He was 'hugely frustrated' and 'is seeking improvements'.

With Mourinho, the spectre of smoke and mirrors is ever present. The same article reported concerns expressed by the Swede Zlatan Ibrahimović, who claimed that his fitness, conditioning and sharpness had been adversely affected by Mourinho's training methods. Was Mourinho's implied criticism of Manchester United's medics an attempt to divert criticism from his own management?

In 2017 Mourinho made further jabbing remarks when accusing England team doctors of injecting his player, Phil Jones, before a game against Germany. His main gripe was that the game was a friendly. However, refreshingly, Mourinho admitted that he 'was not an angel' and had 'had players injected to play official matches'.

Following his appointment at Tottenham in 2019 the media dissected Mourinho's Old Trafford legacy. 'Mourinho engaged in conflict with the club's physios and doctors,' *The Times* said, adding, 'that time and time again, Mourinho has shown that he regards his players' bodies as an expendable resource that should be exhausted in the pursuit of victory'.

Where Angels Fear to Tread
Novel by E.M. Forster (1905)

Mourinho is not alone.

In May 2006, media outlets reported that Mike Stone had left Manchester United after ten years as club doctor. The official statement from Old Trafford stated that, 'There was a difference of opinion on a non-footballing and non-clinical issue, as a result of which Dr Stone felt it to be in his and the club's best interests for him to leave. The difference was over a non-clinical issue and had nothing whatsoever to do with any medical treatment to a Manchester United player.' The newspapers clearly thought the club 'doth protest too much' and widely reported that a bust-up over Wayne Rooney's metatarsal fracture had occurred between Stone and Alex Ferguson. Fortunately, Stone's expertise was not lost to sport and he went on to work for England Cricket, the English Institute of Sport and Birmingham City FC. Over the years I liaised with Mike and found him to be a most conscientious and well-informed colleague. Meanwhile, Manchester United asked a shoulder surgeon for an opinion on Rooney's foot.

The 2012/13 season for Manchester City was not as glorious as their championship-winning triumph the year before. By November the club had exited the Champions League and by May the team had lost their domestic title and Roberto Mancini, their manager, his job. The Italian's Wikipedia page states that, 'Mancini's public criticism of backroom and playing staff, as well as his distant relationships, alienated the players and the club hierarchy during the last eight months of his tenure.'

One of the earliest casualties of that season was Phil Batty, who had worked at Manchester United and Blackburn before joining City in 2010. He was another very talented sports physician with many strings to his bow and a firm belief in evidence-based medicine. The *Daily Telegraph* reported that 'Mancini expressed his unhappiness with City's medical department last season despite the club having the best injury record in the Premier League (last season they suffered 50 per cent fewer injuries than Manchester United)'. City's loss was rugby union's gain; Batty was appointed to the England senior men's team.

Many physiotherapists have recounted serial 'roastings' from managers. These usually follow one of two lines. A player has come back too early and is clearly not fit – conveniently forgetting pressure from the manager to return to the team. Or the player is taking too long to recover. Physiotherapists are on the horns of a dilemma and scoldings are often accompanied by weekly dismissal threats. I know of at least one physio who jumped ship before the inevitable sacking.

During a Liverpool evening match at Leeds in 1999 Michael Owen suffered a bad hamstring injury. The manager, Gérard Houllier, had ignored the advice of his physio and insisted Owen be brought back from injury quickly. Owen recalled that 'my hamstring snapped in two and it was at that point that my ability to perform unimpeded was finished'. The incident allegedly led to the departure of the Reds' physiotherapist Mark Leather.

Some high-profile sports coaches are aware of the limits of their medical training, however. In 2017, during the Lions New Zealand rugby tour, Scottish full-back Stuart Hogg sustained a facial injury. Head coach Warren Gatland commented post-game, 'We're hoping he'll be OK, but we're just getting someone more qualified than me to assess that.' How refreshing!

Monkey business

Recent managerial miscreants have a role model in the form of a military man.

Major Frank Buckley managed Wolverhampton Wanderers from 1927 to 1944 and was credited with many innovations. In the mid-1920s, as Blackpool manager, Buckley gave pep pills (possibly amphetamines) to players pre-match. He was not alone in doing that but it is his handling of testicles for which he is best remembered.

Following the theories of Russian medic Serge Voronoff, Buckley sought to rejuvenate his players by giving them monkey genitalia. In 1937 he injected his players with monkey gland extract twice weekly for six weeks. The benefits were claimed to last a season and his team's performance improved. Several players refused, though, and one brought his father in to decline consent.

Improving virility by using animals' testosterone had been a matter of speculation for some time. In 1889 French scientist Charles-Édouard Brown-Séquard injected himself with dog and guinea pig extract. He claimed several benefits including the curing of his constipation and the lengthening of the arc of his urine. The following century, famous American baseball player Babe Ruth self-administered sheep testicle extract and became extremely ill. His symptom was described as a 'bellyache' by his club, the New York Yankees.

Back to Wolves. Impressive results led to claims of unfair advantages being gained. After defeating Leicester City 10-1, the latter's local MP, Manny Shinwell, demanded a government inquiry. The mischievous Labour MP suggested that the Tory government would benefit from the injections.

Other clubs did not want to miss a marginal gain including Portsmouth and Tottenham Hotspur who medicated their men with magical monkey measures. The 1939 FA Cup Final was played between Pompey and Wolves and was known as the 'Monkey Gland Final'. However, by the outbreak of war the fad had faded away.

Such potions had no scientific validity and could cause potential harm. One wonders who administered the injections and did they have any ethical misgivings. Throughout my childhood, my parents and their friends would pose the question, 'Are they on monkey glands?' when witnessing an extraordinary sporting feat.

(Touch)lines of reporting

In organisations as valuable and supposedly sophisticated as major sporting teams, one expects a clear line of responsibility. Clubs have a chairman, board, chief executive and director of finance. They carry ultimate accountability for corporate success and financial soundness but additionally function as guardians with ethical and legal responsibilities towards employees and customers.

The exact position of the sports team manager or coach is interesting. It is not one easily identifiable in other commercial, industrial or financial concerns. Managers are directors of operations, acting as the link between the product on the pitch and the wider corporation. Football managers have a short shelf life. Their existence is precarious and entirely results driven. In 2015 the average stretch for a football manager in the senior four English divisions was 15 months. The average survival time of a manager in the Premier League dropped from 3.14 years in 2000 to 1.64 years in 2018.

Football managers' stress is a real and long-recognised phenomenon. Mental and physical health problems are common. Jock Stein, Barry Fry, Gérard Houllier and Graeme Souness suffered serious heart conditions, a problem that claimed the life of Stein. In 2019, Justin Edinburgh's death, at 49 years old, from a heart attack shocked the football world. Two years previously he had been Northampton Town manager. He was one of the most approachable managers I have met.

When the team embarks upon a poor run scapegoats are sought. However, repetitive criticism and the undermining of support personnel is unproductive and contributes to poor morale. Excellent relationships do exist between many managers and medical departments and, rightly, decisions to dispense with peoples' services are not always disclosed publicly. However, the decision-making often centres on the manager with little objective, less emotive input from wiser heads within the organisation.

Building up a successful and functioning clinical team takes time, just as rebuilding the side on the pitch does. This begs the question, why do CEOs and directors allow medical departments to be dismantled on the whim of the manager when, statistically, the latter is likely to be picking up their own P45 a few months later?

Chapter 12

WHAT A LOAD OF COBBLERS

'Wishin' and Hopin''

Top-ten hit for Dusty Springfield (1964)

THE OLD Northampton County Ground, the home of Northampton Town FC, had a rickety wooden stand, permanent terraces at each end and a pub behind one of the corner flags. The aroma of embrocation seeped through the stand's floorboards from the changing rooms below. At the back of the stand was the press box, which was partially concealed by the smog of pipe smoke.

My first visit was during the 1957/58 season – the last of the old Third Division (south). I sat beside Father on the press bench. He made notes, phoned in copy and chatted with colleagues. I sucked in the scene and the nicotine as much as any three-year-old can. We were both happy.

Later, responsibility for getting me to Cobblers' games passed to my grandfather. Carrying an orange box to stand on, we caught the bus to the ground. We had the Saturday habit. One week the first team, the next the reserves in the Football Combination. Youngsters went free if they could be lifted over the turnstile. My ageing grandfather could still manhandle the pedestal and lift me up and over when I was nearly as tall as him.

With programme, rattle and scarf we stood on 'Spion Kop' at one end of the ground and named after a famous British defeat in the Boer War. It was a metaphor for most of Northampton's inglorious football history. Pre-match entertainment included listening over the superannuated tannoy system to Frank Ifield, the yodelling Aussie, crooning 'I Remember You' and to 'Wishin' and Hopin'' by the singer we called Rusty Springboard. There were no merchandising stalls or pie outlets then.

Back home afterwards we were greeted with a plea for silence – Grandmother was checking the pools. *Dixon of Dock Green* would follow shortly on TV. 'Evenin' all.'

Housemates

Cricket and football shared the County Ground where Northamptonshire Cricket Club were the landlords. Football paid rent and due homage. Like Venn diagrams, the playing surfaces overlapped and the Cobblers erected temporary wooden stands for home games. It could lead to a lopsided start or finish to the football season. In 1953/54 the Cobblers' first four league games were all away, to accommodate the cricket team's Championship games against Surrey, Glamorgan and Kent.

In 1985 the stand was condemned after the Popplewell Enquiry following the Bradford City fire. Journalists had to use the cricket press box 100yds away from the action. Heaven knows how they recorded accurately the game against Tranmere on a wet Tuesday night. The Cobblers' new stadium at Sixfields opened in 1994. They were still tenants – this time to the local council.

Something's a-stirring in the neighbourhood

In 1959 the Cobblers appointed Dave Bowen as player-manager. Bowen had played for Arsenal and captained Wales in their only World Cup (Sweden, 1958). He was one of the first Arsenal players (along with keeper Jack Kelsey) to play in a World Cup.

Northampton must have been a culture shock to him. However, the Welsh wizard steered us past Barrow and Bradford Park Avenue out of the Fourth Division in 1961 – attracting home crowds of up to 21,000. Two years later we said goodbye to Brighton, Bournemouth and the two Bristols as champions of the Third Division . Not daunted by the likes of Manchester City and Southampton we strode into the First Division (now Premier League) in 1965.

Even as a child, I knew that teams like Northampton should get nosebleeds in the higher football echelons.

After the Lord Mayor's Show

It couldn't last. It took five seasons for the cream to rise to the top and four seasons for it to turn sour. We were back where we started. Five of the

Fourth Division team had played important roles in our First Division campaign and one player, Barry Lines, played in the old fourth division in 1960 and was back there in 1970 having sampled everything in between.

The golden season provided happy memories. We were relegated, yes, but with a record number of points. We'd done the double over Aston Villa and I'd watched Spurs claim a late equaliser at White Hart Lane through a Jimmy Greaves penalty. How could I not be bonded to such an outfit for life?

The subsequent half-century has been tough for the club and the team have played mostly to the standard of their moniker. They have won two fourth-tier championships and five other promotions from the same division and have made several jaunts to Wembley. Once, famously, in 1970, they were at the wrong end of Manchester United – an FA Cup 8-2 thrashing at Northampton with George Best scoring six.

Northampton have always been a selling club. The best export was Phil Neal, who went on to make 417 consecutive Liverpool appearances and win five First Division titles and four European Cups. Without a hugely wealthy benefactor clubs such as Northampton have a ceiling. In 1998 the Cobblers played Grimsby at Wembley for a First Division place. I operated on one of the club directors a week before and as we anaesthetised him he joked, 'Don't wake me up if we win at Wembley.' The board had done their maths: the club could not survive financially in the second tier. Mid-table mediocrity in the Second Division was a stable financial playing field.

As my father and I and 30,000 others urged our team on, I had visions of the directors sitting with their fingers crossed. We lost 1-0 and haven't seriously troubled the business end of the third tier again.

The hoping goes on, and draws us to Sixfields on Saturdays. It is illogical but 1964/65 could just happen again.

'My Name Is Jack'
Song by Manfred Mann (1968)

During my teenage years, torn hamstrings and sprained ankles were par for the course. My dad had just the cure: Jack Jennings. His part in sporting history risks being lost.

Jennings lived in the street where my father was born and within a good strike of a cricket ball or football from the County Ground. Born in 1902, he played for his hometown, Wigan Borough, then Cardiff City,

Middlesbrough and Preston North End before joining the Cobblers. He was a masseur by training.

Jennings rehabilitated servicemen during the Second World War and in 1943 Cobblers' manager Tom Smith asked if he would reprise the role of trainer-coach undertaken at Preston. Little did Jennings know that at the age of 41 he would be press-ganged into playing 17 times that season, including in a 9-1 home win over Nottingham Forest.

Sir Stanley Rous, FA secretary and future FIFA president, congratulated the Cobblers on Jennings' appointment. 'I am very glad to see you have availed yourself of this man's talents and compliment you on doing so,' he said. Rous believed Northampton to be the country's fittest team because they were under the beady eye of Jennings, who remained trainer to Northampton until 1964.

Jennings persuaded recovered servicemen to take their boots to the Cobblers. Tommy 'Flash' Fowler was on Everton's books before the war but joined Northampton at Jennings' encouragement. Fowler made a record 583 appearances for the club from 1946 to 1961. I still prize the signed copy of his autobiography, *Quite Simply a Flash of Genius*, given to me after I had replaced his hip.

Jennings found himself in the managerial hot seat in August 1963 when David Bowen needed a rest. Jennings' managerial record was played 3, won 3, drawn 0, lost 0, a double over Scunthorpe and an away win at Sunderland in front of a crowd of 39,201. Bowen was reinstated within a fortnight and led the club to the promised land two seasons later. Heaven knows what Jennings did wrong. Perhaps Bowen recognised a rival in the making.

One of Jennings' recipes for healthy living was a daily cocktail of sherry and raw eggs. My father insisted that I try this on more than one occasion. The only thing that made it palatable was Dad telling me that one club was drinking bull's blood as a 'pick me up'. What social services would make of it now, I do not know.

In 1954 Jennings was awarded a testimonial match against a Combined League XI. The great Blackpool duo of Stan Mortensen and Stanley Matthews agreed to appear, but Matthews picked up an injury. Not to disappoint the crowd, the little wizard ran the line. It was the current day equivalent of Wayne Rooney and Harry Kane turning up midseason for a testimonial for Accrington Stanley's physio. A programme of the game is one of my treasured sporting possessions.

Jennings used to emerge on to the field in his baggy tracksuit, elasticated at ankle and wrist. He would hare to the stricken player clutching a rubber bag of water, which was virtually empty by the time he reached his destination. He doubled up at cricket and looked after Northants CCC for 38 years until his retirement in 1983. He even doubled up as cricket scorer during wartime away games.

He worked at three Olympics, from 1952 to 1960, toured with England's amateur football side, acted as Indian cricket team trainer in 1946 and was masseur for the England (aka MCC) Ashes trip to Australasia from 1965 to 1966. It is exhausting just recounting it. Jennings' reputation saw opposition cricketers flock to his treatment table. Sir Leonard Hutton repaid Jennings' curative work by scoring centuries in each innings against Northants. In the 1970s, England bowler Mike Selvey would bypass the Middlesex physio and drive up the M1 to see Jennings.

Jennings ran a private practice from a couch in the lounge of his terraced house, surrounded by sporting mementos. Bob Taylor, the future British Lion and RFU President, remembered his father packing him off to Jennings for treatment.

Jennings examined injuries, applied liberal lashings of Elliman's rub and massaged deep into damaged tissues. After ten minutes he seemed exhausted by his manual work and wheeled out 'Big Bertha' – the heat lamp, which was carefully positioned so that its rays could produce intense redness on the target. Meanwhile, Jennings retreated to his kitchen for 20 minutes to drink tea. His patients had to listen to *Mrs Dale's Diary* on the radio during their treatment. I never dared question his methods, always walking home with a glow on the damaged tissue, which uncannily seemed to make a rapid recovery.

Jennings lived until the ripe old age of 95 – it must have been the sherry and eggs. Thank you, Jack, for treating my various strains and sprains and introducing me to the home life of Dr and Mrs Dale.

From Silverstone to Sixfields

Having returned to Northampton in 1996, I became increasingly re-acquainted with Cobblers players. In August 1999 the club's secretary called, having seen me on TV. 'If you can look after Michael Schumacher, could you become our honorary orthopaedic surgeon?' With due respect to the great Formula 1 world champion, this was the ultimate appointment.

Four decades after my first appearance in the press box I was furnished at last with an all-areas pass. It has been a roller-coaster ride covering two decades of the club's matches. I've seen four promotions and three relegations in the lower echelons of league football and a flirtation with exit from the league itself.

During the 20 years to the end of 2019 the Cobblers have had 16 managers. Unlike the Premier League we have only 'gone exotic' once, in appointing Dutchman Jimmy Floyd Hasselbaink. In the previous 100 years we'd had 29 managers but even in the Football League basement the hot seat gets ever hotter. Chairmen and financial backers have come and gone. Money has arrived and mysteriously disappeared. The show still goes on.

My role has been to support the physiotherapist and club doctor. While many managers have flown the nest there have been only four physiotherapists and four club doctors in the last two decades. This has allowed the development of continuity, teamwork and mutual respect within the medical department, something not to be sneezed at in a club where resources and playing staff are limited. Game-time gives the clinical team an opportunity to assess players together, including fresh and established injuries, and monitor progress after surgery.

Most orthopaedic surgeons only see injured patients after arrival in hospital but seeing the injuries happen in front of you gives a different perspective. Damage is not only sustained by players. I have taken several referees to casualty in my car, with assorted problems. On one occasion, an assistant referee collapsed like a sack of potatoes with a ruptured Achilles ten yards in front of me while I was watching in the stands.

I also see the other side of the strains on the emergency services. Several years ago a visiting player sustained terrible fractures of the tibia and fibula (the two shin bones). Although not a home player, I knew him well and had operated on his knee in the past. In the medical room he was splinted and given pain relief. We waited over 90 minutes for an ambulance. The player was forced to retire following his injury. Goodness knows what Mourinho would have said if it had been a Chelsea, Manchester United or Tottenham player. Sadly, this is life at the wrong end of the football pyramid. I've heard similar stories of amateur and professional players waiting on sports pitches for several hours following fractures and dislocations. I mean no criticism but simply reflect on the ever-growing demands on our NHS.

My position at the club is one that I have clarified with every sporting organisation I have been associated with. Those problems I feel I can deal with competently I will look after. If an injury is better dealt with by another specialist, I will give my recommendation.

Occasionally, players coming down the football pyramid have had to have their expectations recalibrated off the field as well as on it. Things they had immediate access to, such as MRI scanning, may have to wait until tomorrow. Manchester United's Carrington training complex, Sixfields is not.

Players may seek to influence medical matters at a fundamental level. Some years ago the Cobblers experienced what can best be described as a medical coup d'état by the players. One player was prone to supplement the club's medical offerings by travelling north to receive osteopathic treatment. He had a large influence on the changing room and persuaded the manager to appoint his osteopath as the club's head of medicine.

In my view, the manager involved ranked as one of our best over the last 60 years and was usually imbued with enormous common sense. Nobody realised that there was a vacancy and no wider soundings were sought; it was presented as a fait accompli. The appointee had never worked in a sports organisation before. He arrived, and both the long-standing club physiotherapist and doctor promptly resigned. I was canvassed for support by the 'torpedoed two'. The club was faced with a medical mutiny. The osteopath left within the week and life returned to normal. The manager made an appointment to come and see me in my clinic and apologised. It was a magnanimous and unexpected gesture which I very much appreciated.

Over the years, I have seen players from clubs all over the country and from all divisions. I enjoy hearing about their careers, which like all in professional sport are precarious; the players are always one tackle away from never playing again. I have enormous respect for the PFA, which picks up the pieces pastorally, medically and financially when players have been offloaded by their clubs.

Survival of the (un)fittest?

'Victory, however hard and long the road may be; for without victory there is no survival.'

Winston Churchill, speech to the House of Commons (1940)

Care for the local professional footballer has come a long way since the days of 'our Jack'. However, the Cobblers today find themselves in a similar position on the field as they were in the 1950s. For those of us supporting them and involved professionally, we are simply relieved that they still survive in the Football League. I smile at the sound of distraught Premier League fans phoning into radio programmes on Saturday evenings. Their displeasure revolves around their club's failure to lift another major title. There is no entitlement to sporting success. We would be delighted to shade Forest Green in a five-goal thriller.

For myself, I can hardly believe that more than 60 years have passed since I donned the claret and white scarf for the first time. The club's journey has rarely been distinguished and only once touched the heights. However, for me, it has been the greatest pleasure to have supported, been involved with and provided some help along the way.

Chapter 13

THE HEALING POWERS
OF THE PLACENTA

'I conjure you, by that which you profess,
Howe'er you come to know it, answer me.'

Macbeth addressing the three witches in William
Shakespeare's *Macbeth* (1606)

Belgrade-bound

In November 2009 Arsenal striker Robin van Persie injured his ankle
ligaments playing for the Netherlands. Two examining doctors believed
he would be unable to play for around seven weeks. A Dutch journalist
was more optimistic. Van Persie 'could be back in as little as four weeks
if the treatment works'. The Dutch superstar must have been disconsolate
having taken preventative action only months before – he had had some
teeth removed, of which I'll say more later.

Van Persie flew to Belgrade to seek help from someone with unusual
remedies, reporting that 'she is vague about her methods, but I know she
massages you using fluid from a placenta. I am going to try. It cannot
hurt.' He added, 'I've been in contact with Arsenal's chief physio about
it. The club has allowed me to have this treatment done.'

The stampede to Serbia was started by the Liverpool player Yossi
Benayoun. The Israeli explained that 'there were no animal parts used ...
she would be using fluid from a placenta that had come from a woman'.

'Afterbirth', or placenta, sits on the lining of a mammal's womb and
is connected to the foetus by the umbilical cord. It provides nutrition
and oxygen, an outlet for waste disposal and is expelled after the birth.

Speculation began in the media and football circles. The *Daily Telegraph* referred to 'revolutionary new treatment', adding, 'Arsenal physiotherapist, Colin Lewin, has decided that the massage therapy treatment in Serbia cannot cause further damage, although there is scepticism as to whether it will speed up van Persie's recovery. But even if it provides only a psychological fillip to the player, it will be of some help.' The BBC's health correspondent highlighted other uncommon remedies used by famous athletes including 'rubbed oil from the belly of an emu to ease injuries sustained in a collision with a cyclist'.

At some stage it appeared that the 'miracle doctor', Maria (or Marijana) Kovacevic, had swopped horses by moving from human to equine afterbirth. Her qualifications and training varied according to media outlets. The BBC described her as a 'specialist' and the *Daily Mirror* as a 'human placental therapist' before later demoting her, clinically speaking, to a 'housewife'. Van Persie was content that she was a 'doctor' and seemed rather indignant. He was quoted as telling the Serbian newspaper *Alo!*, 'It's good, I'm happy. The woman is a miracle.'

Liverpool manager Rafael Benitez chimed in. 'We heard about her about 15 days ago and the information we got was very positive.' Rafa reassured the public that Ms Kovacevic was a 'doctor with a degree in pharmacology'.

Surprisingly for a medic she had an agent. Star Management Signings informed the waiting world that she was a person 'schooled in physiotherapy'.

In Belgrade a different picture was emerging. A nearby bar owner reported that 'she always wears big lipstick' and 'looks like Morticia from the Addams family'. Alarmingly, Serbia's health minister 'ordered a full investigation into her clinic and whether she has got a medical licence'. 'We are now trying to trace Kovacevic,' he said.

The media claimed she charged £5,000 per treatment. Apparently, the clinic was not registered with the authorities and had never paid taxes. One Serbian doctor claimed, 'It just makes us a laughing-stock.' The *Daily Mirror* reported that 'locks were put on the office and it appears the clinic has been shut down until the investigation is complete. The [health] department says there is a widespread problem of unlicensed therapists.' However, *The Times* entitled an article, 'Robin van Persie's treatment the embryo of a brilliant idea'.

Why don't you join us?

Elite clubs were not put off. *The Times* reported, 'Manchester City tried to take her on to their full-time staff,' adding that 'just because City have got more money than sense these days, we shouldn't infer anything about the practices – effective or otherwise – of Ms Kovacevic'.

There was a scramble for her signature. Romanian club CFR Cluj tempted her with a £190,000 annual salary. The *Daily Mail* reported Liverpool's interest under the headline 'Rafa Benitez pulls a Christmas quacker!'. The imminent arrival of Morticia on Merseyside proved too much for some fans. One reported to the *Daily Mail* that 'all the players treated so far with the horse placenta were in a stable condition!' Another pleaded, 'Rafa, please contact me about some magic beans I have for sale.'

The denouement

Van Persie's injury did not heal and he travelled to the Netherlands for surgery. He returned to play five months after the injury.

Onwards, upwards and eastwards

Would this much-hyped therapy die a natural death? No.

Elite footballers Frank Lampard, Alberto Aquilani, Albert Riera, Glen Johnson and Fabio Aurelio among others beat a path to Kovacevic's door. She was used by Serbia during the 2010 World Cup in South Africa. During the 2012 African Cup of Nations football tournament it was reported that she used equine placenta to heal Ghana's Asamoah Gyan. The recovery from the injury was supposed to take four weeks but in fact took four hours.

In 2014 Atlético Madrid played Real Madrid in the Champions League Final. Their star striker, Diego Costa, was injured and the *Daily Telegraph* stated that he 'travelled to the Serbian capital earlier this week to meet with "miracle doctor" Marijana Kovacevic … for horse placenta treatment for his grade I hamstring tear'.

The BBC reported the outcome. 'It was only nine minutes before the answer was delivered as a clearly unfit Costa signalled to the bench that he could not continue.' Atlético Madrid's coach, Diego Simeone, said afterwards, 'No doubt the fact Diego played was my responsibility and I made a mistake.' It was a refreshing admission in a sport not awash with reflective statements.

Social media was quicker off the block than Costa proved to be. Those on Twitter reacted pithily. 'Only fools and horses,' said one, 'Sales of horse placenta have just nosedived,' another, while a third commenter tweeted, 'Horse placenta. Foal's Gold.'

Undeterred, the 'miracle doctor' moved to Dubai, where the great and good flocked. Soon after Real Madrid *galactico* Christiano Ronaldo injured a knee in the 2016 European Final. He sought Kovacevic's intervention for a problem described as a 'partial anterior cruciate ligament injury'. *The Sun* described her practices as 'oddball'.

Ms Kovacevic's own website clarifies that she has a pharmacology degree (the study of drug actions) and that she worked in laboratories and pharmaceutical institutions before starting a 'medical practice' 15 years later. I cannot find any evidence that she is a 'doctor' in terms of being medically trained or possessing a PhD.

'I've looked at life from both sides now'
Joni Mitchell, 'Both Sides Now' (1967)

Has this account been unfair to Ms Kovacevic?

In the early 1980s I worked as a dermatology junior doctor at the Royal Free. Regularly I went to the labour ward to secure a fresh layer of afterbirth, (the amnion – a protective sac for the foetus) from a plastic bag full of placentae. It was to be used on leg ulcer patients. The amnion is rich in protein and nutrients and promotes ulcer healing. However, after two to three days it has to be replaced because of the smell emitted as it decays. Placentae have been used in surgical reconstructive procedures since the early 1900s and today their uses include burns therapy and forms of eye and dental surgery, as well as the treatment of ulcers.

As doctors we are encouraged to seek evidence for treatments we prescribe and to keep an open mind. The adoption of any new treatment should be associated with proper research. But such carefully designed trials are a rarity in sports medicine – especially soccer.

Arsène Wenger was quoted as saying he was doubtful about the Kovacevic treatment but gave his permission to van Persie. 'I'm not a fan, but I'm not a doctor either,' Wenger said, which begs the question, why didn't he ask one of his medics?

We must acknowledge some truths in sport. There is an impatience to return to play and athletes' careers are short. No treatment carries a 100 per cent guarantee of full recovery. Ms Kovacevic's website doesn't mention placental fluid and an extensive literature search found no publications about her methods in recognised scientific journals. Her other methods, including massage and electrical therapy, appear to mirror methods used by clinicians in this country.

Nevertheless, many footballers have sought her help. Does their presence in her clinic legitimise her methods even if they did not effect a cure? Most sporting soft tissue injuries heal on their own; we just tinker around the edges. The fact that an injury has had a treatment during the normal healing cycle, whether it be drugs, physiotherapy or equine afterbirth juice, does not imply that the intervention per se has been successful.

Why have other sports doctors and physiotherapists not rushed to human or equine birthing units? Could it be that there is no clear advantage over what is already offered? The next chapter will explore further what these episodes teach us about ourselves as doctors and the way we operate.

Chapter 14

THE WISDOM OF TEETH

Roots that reach the parts that others cannot
'It is very vulgar to talk like a dentist when one
isn't a dentist. It produces a false impression.'

From Oscar Wilde's *The Importance of*
***Being Earnest* (1898)**

ATHLETES FIND injuries frustrating. They fret if they recur or become chronic. At times they seek help from unusual sources, including dental intervention to cure leg ailments.

In 2009 Jamie Redknapp told the *Daily Mail* about his knee. He played for Liverpool from 1991 to 2002 but made only 17 England appearances. Injuries ruled him out of the 1998 World Cup. By the age of 26 he had undergone 12 knee operations in America and Europe.

Redknapp admitted that 'footballers have always been desperate to chase any miracle cure that can help prolong their careers'. He confirmed that he 'had a passport stamped with unlikely destinations that were filled with promises' and 'went to France, where I travelled with a knee injury and the osteopath wanted to take my wisdom teeth out. Apparently, it is to do with clear pathways around your body.'

He felt that 'instead of sitting around and waiting for the injury to heal, seeing different physios, medics and healers at least it makes you feel as if you are being proactive'. Redknapp added, 'In that respect, it's good for the mind ... even if it doesn't always help the injury.'

The player sought advice from faith healer Eileen Drewery, who was controversially appointed by England manager Glenn Hoddle to the 1998 World Cup coaching staff. Redknapp reported that Drewery 'was promising to help me and, for a while, it felt as she was making a difference'. Sadly, Redknapp's problems continued and he missed the final four months of the 1999/2000 season and the 2000 UEFA European Championships. In July 2000, the BBC reported that he would be returning to Colorado for a 'final knee operation'.

Redknapp missed the 2000/01 season and played only eight games of the following season before injury struck again. After a further 84 games over four years for Tottenham and Southampton, he bowed to medical advice and retired.

Dutch dentition

Was removing teeth to cure injuries dismissed as a treatment following its failure to resolve Redknapp's chronic knee problem? Of course not. In 2014, the *Sunday Times* ran the headline, 'Dutch left with less bite'.

The Netherlands World Cup coach Louis van Gaal wanted his players' wisdom teeth removed, believing that poor contact between teeth affected posture and increased injury risk. Ten days earlier, Dutch fitness coach Raymond Verheijen had complained that Van Gaal's over-training regime had caused injuries, including Robin van Persie's groin strain.

But Van Persie had had wisdom teeth removed in 2009 after blaming them for his injury-prone season at Arsenal. He was following in the dental tracks laid down by Steven Gerrard and Florent Malouda. Unfortunately, Van Persie sprained his ankle only months after the teeth were extracted, which triggered his pursuit of afterbirth juice therapy. Did Van Gaal know that his star striker had been without his wisdom teeth for five years prior to the announcement of his own dental solution? Clearly the extractions had not rendered Van Persie immune from further injuries in the interim.

Looking gifted horses in the mouth

Poor dental hygiene in athletes should come as no surprise. In 2015 it was reported that most professional footballers had dental problems. Four years later the same researchers found half of Olympic and other professional athletes had untreated tooth decay. Worryingly, one-third claimed that problems with their teeth had interfered with their training. Footballers were twice as likely to develop cavities than other sportsmen. Sugary energy drinks were a potential culprit.

Dental disease is painful and debilitating and affects training and performance. Eradicating poor oral health should be a footballer's goal. It may indicate other health shortcomings. A laissez-faire attitude to welfare might increase injury risk and a resistance to following rehabilitation guidelines diligently. Preventative dental strategy is laudable, but is inflating it as a panacea for most ills far-fetched?

Some senior physiotherapists feel that bite problems caused by a misalignment of the teeth (malocclusion) can create tension around the head and neck. Some preliminary work suggests that cranial osteopathy in footballers with dental concerns can improve balance. However, there is little evidence that dental extractions will cure chronic joint and muscle problems in the lower limbs, particularly if the removed teeth are healthy. Doing this creates false hope in sportsmen desperately looking for solutions to career-threatening injuries.

This has not prevented the development of an industry dedicated to such issues. Companies claim that their products and services will cure injuries and prevent future problems. The combination of dental issues and leg injuries is common in athletes but one is not necessarily caused by the other.

Are the lunatics running the asylums?

These examples raise wider concerns relating to the status, behaviour and relationships of clinicians and coaching staff within large sporting organisations.

Medical departments in elite clubs have massive budgets and huge numbers of intelligent and expensively assembled clinicians. Those medics should have the experience and scientific objectivity to assess new treatments and the courage of their convictions to advise players, managers and agents of when an athlete should not pursue particular avenues of intervention. The fact that players are chasing dubious treatments from individuals of limited, relevant clinical experience deserves closer analysis. Is the club's medical team fully exercising their duty of care to a player? Is it enough to say 'it probably won't do you any harm' when giving the green light to such interventions?

Such treatments are not without hazard, including surgical site infection and reactions to anaesthetics and other medicants. It is rare, but dental interventions can have catastrophic consequences – in 2017 the great ballet dancer and choreographer Sergei Vikharev died in a dental chair.

Does pursuing dubiously effective 'treatments' delay the start of more suitable and proven injury-management options? There are extraneous pressures on these doctors from many directions, from managers, coaches, the collective changing room, agents and parents – even before they start looking after the patient.

The many individuals situated on the periphery of the sporting world and attempting entrée into its seemingly attractive life create dangers for sportspeople. Redknapp saw a French osteopath. Presumably they had not long been acquainted. Did the osteopath have the knowledge and education to understand the player's long medical history, or have superior experience of treating such conditions compared to surgeons across two continents? Unlikely. Instead the osteopath wanted to prove their worth by advising 'try something different' but with no logical likelihood of success.

What should the position of the employing sporting organisation be in such circumstances? Should it agree and condone treatment by underqualified persons and fund jaunts to visit them? What is the responsibility of the media in lauding such treatments initially but lacking later reflection on their effectiveness?

Parents, agents, employers and the media should try to protect athletes. All have a responsibility to examine critically new and fantastical treatments. Finally, we should trust the appointed, experienced medical staff to do their best for the athlete.

Chapter 15

THE FEUDALISM OF FOOTBALL
... AND MOST OTHER SPORTS!

Medieval lords, vassals, peasants and fiefs

'I dreamed that I dwelt in marble halls
With vassals and serfs at my side.'

Alfred Bunn (1796–1860), English theatrical manager and
writer of librettos, from the opera *The Bohemian Girl* (1843)

THE MEDIEVAL feudal system was used to organise society across large swathes of Europe from the 9th to the 15th centuries.

The lord owned all he surveyed – his fiefdom – but owed allegiance to the monarch. The vassals, or knights, contracted with their lord to provide services in exchange for protection and use of land (fief). Obligations included going to war in the lord's colours or fulfilling non-military tasks. They might fight for the crown or embark on holy wars abroad. The peasants were at the bottom of the pile. They worked the land and made tools in return for protection. Everyone knew their place. By 1500, feudalism had died out across most of Europe, although serfdom lasted in Russia until 1861.

Modern lords, vassals, peasants and fiefs

'The greater the power, the more
dangerous the abuse.'

Edmund Burke (1729–1797), Whig politician

Football retains many of the vestiges of the feudal system – 500 years after it died out in most of the rest of Europe.

Powerful lords (club owners) own personal fiefdoms – the stadia are their castles and the pitches their land. They owe allegiance to the monarch – the Football Association or Premier or Football League. As warring nobles, they desire glory. They need an army of vassals – knights in shining armour (or players in expensive livery). Armour is redesigned annually with different attire for home and abroad. The peasants must dress similarly.

Vassals are remunerated handsomely. They are granted a fief – a flank, goalmouth or churned-up midfield. Vassals need to be teak hard, skilled, regimented and trained to respond to opponents' sallies during battle. Lords will replace underperforming or badly injured vassals. Lords have nurseries of aspiring young warriors and sieve through thousands until Sir Galahad appears. Soldier-cadets may be loaned to lesser fiefdoms to win their spurs and many remain non-commissioned officers forever. During crises, mercenaries from far away are engaged to add backbone to their attack or defence positions.

Vassals perform in a range of meteorological conditions and compete when fatigued or carrying nagging aches. One cold Wednesday night, they might re-enact the Battle of Stamford Bridge and afterwards trudge wearily to deepest, darkest Wales to repel Swansea four days later.

The altruism of the lords is stretched if vassals are selected to represent the crown. Mysterious injuries contracted on home jousting fields lead to unexpected withdrawals from the royal ranks. Lords seek victories on the European mainland and during domestic truces ask vassals to travel abroad on goodwill missions to convert foreign peasants to the fiefdom's religion and sell replica armour. Local peasants may be offered employment at the castle as programme sellers, turnstile operatives or as launderers of the vassals' clothing. Outside the castle walls, more peasants provide goods and services for the lord. The majority, however, simply pay homage and swell the coffers by attending encounters at the castle.

Lords may overreach themselves searching for the Holy Grail (or FA Cup), causing insolvency, and take on a very *un-noblesse oblige* posture during financial collapses. The monarch requires that 'football creditors', including wealthy footballers and their agents, are reimbursed in full following bankruptcy. The peasants, including HMRC and local tradesmen, go to the end of the queue as 'ordinary creditors' receiving a fraction of owed bills.

I have been a helpless peasant more than once, when football and rugby teams of my professional acquaintance used the 1986 Insolvency Act to go into administration. In such cases, creditors can go hang, leaving outstanding bills for knee surgery on the centre-half or loose-head prop.

Out of this mess they 'phoenix' and re-form as a new company unencumbered by previous debts.

In 2010, Baron Brian Mawhinney, a former personal mentor and later Football League chairman, asked during his time in that post, 'Talking about the moral strengths of the brand, are we all comfortable that, in financial and debt terms, we treat football clubs more favourably than we do our local communities and businesses, other taxpayers (to whom we have a civic responsibility) or St John Ambulance?' In the 2018/19 season eight of the 72 Football League clubs experienced winding-up petitions.

But their players were still paid while others such as HMRC, doctors and local tradesmen were not. In such situations clubs can then rename themselves and continue playing – it is the continuing power of the modern medieval lord.

Where does the medical team fit into the hierarchy of this contemporary Camelot? As a modern-day apothecary or physic? Clubs' medical departments are specialised occupational health (OH) units for which no equivalent existed centuries ago, but their clinicians still inhabit the peasants' stratum. Football is not alone in this; other sports have followed similar models.

By making UK Sport the distributor of Lottery funding a new hierarchical feudal system has been created. It has ensured Olympic successes but has come with strings attached. Athletes have access to equipment, facilities, coaching and clinical support but their freedom to train and compete at times and venues of their own choosing is curtailed.

The 'Olympic council of lords' is ruthless with underachieving units in battle. Basketball found itself with little funding following a poor 2012 Olympic campaign, despite being the second most popular participation sport among British youngsters.

Evidence that feudalism is alive and kicking in modern British sport is clear from a consideration of its key pillars: player contracts, athlete welfare and the ruthless search for young talent.

Contracts

> *'There is some ill a-brewing towards my rest.*
> *For I did dream of money-bags tonight.'*
>
> **William Shakespeare, *The Merchant of Venice***
> **(1596–1599)**

A frequent fly in the sports medicine ointment is a player's contract.

From 1893 English footballers were bound by the 'retain and transfer' system. Players' registrations were retained by clubs even after contracts were up. Theoretically, they could be bound to a club for life but if their team condescended they could move clubs in return for compensation – later known as a transfer fee. The system was designed to stop poaching by bigger clubs but severely capped wages.

English football emerged from the dark ages in 1961, when the maximum weekly wage of £20 was scrapped as a result of the pioneering work of PFA chairman Jimmy Hill. The 'retain and transfer' system was weakened by the introduction of transfer tribunals. Intimately involved in these seismic changes, with their ground-breaking stands, were two idols of my childhood, Johnny Haynes and George Eastham. Fulham made Haynes the first £100 per week footballer.

The next major milestone was the 1995 Bosman ruling. Jean-Marc Bosman took on the Belgian authorities and his club, Standard Liège, who blocked his move to French club Dunkerque after his contract ended. Liège demanded a transfer fee beyond the finances of Dunkerque. Bosman could not leave and was offered a new contract with a 75 per cent salary cut. The landmark ruling confirmed that players could leave a club within the EU without a transfer fee at the end of their contract. The judgement also outlawed quota impositions on the number of foreign EU players within a team.

The Bosman ruling and the advent of satellite TV funding caused player power and players' earning potential to skyrocket. 'All hell broke loose. Suddenly it was a free-for-all,' explained Sir Alex Ferguson. Elite footballers held out to the end of their contracts to secure lucrative moves elsewhere or to wring more money out of their existing clubs.

However, football reality outside the Premier League goldfish bowl is different and here few clubs can boast stable finances. Players' contracts are often short and there is a constant churning of players during transfer windows, accelerated by the inevitable manager merry-go-round. The

2020 COVID-19 pandemic has further exposed the gulf between the Premier League and Football League clubs.

Each August half the team are introduced anew to club supporters. Do fans consider the Theseus paradox, which, in their case, would ask whether their beloved club remained the same if all the important components parts (the players and coaching staff) had been replaced. Consider Trigger's 'new broom' in *Only Fools and Horses*. Trigger possessed a road-sweeping broom for 20 years. During that time, the broom needed 17 new heads and 14 new handles. This reminds us of most football teams and the flux of managers and players.

Players face uncertainty in their finances and in planning life for their families. Injuries occur at the most inopportune time. They want to maintain their form throughout a season, but the most important time is after Easter, because their clubs may be fighting for honours or to avoid relegation, or because they may need another contract. The late-season hamstring tear can be a killer; non-appearance at the season's sharp end may mean the player is ushered through the exit door.

Hard-won players' rights to make them masters of their own destinies have in some ways loosened the obligations of their clubs. Career-ending injuries at any time are distressing for all concerned. However, a less serious injury, occurring at a critical juncture in a player's career, can be just as significant in terms of sporting progression. Support mechanisms, including the PFA, are helpful in softening the psychological and financial blows for the player.

During clinics, I ask the player about their contract position – if it seems appropriate to injury management. Players will tolerate discomfort when a contract is up for renegotiation. A new manager or coach produces similar stoicism because each player wants the good opinion of their new boss. Once the new contract is signed, the player wants the injury resolved.

Bonuses triggered by appearances and results can be troublesome. One player delayed surgery for one further game because it would trigger such a windfall. I was at the game and aware of his internal joy as he ran on to the pitch. His elation was short-lived. The match was abandoned following a first-half monsoon and the game declared null and void for contract bonus activation. The player knew that he could not defer his surgical assignation further.

A new manager means a large player turnover; managers want to create a team in their own image. The next transfer window is the new coach's opportunity to make their mark. Money can be showered like confetti as a statement to the club's supporters. Sensible rules for a prudent transfer policy are thrown to the wind.

What does the new manager of an English League One or Two outfit do? Buys an ageing centre-forward who is sliding down the leagues and wants a few more pay days. Woe betide any sports doctor who might try to raise concerns based on an objective assessment of the player's medical records and recent appearance history. Even at the bottom of the football food chain it might seem sensible to peruse the evidence, examine some ankles and even spend £500 on MRIs of the dodgy knees that carry the career prospects of the player and his new manager with them.

Premier League outfits are diligent in new-player assessments. One could argue that smaller clubs with less cash to splash should be even more careful. They rarely are.

Many years ago I attended a game in which the opposition's senior striker looked as if he could lead the line for Brazil. He terrified the opposing centre-backs and scored a hatful. What did the opposition do? Sign him in the summer transfer window and break their salary ceiling in the process. I got to know the player well. He was an extremely likeable and intelligent athlete. Why did I know him well? His knees were shot. He was an honest pro who worked selflessly for the team but his legs could not do the work they previously had. In the first two seasons with his new team he scored less than a third of the goals he had scored in the previous two years with his old club.

In the January window, clubs seek to strengthen squads or offload players deemed surplus to requirements. Into the middle of this mayhem drops an injury to a player about to be transferred. The selling club wants the transfer fee but the club bidding for the player's services want him sprinting straight out of the blocks; they want someone to enliven their faltering promotion bid in the 12 to 14 games left. Will that ankle ligament injury from two weeks ago hold up? Situations like this can be a potential medical minefield and it is important to put the blinkers on, assess the problem in front of you and try to exclude all the 'extraneous noise' – even if it is the player's 'dream move'. A reasoned prognosis based on a sound medical history, examination and review of the scans is all that is required.

Let the parties involved interpret your opinion and come to their own decisions accordingly.

Flogging the prized stallion

'O, for a horse with wings!'

William Shakespeare, *Cymbeline* **(1608–1610)**

Biennially, much of the country dreams that its national football team will triumph in a Continental or global tournament. It has been half a century of hurt and counting … since 1966.

Players need to be ready, physically and mentally, for challenges such as these. Track and field athletes peak for isolated major championships; Ireland's rugby union team punches above its weight due to careful game management for its star performers. What does English football offer? Relentless soccer from August to May.

This issue comes into focus each January when the top teams must play their FA Cup 3rd round tie on the sloped mudbath pitch of a non-league side. In 2018, Pep Guardiola, the Manchester City manager, said the holiday schedules were 'killing' players. In the same period, Leicester City played four games in under nine days. Social media commentators varied in their opinions. Some were sympathetic while others compared the players' workloads with other sportsmen such as Roger Federer and told them to get on with it. Clubs still travel to the Far East or North America for meaningless pre-season tournaments. Of course players need to regain condition and fitness prior to the August kick-off but does that require 10,000 miles of flying and crossing many time zones?

BBC Radio 5 Live interviewed sports scientist Matt Dinnery, who revealed that December 2017 saw a 32 per cent increase in injuries compared to earlier months of the season. Injuries to muscles, tendons and ligaments rose by 45 per cent. Yet in the post-war years football had been played on Christmas Day and Boxing Day on unsuitable grounds where there was little understanding of sports science or the latest aids to recovery. Additionally, modern major clubs possess much larger squads who can be rotated. Northampton Town turned out on Christmas Day morning (unless it was the Sabbath) until 1956. Up to 17,000 locals were excused Brussels sprout-peeling duties to watch. Thousands more attended the next day for Boxing Day matches. Dinnery said the problem was that modern players were fitter and the game quicker. Is being too fit a risk factor for injury? Are the sports science and medical departments doing their work too well?

Football's problem is the media. Satellite television pays enormous sums to broadcast football matches – the average cost to BT for showing a Premier League game between 2016 and 2019 was £7.6m. Naturally, the paymasters want wall-to-wall football on their channels during the festive period. On top of this, clubs have huge overheads, mostly players' salaries, which commonly consume between 40 and 85 per cent of total income – sometimes even more. The threat of losing television income during the COVID-19 crisis highlighted Premiership clubs' dependence upon this revenue stream.

Premier League winter-shutdown talks were first held in 1995 but in England, unlike other European countries, the proposal was not popular. In 2018, researcher Jan Ekstrand demonstrated that between January and March players in European leagues without a winter break missed 64 per cent more training and playing days due to injury – an increased injury burden – and that increased injury rates continued into the start of the next season. Ekstrand had been producing this kind of evidence for a decade. In addition, in seasons ending with major championships, the last weeks of domestic campaigns are condensed. Is it any wonder that our international players go down like skittles or fail to perform? Within four months of the 2018 World Cup ending two-thirds of returning English league players were injured; the 'big six' Premier League clubs were, at some stage following the tournament, stripped of the services of 41 players in total.

In 2018 the English Premier League finally acted and announced an annual two-week winter break from February 2020 (taken by different clubs at different times) – 25 years after the proposal was first put. Sense had prevailed and not before time. But even before that, the 13-day 2019/20 festive fixtures brought about injuries to 74 Premier League players. It seems ironic that this break occurred immediately before the coronavirus lockdown.

What can be done to improve player welfare? Playing less is the obvious answer but could entail dropping a domestic cup competition (or excluding Premier League clubs from it) or reducing the Premier League size. However, most leading clubs already treat the early rounds of the League Cup with disdain and field weakened sides. Reducing Premier League club numbers, on the other hand, requires the approval of teams who might often face relegation. There is too much vested interest.

Fixture scheduling needs optimising and players need at least 72 hours to recover from matches. Better use of large squads would reduce an individual player's game-time, but even though peripheral squad members are paid a king's ransom there seems little appetite to blood some of them. Maximum playing minutes per season, imposed by league management, might help. It is used in other sports and would could make clubs make better use of all their players.

Other sports face a similar problem. Rugby union tries to balance the competing interests of clubs, country and fans while protecting players. In England, players are not centrally contracted and clubs and their owners have legitimate interests in how their employees are used. Inevitably, problems revolve around summer tours and the four-yearly World Cup, which has pride of place in the international calendar. Southern hemisphere tours build experience and teamwork but leave players with inadequate recovery time. Ireland, where unions have more influence, has a more enlightened approach to managing player exposure than nations such as England, where the clubs have greater power.

The quadrennial Lions tour seems the most endangered event. This trip is the highlight of a British player's career, the ultimate tour experience for fans and a financial bonanza for the host nation. But many of rugby's leading administrators see it as an outdated and unwanted trek. In amateur days, concerns didn't arise because returning Lions could rest for months before returning in late autumn to the club game. The 1881 Lions enjoyed a 35-game, 249-day tour, and while the 2021 South African tourists will play just eight games, they will stay no more than five weeks and have only one week after the domestic season ends to adjust to the high veldt. This comes after the COVID-19-related late finish to the 2019/20 season and the squeezed 2020/21 pre-season. This wonderful institution that is the Lions is threatened not by neglect but by strangulation and increased player risk.

The 2018 spat between the English rugby coach Eddie Jones and Bath Rugby owner Bruce Craig over injuries to Bath players while on England duty epitomised the feudalism of sport. Jones is an experienced general and knows his troops need to train as they will fight, but his approach risks casualties from friendly fire; it is the sporting equivalent of the Americans using live ammunition on their own troops as they practised for the 1944 D-Day landings on Slapton Sands in Devon. For Jones's platoon to reach their goals they would have to scramble over injured colleagues who did not make the final cavalry charge. Unfortunately, they came up just short in the 2019 World Cup Final.

However, injuries were sustained in training and for one player from Wasps a career was finished before it had hardly started, while five Bath players were hurt. Craig spoke of a 'duty of care' and Jones retorted by describing Craig as the 'Donald Trump' of rugby. It is a personality type that clearly intrigues Jones: a year later he described the entire US national team as '15 Donald Trumps'. The England–Bath quarrel continued over the alleged care of winger Joe Cockanasiga during the 2019 World Cup campaign. The 2019 RFU injury audit supported Craig's position: six times as many days were missed from training and playing under Jones than at any time under his predecessor Stuart Lancaster. Commentating on over-training, over-coaching and rest management, Ben Ryan, coach of the 2016 Fijian sevens Olympic gold medallists, said that 'thicker play books make thicker players'.

When Olympic-centred sports were amateur, the bond between governing bodies and athletes was looser and principally involved selection, coaching support and the arrangement of events. Centrally supplied funding altered this relationship. In 2016, Jess Varnish, the British cyclist, alleged bullying and sexism by UK Cycling staff and investigations found evidence of discriminatory language and 'a culture of fear'. During an employment tribunal Varnish claimed that the 'extreme control' exercised by British Cycling and UK Sport created an employee–employer relationship rather than one that made those bodies enabling service providers for freelance athletes. If the tribunal had upheld her allegations it would have had serious ramifications for the funding model for such sportspeople. However, in January 2019, Varnish lost her legal battle and lost the subsequent appeal in July 2020.

Whence the medic in all this?

> *'God and the doctor we alike adore*
> *But only when in danger, not before;*
> *The danger o'er, both are alike requited,*
> *God is forgotten and the Doctor slighted.'*
>
> **John Owen (1563–1622), epigrammatist**

In the not too distant past the local GP attended professional sports clubs weekly, went to home games and saw players in their own clinics. They worked with part-time trainers or physiotherapists. The GP's livelihood did not depend on a stipend, if there was one, from the club and the doctor retained their independence. Their work predominantly involved caring for other patients and their activities were influenced and monitored by local colleagues – not by the sporting organisation's culture. They had an encyclopaedic knowledge of the regional health scene and the strengths of local specialists. Many lower league football, rugby and cricket clubs have similar models of care to this day.

In the 1990s Premier League football began employing full-time doctors. Bringing in previously independent, and often volunteer, doctors required significant changes to those practitioners' relationships with organisations now acting as their employers.

Outside of sport, major companies have OH units concerned with the workplace. They deal with the prevention and management of injury and illness and have a responsibility to the employee and employer. They advise employees on their readiness, or otherwise, to return to employment, manage minor injuries and work in a multidisciplinary fashion with nurses and physiotherapists. Doctors within major sporting organisations have similar responsibilities. Their employers want success, and maintaining a healthy workforce is essential to that aim.

In industry, doctors might visit the factory floor to assess safety or provide first aid, but their primary place of work is usually separate and where records are securely held. Senior management do not make uninvited visits to clinical areas and it is rare for doctors to perform duties away from their base. Management is unlikely to bypass their own OH unit's views in acceding to employees' requests for fantastical health remedies.

Conversely, sports physicians work in many locations (often in less than optimal conditions) and are constantly busy. The injury risk in soccer has been estimated to be 1,000 times higher than high-risk industrial occupations. In major companies, the OH unit provides care to all employees – often hundreds or thousands. A major sporting organisation might employ similar numbers but its clinicians are tasked with caring for the chosen few – the athletes – unless there is an emergency.

Clinical line management in sport can create difficulties and there are increasing tendencies for non-medical staff to act as overseers. In sporting organisations with poor structure and governance, line management may not be clear at all. Elsewhere, the hierarchy may be obvious but strong-minded individuals, such as coaches and managers, may cut across clear lines of responsibility. I know of Football League doctors with no contract or idea of lines of responsibility and defined roles and responsibilities. Clashes between clinicians and coaching staff over player care have led to the dismissal of medics, such as Carniero.

Aligning clinical staff closely to coaching and performance personnel comes from a desire to improve communication. Dangers arise when clinicians become embroiled in the 'grey zone' – when their welfare responsibilities become blurred and attempts to enhance individual or team performance and pressures to reintroduce players before they have recovered can become overwhelming. The central question is, are doctors there to look after the employee's health or are they part of the machine geared towards winning?

A physio friend exemplified the dreadful dilemmas faced by some clinical staff. A new head coach had arrived where he was employed and explained how things would work in future. The physio was forbidden from discussing a diagnosis with an injured player – it was only to be divulged to the coach who would decide whether the player was fit to train or play. If the physio refused to do this he would be replaced. Inevitably a flare-up occurred. An injured player came to the edge of the pitch with a torn muscle and was led off for assessment and advice. The coach arrived in the treatment room and the player was told to return to the game. When the physio objected, he was grabbed by the collar, lifted off his feet and had his head banged against the wall. Relationships were never rebuilt and the physio left.

The coach was ordering the physio to break his professional code of conduct. To disrupt the clinician-patient relationship by withholding diagnoses and releasing confidential information to a third party without specific consent risks disciplinary action by higher parties than a bullying coach. I had telephone dealings with the same coach requesting medical details of an injured player. I refused to give them.

Coaches may decide to query injuries and an athlete's desire to play and train. In 2018, Stephen Ward, an Irish international footballer, reported that the assistant manager, Roy Keane, had burst into the medical room and asked the injured Harry Arter, 'When are you going to train, you f***ing pr**k? You're a f***ing pr**k, you're a c***, you don't even care, you don't wanna train.' I write this as a surgeon who was asked if I needed anger management training for using the word 'damn' in the operating theatre (I replied that I thought not). I had asked where my missing instruments were during a difficult surgical case on a child. I wonder how major non-sporting organisations would deal with the likes of Keane.

In 2019, former international footballer Micah Richards announced his retirement. At 31 his knees had had enough. He made a revealing statement: 'The ugly side of the game that many of us are exposed to has had a hugely detrimental effect on my mental health. I witnessed and was on the receiving end of racism on several occasions and have seen an incredible amount of bullying, manipulation and verbal abuse to an extent which, for many, leaves a dirt stain on this industry.' Such intimidatory behaviour would lead to instant dismissal in 99 per cent of places of employment. Why is it still permissible in certain sports?

In January 2020, Ole Gunnar Solskjaer reported that his Manchester United player, Paul Pogba, had been 'advised to have an operation by … his people'. Solskjaer backtracked later but it was clear the player had decided to seek an independent second opinion. This is not unreasonable, but the real question is whether the choice of a suitable specialist is likely to be better in the hands of the player's advisers than the club's medical department. I have witnessed the most bizarre medical choices of 'football people' and have received hair-raising accounts from colleagues of players diverted from experienced surgeons to less suitable alternatives on the whim of managers and agents.

Sports doctors need to risk-assess for medical conditions such as concussion and previously unsuspected underlying problems, including congenital heart problems. They might need to review training schedules that could identify reinjury risks for a player. If reporting structures for the doctor lead straight to the manager there is potential for conflict.

A footballer re-attended my clinic 18 months after a serious injury and surgery. He had been progressing on schedule but in his playing absence a new manager had arrived and had told the player he had no future at the club. The manager tried to accelerate rehabilitation to facilitate a transfer. This led to depression, failure to achieve recovery goals, significant weight gain by the player and his ultimate dismissal. He applied for compensation for medical retirement. With no clear insurmountable physical impediment, a more considered attitude towards the player would probably have salvaged his career.

Concerns over these strains has been the subject of investigation, innovation and comment in recent times. In 2017, the ex-Manchester United doctor Michael Stone reported that it was not unusual for the club doctor to be appointed by the football manager. Stone urged the club to take responsibility for the appointment, contracting and appraisal of medical staff. If the manager plays a central role in the hiring and firing of medical staff there is a risk that the welfare aspects of medics' jobs will be compromised. I was asked to sign a 'contract' as a voluntary doctor for a sports team and insisted that the wording reflect that I was directly responsible to the chief executive.

Alternatively, clinicians could be appointed independently by the overarching sporting authorities, such as the FA, RFU or ECB. However, the introduction of non-aligned doctors in rugby to assess head injuries to avoid 'gaming' by coaching staff has not been an unqualified success. This subject is discussed in a later chapter.

In 2017, Baroness Tanni Grey-Thompson chaired an independent review into athletes' welfare. At that time two controversies were prominent in people's minds: the 'jiffy bag' mystery involving Dr Richard Freeman, British Cycling and Sir Bradley Wiggins; and Mo Farah's undocumented intravenous infusion of L-carnitine by Dr Rob Chakraverty. The review concluded that rules should be established to separate a team's medical staff and coaches. 'Consideration should be given to a separation within a performance team of the medical and safeguarding staff and place them under the assurance regime of the duty of care guardian, as opposed to performance coaches,' it said, adding, 'This would provide a clear line of demarcation and separation of potentially conflicting advice.'

The message was an admirable and compelling position statement but I am concerned about its implementation in modern professional sport. An isolated physio on the team bus to Carlisle would find it hard to establish physical or professional distance between themselves and the manager sitting in the row ahead.

Fifty years ago it was much simpler. The personnel involved were tiny in number and roles and responsibilities were clearer. The local GP, doubling up as club doctor, sat squarely within the welfare circle, alongside others such as the club chaplain. Grey-Thompson has argued for a return to this position.

The performance circle was also smaller in the past and occupied only by the manager and trainer. This area has widened enormously, with an army of coaches, performance directors and, more latterly, S&C staff now involved. The latter are usually embedded within an expanded sports medicine and science department. This can create mixed priorities if the performance circle threatens to overwhelm its welfare counterpart and at the very least overlap and create the 'grey zone' previously referred to. Perhaps the real issue is the merging of medicine and sports science into one department – it blurs goals.

Where do other key staff fit – physiotherapists, nutritionists, psychologists and psychiatrists? Physiotherapists are primarily responsible for recovering injured players. However, their close, daily proximity to the performance team can distort decision-making. Nutritionists help players recover from games and training, and prescribe diets and supplements to support strengthening programmes. They have both welfare and performance-enhancing roles. Mental welfare in sport has been highlighted in recent times; when a psychologist or psychiatrist counsels athletes on issues such as substance abuse, anxiety and depression they are performing a welfare role. When they develop strategies to reinforce concentration and confidence during activity, they move into performance-optimisation territory.

Orthopaedic surgeons should not be drawn into this tangled web. Many injuries have surgical and non-surgical options – for example, several months of rest and physiotherapy might be advised for non-elite athletes and have an expectation of injury resolution. Many protocols encourage a period of six months of conservative treatment. If problems continue, surgery can be embarked upon knowing that all other avenues have been exhausted. Indeed, we are failing in our duty of care if we do not inform patients of all the 'rungs' on the injury-management ladder. Such an approach may be alien to professional athletes and coaching staff. Their priority is a return to sport – as soon as possible – and the scalpel is reached for earlier, while acknowledging that any form of surgery carries risk to the patient. By applying different strategies to the elite athlete, surgeons may be stumbling into the grey mist.

There are two key elements that should ensure proper clinical governance within a sporting organisation: the performance of its board, and the bond and common ethical standpoint of the members of the medical department.

The board of a sporting organisation, like any industrial or commercial entity, has ultimate responsibility for the health and safety of its employees. It should demonstrate knowledge and the willingness to implement safe systems within its establishment. It should be prepared to listen and act upon concerns expressed by employees, including medical department members. A designated board member with responsibility for liaising with the medical lead can facilitate this process. A clear demonstration of these principles sets the tone for the entire club or sport.

Many professionals contribute to sports medical departments. Most are highly qualified practitioners aware of the conventions of their calling, including their primary responsibility to their patient. Doctors no longer recite the ancient Hippocratic Oath, but its ethical basis remains central to our work. Ideas about patient confidentiality, beneficence and non-maleficence are key components of this. The latter two involve balancing benefits of treatment against risks and costs, and avoiding causing harm.

In my experience, small, tight medical units find it easier to maintain uniformly agreed high standards and teamwork. Larger expanded departments containing people from multiple allied health professions must work harder to gel and operate by common governance standards. Rapid staff turnover and the importation of members unused to national guidelines potentially increase difficulties. The larger the department, the more likely it is to leak in matters such as patient confidentiality.

The needs of the employer and employee must be considered. Employee consent must always be gained before discussing medical matters with employers. The latter has a right to know if an employee is unfit to perform their specific job, but not an automatic right to access confidential information. I am aware of one coach who was dismissed for removing confidential medical records without consent.

In 2019, the United States Anti-Doping Agency (USADA) published its findings on the Nike Oregon Project and banned coach Alberto Salazar and his personal physician, Dr Jeffrey Brown, for four years. USADA took four years to report and highlighted the problems arising when a doctor and trainer form an unholy alliance. Brown was accused of delaying the release of records. 'Salazar and Dr Brown communicated repeatedly about the athletes' medical conditions, exchanging information without any apparent authorisation by the athletes,' the report said, adding, 'Salazar and Dr Brown shared information with the aim of improving the athletes' performance via medical intervention.' It continued, 'Mr Salazar and Dr Brown demonstrated that winning was more important than the health and well-being of the athletes they were sworn to.' Salazar had no medical training but was accused of giving his athletes prescription drugs. He denies wrongdoing and has appealed to CAS. If the findings are upheld Salazar and Brown will have been shown to have lost their moral compasses.

Good communication does need to be maintained between coaching and medical staff, however, and if confidentiality concerns are resolved, internal interactions are beneficial. Ekstrand studied this (in addition to injury prevalence in winter) and reported that in football clubs with poor dialogue between managers and medical teams, player availability was 6 to 7 per cent lower and the injury burden 50 per cent greater compared to better-interacting organisations. He said that one newly appointed manager told the team doctor, 'I don't want direct contact with you. Talk to my assistant.'

Expensively resourced and staffed elite sporting medical departments can appear as lavish tropical islands separated from the surrounding normal health community in which they are located geographically. Healthcare provision provided by sporting organisations is not subject to the scrutiny of the Care Quality Commission (CQC), which oversees standards in all other clinics and hospitals in the country. Instead, it falls to the Health and Safety Executive (HSE).

High-profile lawsuits and unseen work by groups of committed senior sports physicians are bringing change. Sport will never be a risk-free occupation but doctors in sport have an obligation to identify and minimise danger and support injured and ill athletes. Continuous dialogue with coaching staff relating to roles and responsibilities and overt support at boardroom level are vital elements.

Chapter 16

CHASING THE EGG

*'Egg Chaser: someone who plays rugby – usually
what people who play football call them.'*

The Urban Dictionary

THE 1995 Rugby World Cup in South Africa preceded the end of 'shamateurism' at the highest echelons. Within a year, the northern hemisphere game had embarked on a fully professional sport for its elite.

The black, green and gold

Northampton Saints colours

Six months later I returned to Northampton after 23 years away. One of my first ports of call was Franklin's Gardens – home of the Saints. The ground was part of my youth and is where two of my front teeth lie buried in the pitch having been 'removed' during a 1977 junior club final.

The rickety wooden stand, the pond behind the goalposts, where conversions invariably landed and a man with a boat fished out the ball, were familiar. At the other end was the Sturtridge pavilion, named after an ex-club captain and local gynaecologist. It was a reminder of days when the two careers could be successfully combined. The East Midlands had played the Barbarians at Franklin's Gardens on a Thursday afternoon each March, and every local schoolboy had attended to follow their heroes.

Rugby success was engrained in my school's psyche and schoolboy international honours were expected annually. As we filed into morning assembly we passed beneath the honours boards of ex-pupils such as

Bryan West and Bob (R.B.) Taylor – both of England and the 1968 British Lions. The latter become RFU president in 2007. More recent luminaries include Steve Thompson (2003 Rugby World Cup winner) and Courtney Lawes.

I captained the town's schoolboys and represented the county. During undergraduate life I ventured to the Gardens but accepted that I was somewhat short (literally) of 'what was needed'. My ability to cover 100 yards in ten seconds couldn't offset the fact that my 5ft 8in and 9st-something frame crumbled like a twiglet when tackled. Memories of training nights include piggy-backing the sizeable frame of England prop Gary Pearce in shuttle runs. It scarred me for life. I returned to my junior club, Old Northamptonians, and concentrated on my surgical career. But one Monday morning I appeared in theatre with a black eye and stud imprints on my torso. My boss took one look at me and said it was time to decide – 'sport or scalpel'.

Can I be of assistance?

At the end of a game in January1996 I introduced myself to the Saints coaching and clinical team. The latter comprised a local GP and physiotherapist Phil Pask. My offer of help was, surprisingly, welcomed.

My retired surgical predecessors at Northampton Hospital had not been involved. One was a season ticket holder and saw the game as a source of relaxation away from work. Perfectly reasonable. Another met an enormous forward in a clinic and asked what he did. 'The Lighthouse' replied that he was a rugby player (not revealing that he was an established international). The surgeon retorted, 'No, what do you really do?'

The Saints started 1995/96 in Division Two following relegation. However, they retained the likes of Tim Rodber, Martin Bayfield, Matt Dawson, Nick Beal, Budge Pountney and Paul Grayson, all of whom would form the nucleus of later great sides. The mercurial star Gregor Townsend was added but most importantly the Saints appointed the brilliant coach Ian McGeechan. The club were unbeaten that season and were promoted.

The following campaign was the first fully professional season in England. Medical teams struggled to become organised – we were ill-equipped in terms of personnel and equipment to embrace the change and struggled to parallel off-pitch treatment with the improved on-pitch standards.

In early 1997 the medical teams of England's elite clubs met and the experienced Bath team doctor commented, 'Until last season, I was the only professional in an amateur sport. Now I feel as though I am the only amateur in a professional sport.'

Prior to professionalism, players joined long NHS queues; forget flying off to America for a medical opinion. The Saints had used a therapist but there had been little liaison between injured players and the club – players would let the club know when they were available for selection once the hamstring had mended. More serious injuries might warrant a lift to casualty. After that, it was a case of 'see you when your plaster is off'.

Phil Pask multitasked as the Saints' physiotherapist, rehabilitation specialist and S&C coach, while also doing his daytime job in his physiotherapy practice. Phil had played for the team and during his career the side had fielded more qualified physiotherapists than there were on the touchline. One of these touchline 'physios' worked as a security guard during the week and had learnt his basic 'clinical skills' from weekend courses. Phil graduated to England duties in 1997.

I provided surgical and medical back-up for all home and many away games and received excellent support from colleagues Nick Birch and David Stock. Our time and expertise were given for free and we still paid for a season ticket to gain entry to the ground. My honorary status preserved my independence and made it easier for the club to seek alternative opinions if they wished. My modus operandi was straightforward: those injuries I felt well-qualified to deal with I would. Alternatively, I would advise the player which clinician's opinion to seek. Such referral pathways were not known, let alone established, at the advent of professional rugby.

Over the ensuing years I undertook surgery on shoulders, elbows, wrists, hands, knees, ankles and feet – approximately 80 operations on the first-team squad alone. Head injuries were assessed and there were numerous trips to casualty with injured home and opposition players, mostly using my car. Other injuries included traumatised testicles, disfigured dentition, and bleeding eyes and ears. All needed first aid and onward referral.

Pitchside clinicians see a slightly different game to the paying public. Your first concern is player welfare. You are aware of players carrying injuries into the game and watch for early signs of hamstring tightening or shoulder stiffening. You have one eye on the action that has just taken place. Who hasn't got up or is looking sluggish? You also watch those players with fresh injuries. You scan the field looking for signs that they are not as fit as they may think they are. Sometimes you miss the key points of the game and even lose track of the score.

Incidentally, Eddie Jones's England has evolved the mantra of 'reload and reform', which looks at how quickly players rise from the breakdown; how rapidly they take position to defend or attack is measured in seconds. If a player fails these targets through injury or fatigue, their game impact is reduced.

Ian McGeechan had a rugby brain few could match for innovation and tactical appreciation yet was implacably polite and mildly spoken. From 1996 to 1999 I would sit as close as possible to 'Geech' on the Saints team bench during matches and tune into his running commentary on the game. It was a masterclass in interpretive and tactical appreciation and needless to say I just listened. It was ironic that it was only after McGeechan's departure that the club achieved its single greatest success – winning the 2000 Heineken Cup by defeating Munster 9-8 at Twickenham. John Steele, the club's former fly-half, had taken over coaching duties.

Both McGeechan and Steele understood the entire workings of the club, as did Steele's successor Wayne Smith, a future All Blacks coach. All three knew everybody's roles and responsibilities and not a Christmas would go by without a handwritten note from them thanking you for your time and commitment. These were treasured letters that meant more than any financial reimbursement.

The season 1999/2000 was truly memorable, with the Saints fighting for honours on several fronts and trying to lose their tag as serial bridesmaids. We won all the cup cliffhangers, due in no small measure to the accuracy of Paul Grayson's kicking. The five fixtures leading to the Heineken and Tetley Bitter cup finals were won by an aggregate of only 24 points. Then we had two Twickenham finals in two weeks with a league game at Newcastle in between.

The effort had been attritional. Matt Dawson dislocated his shoulder in the Heineken Cup semi-final against Llanelli. It required manipulation under the stands at Reading's Madejski Stadium. We lost to Wasps in the Tetley Bitter Cup Final so then had to ensure we did not finish such a season of derring-do empty-handed. Our patched-up team hung on in the Heineken Cup Final at Twickenham with three more penalties from Grayson.

It seemed the whole town celebrated back at Franklin's Gardens later that night. An ultimately triumphant season was over but not without its toll – several of the squad needed surgery in the weeks following Twickenham.

My seasons with Northampton Saints enabled me to forge strong ties with many of the players, which survived beyond those players' rugby retirement. Experiencing the ups of club and individual successes and the downs of injuries bonded the squad and medical attendees. The Saints captain, Pat Lam, subsequently agreed to open our local summer village fete and brought along the European Cup for the kids to be pictured with.

Another of those players, Budge Pountney, captained his club and country, Scotland. We shared many good times. Once, he was seconded to Sunday morning sprint practice at the local athletics track to sharpen his speed alongside the promising young runners, including my teenage daughter. He retired from international rugby in 2003 after winning 31 caps, concerned at what he perceived to be less than optimal support for the players. As a result, he missed the 2003 World Cup, instead playing in a pre-season club match and dislocating his ankle, which led to his retirement from playing. Pountney coached the Saints and asked me to be the patron of his benefit year, 2004/05. It was something I accepted with pride. I reprised the role by being on Ben Foden's testimonial committee in 2018.

Northampton Saints 1st XV squad usually numbered no more than 30. I got to know their ailments well. At times, I felt I could recognise an individual's knee in the dark, from its characteristic mobility, size and pathology. I also got to know the eccentricities of individuals. For example, Matt Dawson had a needle phobia and I wrote in his testimonial brochure of one escapade when he was scheduled for knee surgery. My anaesthetist approached Matt with a large needle and broad Scottish brogue. 'Daws' took fright and ran out of the anaesthetic room with his theatre gown flapping open behind. He refused to come back.

'The party's over, it's time to call it a day!'

Nat King Cole, 'The Party's Over' (1956)

Saturday, 21 June 1997 was a pivotal day in my rugby life. As recalled in Chapter 3 it was the day I hung up my boots just before the British Lions played the Springboks in the first Test at Newlands, Cape Town.

Ian McGeechan was coaching the Lions and five Saints were on the tour – Matt Dawson, Tim Rodber, Nick Beal, Paul Grayson and Gregor Townsend. This magical tour capped the end of the first full season of the professional era.

Our 'Saintly Lions' carried the scars of the domestic season into the matches. One player relied on tackling virtually one-handed because of a shoulder/neck injury at the start of the tour, and Paul Grayson sadly lasted only one match, against Border, before being sent home with a thigh problem.

Matt Dawson's appearance in the first Test was particularly poignant for me. He had sustained a significant knee injury earlier that year which I thought would bar his selection. His determination and Phil Pask's excellent rehabilitation programme was pivotal to getting him on the plane. He was not first choice at scrum-half before the tour but Rob Howley's shoulder injury gave Matt his chance and he took it with both hands. Pask went on to be a Lions physiotherapist four times from 2005 to 2017.

The Lions forged a wonderful victory in that match. The highlight was Dawson's outrageous dummy to the Boks captain Gary Teichmann, before diving over at the corner close to where I was sitting. It was triumphant end to a difficult few months for him.

After the game I went to Pretoria with my friend Daan du Plessis, who followed his own international rugby career by becoming a master knee surgeon, spending many years rebuilding Springbok joints. We spent the next week operating on knees punctuated by a midweek trip to Bloemfontein to watch the Lions take on Orange Free State. It was the match in which Will Greenwood's terrible head injury finished his tour.

At Durban, in the pivotal second Test, Jeremy Guscott's coolly taken drop goal secured the series for the British Isles. The champions crowned, I decided that I had outstayed my host's hospitality and headed for the airport.

Your country calls

The modern England rugby medical set-up is extensive and multilayered but was not always so. Home matches saw an honorary orthopaedic surgeon complementing the physiotherapist and team doctor. My colleague Nigel Henderson, the excellent Aylesbury spinal surgeon, undertook the role for many years. Occasionally I filled in when he was unavailable. Before my first game Nigel told me that usually my duties would mean no more than being present and watching from the stands. Perfect. An enjoyable afternoon watching from one of the best seats in the house.

That game took place on 4 April 1998 and England comfortably beat Ireland 35-17. An 18-year-old called Jonny Wilkinson made his debut as a right-wing substitute. In the second half, two Irish backs clashed heads and collapsed like a sack of potatoes in the middle of the pitch, a collision described as a 'sickening crunch' and 'appalling clash' by the media. The Irish doctor was out of the traps fast but there was only one of him and two of the Emerald Isle's finest were prostrate on the sward. I leapt out of my seat and on to the pitch towards the stricken but unattended player. I passed the English half-backs, the Northampton duo of Dawson and Grayson. They both looked at me quizzically and asked what I was 'doing on the pitch'. I replied, 'Looking after you bu***rs!' I thought that this would be, in all probability, the only occasion that I would find myself in the full gaze of the crowd at headquarters and momentarily took a 360° panoramic view.

The player was awake but clearly disorientated. An Irish voice said, 'Come on *****. Get up and get on with the game!' I replied, 'This player has sustained a head injury. There are 80,000 people watching here and countless millions on television. We are doing this by the book.' The player was still groggy in the medical room and unable to pass the return-to-play protocols. His club side were due to play Northampton at Franklin's Gardens the next Saturday. My concussion advice included rest and not playing that game.

Being England's honorary matchday surgeon was indeed honorary. Your seat was allocated behind the coaching staff in the West Stand but you had to walk to the ground. There was no car park pass. At the game's end, I was given a cup of tea ticket as a thank you for coming. Of course, it was an enormous honour to fulfil that role.

'I guess that's why they call it the blues?'

Elton John, 'I Guess That's Why They Call It The Blues' (1983)

Oxford and Cambridge travel to Twickenham for their annual rugby match in early December.

In the late 1990s the nearby West Middlesex Hospital used the occasion for a morning conference on managing rugby injuries and invited me to lecture on my medical experiences in the early seasons of professional rugby. After lunch I was walking to the ground when an old medical friend rang and asked if I would pass a breathalyser test and was I willing to take on pitchside duties. The appointed game doctor had been 'detained in hospitality'. Like other Twickenham encounters of my experience, the game was not without incident with lacerations and dislocated digits to be dealt with.

Men at work

'Down Under'

Men at Work, 'Down Under' (1983).

On 22 November 2003 England beat Australia in the World Cup Final in Sydney.

Leading up to the tournament it had felt that England's coach, Clive Woodward, was turning a very special blend of individuals into a world-beating team. The side's wonderful performance in Ireland in March 2003 whetted our appetites, and was followed by an astonishing victory in Wellington against the All Blacks, which raised expectations that the Australian World Cup campaign would be different – one not to be missed. I packed my bags.

The bars in Sydney's Darling Harbour were packed with England supporters in the days before the final. The English team stayed in Manly at the Pacific Hotel – where I had stayed on a previous visit to Sydney. Away from training, the players shopped in town and those not involved in the final could be found in the local hostelries enjoying banter with the fans. As in South Africa in 1997, team hotel security was minimal and you could walk up to reception and ask them to phone a guest's room number. How times have changed since then.

Northampton Saints had Matt Dawson, Paul Grayson, Steve Thompson and Ben Cohen in the squad. The final was a magical night with Wilkinson's extra-time drop goal sending England fans into raptures. The sporting reception from the Australians at the end of the game was fulsome and memorable.

Mod cons

England's base at Pennyhill in Surrey was chosen by Clive Woodward. It is a rugby heaven and lacks nothing in facilities for a team in training.

I visited in March 2013 and was fascinated by the scientific analysis available to back up the coaching expertise on the paddock. Players' physiological parameters were monitored as they trained. Injured players had excellent rehabilitation facilities and the hotel had plenty to offer during recovery time. I found Stuart Lancaster's team welcoming, open and inclusive. It was a privilege to sit in the team room as the senior coach outlined the plans for the week ahead.

A place for all?

Rugby union's traditional boast was that, whatever your size or shape, there was always a position on the field for you. Modern elite rugby is nowhere near as inclusive. Power is king. The ramifications for the naturally smaller player are clear: beef up or be blown away.

A life-size cardboard cut-out of the late Springbok Joost van der Westhuizen clutching a large bottle of creatine supplements greeted my arrival to a Pretoria gym in 1997. The potential long-term complications from the use of these tablets was still unknown. Supplements and drug abuse were commonplace in young South African rugby players – one in 11 male teenage players were later found to have doped with anabolic steroids.

In 2018, 5 per cent of teenagers playing in the South African annual schools' rugby tournament (Craven Week) tested positive for anabolic steroids. Coaches and parents were implicated, even to the extent of injecting their own offspring. The actual numbers were probably much higher – the smart ones knew when to stop taking the drugs pre-tournament.

Young players can bulk up by tapping into improved sports science knowledge. Others take short cuts. In the 2013/14 season three under-18 British junior players tested positive for testosterone. The case of one, Sam Chalmers, should be a warning to all. Sam was a fly-half like his father, Craig, who played for Scotland and the Lions. In 2013, Sam was advised he needed to bulk up to become a professional rugby player. He took nutritional supplements for just five days. That was enough. He tested positive for unsuspected illegal elements in the tablets and was banned for two years. He campaigned to warn other young players of the dangers. Was he too small? Pre-supplements, Sam was already too big for his father's 1989 British Lions blazer.

In 2018 half of all athletes serving UK drug bans came from just two sports – rugby union and rugby league. The RFU's 2018 annual anti-doping report revealed that 95 per cent of school players had used sports supplements.

Smaller players on the pitch often look as though they have been blown up by a bicycle pump, yet in the 1960s England fielded players struggling to get over 10st. Willie John McBride is perhaps the greatest Lion of all, appearing in five tours between 1962 and 1974. He was a second row forward but only 6ft 3½in in his rugby socks.

I have had the pleasure of spending skiing holidays with Barry Llewelyn, the ex-Wales prop-forward. In October 1972 Barry played for Llanelli when they defeated the All Blacks. The game was immortalised by the Max Boyce poem '9-3' – it was 'The day the pubs ran dry'. The All Blacks claimed that a joint XV from the two sides would contain only one Scarlet – our Barry. He refused 1971 and 1974 Lions invitations because of family and work commitments but a programme of the 1972 Wales–France international makes interesting reading. Llewelyn, at 16st 4lbs, was the second-heaviest Welsh player.

The average height of the Welsh pack was 6ft 1in and the team's legendary back row of Dai Morris, Merv ('The Swerve') Davies and John Taylor weighed on average 13st 13lbs. In the 60 years from 1955 to 2015 the average British international player has increased his bulk by 24 per cent.

Llewelyn was a PE teacher and a naturally fit and strong man. Llanelli trained two evenings a week and Llewelyn claimed never to have lifted a weight in his life. Wales would meet on the Thursday before an international – obeying International Rugby Board (IRB) regulations – and work on set moves, scrums and line-outs. Friday would be for relaxation – often including golf – before the big event on Saturday afternoon. They appointed their first national coach only in 1968.

Those legends of my youth seemed to play rugby from a different planet. The players sought to create half-gaps and beat defences with sidesteps, mis-moves, scissor calls and off-loads rather than taking the ball into contact. Law interpretation at the time made ball-retention much more of a lottery in the tackle area. Collisions did not reach the impact level achieved by today's behemoths. Injuries happened but not on the scale of today.

Players were mostly taken by the legs rather than the range of tackling heights witnessed in recent years.

'I played ten injury-free years between the ages of 12 and 22. Then, suddenly, it seemed like I was allergic to the twentieth century.'

Nigel Melville, England scrum-half and captain who spent much of the 1980s injured. Director of professional rugby at the RFU since 2016

Rugby authorities were slow to keep up with developments within the game, and then real tragedy struck. In 2018 four young French players died from rugby injuries in eight months, finally waking the authorities from their torpor. The following year World Rugby (formerly the IRB) met in Paris and convened medics, legal eagles, player representatives and officials. Eight proposals were made to improve player welfare.

When had it gone wrong? It could be argued that the game turning professional in 1996 was the worst thing that could have happened in terms of player welfare. Rugby always had the potential for physical harm but, when training fitted around full-time jobs and was confined to a couple of evenings a week and a weekend game, the emergence of leviathans was kept in check. In parallel with the growth in size of the general population, rugby took the brakes off and allowed its elite to train full-time. Coupled with the advances in sports science and nutrition, the end result was inevitable: monsters. Once one coach had unveiled a mobile one-man wrecking ball, every other coach wanted 15 of them.

Since 1995, grounds and facilities have improved out of all recognition. The game is faster and has improved as a spectacle. The players have received reasonable remuneration from the revenues earned by rugby organisations. However, in terms of injuries and long-term disabilities to the participants, professionalism has not been an unqualified success.

The 2005 RFU audit was published at the end of the first decade of professionalism. It stated that from 1991 to 2003 the average size of English international forwards increased by 21 per cent and backs by 20.5 per cent. In 2003, Premier League clubs had on average 24 per cent of their players requiring daily treatment for injuries at any one time. Each player was likely to sustain a significant injury once in every eight games and spend 19 per cent of the calendar year injured.

In the mid-2000s I supervised PhD research on comparative injuries in various professional sports. The student spent several seasons attending weekly Northampton Saints, Northampton Town FC and Northamptonshire cricket games. The disproportionate scale of injuries sustained by the rugby team shocked us all, even those engaged in professional sport for many years.

The pattern and intensity of rugby has changed out of all recognition at the elite end of the sport since professionalism. The following World Cup statistics provide some clues.

In 1991 Britain and Ireland hosted the second Rugby World Cup. It was a great success. All seemed well with the world until the Aussies beat England in the final and as a Twickenham spectator that day I was devastated. The paying punters saw an average of just 24 minutes 48 seconds playing time per game in 1991. When the World Cup returned to England in 2015, that figure had increased to 34 minutes 55 seconds – over 40 per cent more action.

The game had become more dynamic. Between 1995 and 2015 the world cups witnessed an increase in passes by 40 per cent and rucks and mauls by 90 per cent. Conversely, the number of kicks fell by 34 per cent, scrums by 43 per cent and line-outs by 30 per cent. In 1995 the number of scrums was equal to the number of rucks. By 2015 the scrum-to-ruck ratio was 1:14.

Those guaranteed breathers during endlessly reset scrums were disappearing – even prop forwards began to resemble perpetual-motion machines. Translating this increased activity into domestic professional rugby gives players a 40 per cent greater chance of injury compared to the amateur era. The players are conditioned to absorb the bigger hits – and there are a lot of them. A researcher from New Zealand recorded more than 3,000 impacts in one 2013 club game.

Improved muscular development helps players resist increased forces when they're being tackled. But this extra strength also makes them more effective missiles when they become the tackler. Forces taken on a shoulder during a tackle have been calculated to be one-fifth of a tonne.

The decision in 2019 to limit English-based professional rugby players to no more than 30 games annually came not a moment too soon.

Practice makes perfect patients

In rugby, between 89 and 95 per cent of the time is spent preparing rather than playing. Match injury rates are 27 times higher than those of training, but because of the time spent, training accounts for nearly a quarter of the damage. Training intensity and load have come under scrutiny in recent times, with World Rugby trying to encourage reduced amounts of training time.

Returning from injury, playing and training with injuries, older players, moving up to a new level of play, and rapid load increases are the main injury risk areas for players. The last is a concept familiar to all sports.

Stepping up to the next rugby tier brings a player into contact (literally) with faster, bigger, stronger and more skilful opponents and training intensity must be commensurate with the challenge. This issue has come into sharp focus at England training camps under Eddie Jones because 19 players were injured during England training in 2017/18. The RFU's Premiership injury audit recorded 2.9 injuries/1,000 hours. Best estimates for England training are rates two and a half times higher. Something must give – hopefully not another scrum-half's stretched sinews.

The Pr(a)etorian Guard

I hoped that attitudes might be changed after the 2009 second Lions Test against the Springboks in Pretoria, which journalist Stuart Barnes rated as the greatest rugby game he had ever seen.

At the team hotel on the morning of the game I had caught up with the medical team and afterwards had the surreal experience of standing in the hotel car park watching the coaches putting the team through final drills, including line-out work. Hotel guests passed nonchalantly by and cars manoeuvred around the periphery of the action.

The game was brutal. Loftus Versfeld Stadium seemed bathed in the red of the visiting fans' shirts and the on-field action. I had a ringside seat alongside Daan du Plessis, who had led his side to many great victories on that ground.

In the early minutes, on the touchline right in front of us, the Springbok Schalk Burger's fingers contacted a Lion's eyes. It seemed a clear red card to all except the referee and the poor recipient rubbing his smarting sense organs. While the injured were removed to the changing room in a steady sequence, the Lions appeared to be heading for a famous victory that would square the series at 1-1. However, the Boks hit two late penalties to claim victory, and the series, by 28-25.

Five Lions players out of a squad of 22 were detained in hospital afterwards. Was it right to call the contest sport? As the dust settled on the high veldt, Dr James Robson, the Lions doctor (on six consecutive tours from 1993 to 2013) gave his views. 'The balance is wrong between power and skill. We are reaching a level where the players have got too big for their skill levels. [They are] too muscle-bound and too bulky.'

Lessons learnt?

Have lessons been learnt since 2009?

'Everywhere I look I see players artificially inflated in size, whose additional bulk doesn't appear to fit their body shape ... I see "impact" players bred to come off the bench and wreak physical havoc ... I see a game that has moved away from aerobic fitness to celebrate unadulterated power ... Even the so-called little men are monsters ... The future looks bleak.' These were the words, six years later, of Paul Ackford, an ex-England and British Lions forward and former Metropolitan Police Inspector.

In 2018, Wales and Lions captain Sam Warburton retired at 29 having suffered 20 major injuries. 'My knees were so sore – my body just couldn't cope any more,' he said. Two great ex-scrum-halves expressed concern. Gareth Edwards hoped the news of Warburton's retirement would be the final push rugby needed for a major revision of its laws, while Agustin Pichot, World Rugby vice-chairman, warned, 'The red flags are there.' Warburton subsequently issued mixed messages. Within six months of his retirement he was encouraging England to double-team at tackles and smash mauls and contact areas because 'at its heart [rugby is] a collision sport'.

In October 2017 Harlequins had 25 of their players unfit for their game against Northampton Saints. Harlequins' player and qualified doctor, Jamie Roberts, described the treatment room as a morgue. The same month, Welsh side Gwent Dragons had 29 players hors de combat. In early 2018 *Sunday Times* journalist Stephen Jones reported that Premiership Rugby had asked clubs not to divulge the number of injured players.

Calls for change were becoming louder. Professor John Fairclough, an eminent Welsh orthopaedic surgeon, said, 'Rugby is no longer the sport it once was.' Like Ackford, he had concerns over the damage caused by fresh replacements. 'Substitutes should be for injury not for impact.'

At the same time, Warburton appeared to have reconsidered, warning in his 2019 autobiography, 'If something isn't done soon, then a professional player will die in front of the TV cameras and only then will people throw up their hands and demand that steps must be taken.'

The RFU injury audit for 2017/18 revealed that recovery from the average match injury took 37 days compared to 23 days 12 years earlier. 'Match burden' – the number of days a side loses players to injury after each game (calculated by multiplying individual injuries by the recovery time for each) – doubled between the 2005/06 and 2017/18 seasons, from 32 days to a shocking 66 days. What other sport would tolerate two months of player downtime after every game?

Edwards, Ackford, Pichot, Robson and Fairclough are not a group of prosaic health and safety experts. They are rugby men down to their bootstraps. The clamour to improve safety and curb the celebration of size and power over skill has been there for years. Only now are authorities beginning to take decisive action.

In the future, 2018 may be viewed as a watershed year. A Canadian, a South African and a Samoan also died that year in addition to the four Frenchmen. Head injuries, broken necks and heart attacks were to blame. *L'Equipe* commented, 'Rugby kills because it believes preparation protected everything, that the players' bodies could take more tackles, could take harder, higher tackles often made by two defenders simultaneously.'

On a wing and a prayer?
Rugby has always had a special respect for hard-tackling men.

Brian Lima, the Samoan centre from 1990 to 2007 was named 'The Chiropractor' for rearranging opponents' articulations with the force of his tackles. In 1997 he managed to knock himself out while tackling. The game's hard men are still celebrated – the likes of Sébastien 'The Caveman' Chabal of Sale Sharks and France, and Jacques Burger, the fêted Saracens and Namibian hitman.

Even doctors can dish it out and receive it. I recall two bone-shuddering tackles in my youth, both involving J.P.R. Williams. The first was the thundering tackle of St Mary's Hospital's finest on French wing Jean-François Gourdon in Cardiff in 1976, and the second was when England wing debutant and Guy's Hospital medical student John Novak stopped J.P.R. in his tracks at Twickenham in 1970. World-leading heart surgeon Stephen Westaby credited a brain injury during a student rugby match for his successful career. The damage altered his personality to leave him 'disinhibited, bold and aggressive' – perfect for the *mano a mano* world of cardiothoracic surgery.

In 2017, the All Blacks' Sonny Boy Williams was sent off for a shoulder charge into the face of winger Anthony Watson during a Lions

Test match. The incident involved double-teaming – first, Watson was held by Waisake Naholo, who inadvertently shepherded him into the onrushing Williams, an ex-New Zealand heavyweight boxing champion. The incident risked not only facial but also neck damage. Fortunately, Watson survived.

One year later, in New Zealand again, a French winger was not so lucky. Remy Grosso was double-teamed by Sam Kane and Ofa Tu'ungafasi, the latter bringing his shoulder into the Frenchman's face with no attempt to use his hands. Grosso had nowhere to go except the Auckland maxillofacial surgical unit with a double skull fracture. A penalty was awarded but no retrospective action taken against the players.

'Ten scars make a man.'

My dad, after I'd suffered another injury

Toughening up young players for the trials ahead can be misguided at times.

The parents of two young academy players came to me with concerns that their sons' symptoms were not being heeded.

One had recurrent pains in both feet disregarded. He was even told off in front of his peers for letting the team down. He was seconded to a lesser club, where bilateral midfoot stress fractures were diagnosed. Another player was returning from surgery on a broken ankle. He was asked to repeatedly jump from a pillar on to a concrete floor to increase his toughness. He told of continuing pain but was not listened to. The fracture had not healed and required another operation.

The game's laws have gradually evolved and most of those involved in the modern game regard most changes as positive in terms of the 'spectacle'. Medically, I feel some changes have diminished player welfare.

In 1996, the line-out jumper could be supported but a 'pre-grip' was not allowed. It was only in 2008 that lifting was officially recognised. We all thrill at the site of players such as Courtney Lawes soaring into the stratosphere, but losing support so high off the ground and falling without control is a prescription for damage. Landing heavily (often on somebody else's outstretched limbs) produces a fair number of ankle, foot, and head and neck injuries in our clinics.

Rugby union has traditionally worked on the principle that the tackled player must release the ball immediately on hitting the ground. Law 15.3(a) defines this as when one (or more) knee contacts the ground.

Modern players can roll, turn away from an unpromising body position and delay a pass from the ground until a colleague arrives. They can assume more positions than are outlined in the Kama Sutra to ensure the ball is recycled on their side. Law 15.5(a) states that 'a tackled player must immediately pass the ball or release it'. The only other actions a player can do legally is place the ball on the ground (15.5(c)) or push the ball along the ground – not forwards (15.5(d)). The near certainty that the offensive team will retain possession leads to the attack and defence committing fewer players to the breakdown – players whose role in a previous life was to beaver away at the coalface clutter the midfield instead. Accordingly, there is less room for back play and more risk of double-teaming on tackles, with all the attendant injury risk to the ball carrier. The vogue for charging into the nearest defender like a demented, rutting wildebeest would be muted if turnover risk was increased by a reversion to the previous interpretation of tackling. Who knows – it might reduce the mounting injury crisis and make the game less like rugby league with line-outs.

What about the health benefits of tactical substitutions?

At elite level half the team play the full game while the other half are replaced by what Eddie Jones terms the 'finishers'. The front row is the most common unit to play no more than 60 minutes.

Do Ackford's fresh players wreaking physical havoc represent a risk to tiring opposition players? The 2005 RFU injury audit recorded a disproportionate number of injuries in the final quarter of a match with 'starting players' most at risk. It might alter how players are prepared for action if they had to last 80 minutes.

Former fly-halves have been prominent in the call for change. Michael Lynagh and Rob Andrew have advocated exploring maximum weights for players in each position. Stuart Barnes has bemoaned the game's obsession with size.

World Rugby put forward proposals to improve player welfare in 2019, including fewer substitutes, retaining possession for the kicking team after bouncing a ball into touch in the opposition '22' (to force more players deeper), and outlawing the 'jackal' (players who steal the ball in the tackle to slow ball recycling).

As Richard Burton, the late Welsh actor, said, 'Rugby is a wonderful show: dance, opera and, suddenly, the blood of a killing.'

Recently, as much media space has been devoted to player health as the games themselves. This indicates that the sport is in urgent need of major change from statesmen-like leaders. Would a construction company, with the same number of injuries to its workforce as Harlequins and Gwent Dragons, escape a visit from an HSE representative?

Rugby is an exhilarating game that has changed and we must change with it. Player welfare is the most important consideration. There is a fine line between maintaining a box-office spectacle and increasing the risk of long-term disability to its protagonists. Greater men 'than I am, Gunga Din' have been pleading for change. Now is the time.

Chapter 17

SCRAMBLING THE EGG

'I'm so dizzy my head is spinning,
Like a whirlpool, it never ends'

Tommy Roe, 'Dizzy' (1969)

MANY SPORTS have head problems.

American football, boxing, equestrian sports, alpine sports, motor sports, ice hockey, cycling, rugby, soccer, cricket …

Elements of these sports – whether they be contact with an opponent, a hard ball, tarmac or an icy piste – make eliminating all risk impossible. The long-term effects of such injuries are being studied.

Chronic traumatic encephalopathy (CTE) is the best-known problem. It causes shrinkage of certain brain areas and swelling in other parts. The term 'punch drunk' for boxers (dementia pugilistica) was first used in 1928. Its symptoms manifest in different ways according to the brain areas affected, and its diagnosis can only be made with certainty after post-mortem brain examination. Differentiating between CTE and the effects of prolonged post-concussional syndrome are not precise – especially in the early stages. However, CTE is different from the more common Alzheimer's disease of the elderly.

'Football is not a contact sport. It's a collision sport –
dancing is a contact sport.'

Vince Lombardi, legendary coach of the Green Bay
Packers American football team

American football's experience of CTE has alerted UK authorities to the potential legal and financial impacts of concussion in sport.

By 2013 the National Football League (NFL) had offered $765m for medical help to more than 18,000 ex-players. The NFL allows up to $4m for each CTE diagnosis. Kansas City Chiefs are facing additional legal action from former players.

The NFL Mild Traumatic Brain Committee was established in 1994 and initially denied there was a tsunami building of long-term brain injuries. The wheels started coming off in 2005 when pathologist Bennet Omalu reported that the post-mortem on Pittsburgh Steelers' legend Mike Webster revealed CTE. Doctors estimated that the collisions he had sustained during his career were the equivalent of 25,000 car crashes. Webster died aged 50. His final years were tragic. He spent periods living in his truck or at railway stations and had difficulty sleeping. He resorted to self-administered electroshock weapons to help.

The NFL wanted Omalu's revelations retracted but the doctor responded in 2006 by publishing details of a second post-mortem on a player with CTE. Other cases were made public and Omalu's fight against prejudice and ignorance was turned into the film *Concussion* in 2015, starring Will Smith.

The implications of these cases have spread from the professional game to US schools, colleges and other sports. Millions of dollars are now being ploughed into CTE research and pre-season evaluations are exhaustive.

Rules have changed and there are now controls on the amount of time players can engage in contact during training. Each game must have an independent neurotrauma physician present and players showing concussion signs are removed and must subsequently follow stringent return-to-play protocols. Research on impacts has increased in sophistication. Helmet-on-helmet impact has been measured at around 0.73t or a 730kg force.

Is there a place for headball in football?

The 2002 death from degenerative brain disease of Jeff Astle, the West Bromwich Albion and England player, piqued interest in the potential link between repeated ball-heading and brain injury in football. Astle was a brave and imposing centre-forward during my youth. Many of his 168 goals were headed at a time when, on wet, muddy pitches, the panelled leather balls could mimic concrete.

In 2017, post-mortem findings from the brains of six footballers who had developed features of dementia demonstrated damage from chronic repetitive head impacts. CTE changes were demonstrated in four of them. Two years later, Scottish researchers published their findings from a study of 7,676 ex-professional footballers. It showed that the players were five times more likely to die from Alzheimer's than the general population.

Major concussive and multiple repetitive minor head incidents can cause long-term damage. Individual susceptibility varies and is influenced by factors other than the number of heading episodes. Alan Shearer, the ex-Premier League goal scorer, has announced he will donate his brain to research after his demise.

In 2014 Californian parents and youngsters began legal action against football authorities because they said there were inadequate safeguards against brain injury related to heading the ball in junior soccer. The matter was resolved out of court. A year later, US Soccer proposed new safety guidelines including a ban on under-10s heading altogether and under-13s heading during training. In 2020 British authorities banned heading in training for under-11s. Two high-profile incidents two years earlier had highlighted the problems of dealing with befuddled footballers.

The first involved Loris Karius, the Liverpool goalkeeper, who had an apparent double brain freeze during the 2018 Champions League Final, leading to two Real Madrid goals. It was reported that the player had no symptoms immediately post-match to alarm the club's doctors. The German keeper then left for his American holiday but five days later visited my alma mater, the Massachusetts General Hospital, where visual spatial dysfunction was diagnosed This condition can affect decision-making and is one of the 'broad church' of symptoms related to concussion. Liverpool manager Jürgen Klopp decreed that Karius's performance had been '100 per cent influenced by his concussion'. Three months later, further goalkeeping errors led to Karius being loaned to Istanbul club Beşiktaş.

The second incident occurred at the 2018 FIFA World Cup in Russia for which the medical committee had produced guidelines on concussion management but admitted it had no power to enforce them. The regulations included a minimum of six days post-concussion rest before playing again. During the tournament, the Moroccan player Nordin Amrabat was concussed against Portugal and admitted to hospital.

He had no recollection of the game but overruled Moroccan medics, claiming, 'I am my own doctor,' and played again after five days. The team doctor had later to explain his team's sideline tactics for immediate head injury management. This included spraying the stupefied player with water and slapping his face.

Incidents in 2019 suggested that little had improved. In January of that year Udinese goalkeeper David Ospina sustained a head injury during a game. He continued to play, swathed in bandages, before collapsing and being taken to the local hospital. Two months later Fabian Schär was 'knocked out for a few minutes' after a head clash in a Swiss match. Five minutes of treatment were required before he was allowed to continue, a decision censored by FIFA.

In April 2019 Tottenham Hotspur's Jan Vertongen sustained a head injury in a collision with a team-mate in a Champions League semi-final. He was assessed off the pitch and cleared to carry on. Forty seconds later the player signalled that he was unfit to continue. Spurs' medics argued that he had not lost consciousness and the club claimed that the player was not concussed.

The following October, Welsh manager Ryan Giggs claimed one of his players, Daniel James, was 'acting' and 'streetwise and using his nous' during a game against Croatia. The player's head had been caught in a collision and he lay seemingly unconscious. Such claims make it harder for attending medics, who know they will be censored for misjudged assessments. Giggs was criticised by the Headway charity

FIFA and national associations should review their protocols and fall into line with other sports. Medics have called for a ten-minute concussion assessment period when temporary substitutes would be allowed. The English Premier League already uses a third, independent doctor to support club medics, introduced partly as a result of a concussion incident in 2013 involving Spurs player Hugo Lloris. At the time, FIFA described the club's decision to let the player carry on as 'dangerous and irresponsible'.

The compulsory removal of every player who falls clutching their head might be beneficial and a ten-minute head injury assessment might make everyone think twice before feigning injury.

Are men's brains from Mars and women's from Venus?

Some research indicates that women might be more prone to head injuries and concussion than men.

In a study, American female soccer and basketball players were more likely than male players to suffer concussive episodes and to take longer to recover. Explanations, including hormonal differences and reduced neck strength, have been proposed. In horse racing, British female jockeys are concussed at a ratio of 3.6:1 to males. In soccer, the ratio is nearly 2:1. A Dublin hospital reported a five-fold increase in concussed female rugby players over a ten-year period from 2007. American girls involved in high school sport have twice the concussion rates of boys and are more prone to recurrent episodes.

Trying to put Humpty-Dumpty together again

> *'All the King's horses and all the King's men*
> *Couldn't put Humpty together again.'*
>
> **Late 18th century nursery rhyme**

I spent 25 years as an orthopaedic surgeon assessing and treating head injury patients. Three episodes from my career illustrate the devastating effects of such trauma.

As a second-year doctor I was working in casualty when a 12-year-old girl arrived via an ambulance on a Sunday afternoon. She had been horse riding and had fallen on her head. She was unresponsive and died, despite desperate attempts to resuscitate her. No parent should ever experience their daughter going out for gentle exercise and two hours later being told they have lost her. The anguish of telling them will never leave me.

Four years later, as a junior orthopaedic registrar, a young motorcyclist arrived with a devastating head injury suggesting a significant bleed inside the skull. The nearest neurosurgical unit was over 30 minutes away. My own clinical assessment, supported by telephone conversations with the neurosurgeons, was that such an ambulance dash was futile. I had to undertake my first solo burr hole surgery, which involved drilling into the skull to relieve the pressure. The procedure was performed properly but the patient did not survive.

The post-mortem revealed that the trauma was catastrophic and highly unlikely to respond to any treatment. I was 31. Such an experience never leaves you. It might toughen you for future events but the feeling of impotence and looking after the bereaved family is something you never get used to.

The third episode occurred when I was an established consultant. In the early hours of the morning I was asked to assess a middle-aged male with severe head injuries caused by an assault. The emergency team were already resuscitating him. The facial disfigurement was very bad but I recognised him as a long-standing patient of mine. No central referral system existed to provide bed availability nationally and I spent three hours telephoning to get him transferred to a neurosurgical unit – the onus was on the primary receiving hospital to find a suitable centre. A direct consultant-to-consultant conversation was not permitted and I had to outline the clinical urgency to the on-call junior doctor at each neurosurgical unit and then await the outcome of their conversation with the neurosurgical consultant which, often half an hour later, was a refusal to accept. The process started all over again with the next specialist unit and all the time my patient's clinical status was deteriorating. Eventually I found a willing unit. I felt anger and frustration at the critically wasted time and the absurdity of a system that nationwide failed patients at their time of greatest need. The patient died a month later.

Rugby and head injuries

In 1973, Tony Ensor, the Irish full-back, took a forearm from a French player around the neck to stop him in full flight. He was so concussed he could not remember three-quarters of the game or taking the place-kicks afterwards. He did finish the match, however. Another player, Bill Beaumont, the English and British Lions captain, was forced to retire from rugby in 1982 because of the latest in a series of concussion incidents. He was 29.

In rugby's amateur days, such events were common. Most regular players 'remember' returning home unable to recall the score – including me. Misguidedly it was regarded as a badge of honour and avoided giving the opposition a sense of weakness in the home ranks.

In 2013 rugby introduced the Head Injury Assessment (HIA) programme to guide clinicians assessing players during games. It replaced the less comprehensive pitchside concussion assessment.

However, some players have found ways around this system by avoiding pre-season baseline testing, learning by rote the answers to assessment questions and, during games, denying the need for an HIA, such is their desire to play. A 2018 survey of current international players found that over one-quarter had hidden head injury symptoms to avoid time off training and playing.

Gallic gung-ho

Guy Novès, an ex-international player, was Toulouse head coach from 1993 to 2015. He won nine French national championships and four European Cups and was a clever and vastly experienced coach.

In 2014 his star centre, Florian Fritz, sustained a nasty head injury and had blood streaming down his face as he was led away. To general surprise, Fritz returned to the field at the apparent behest of his coach. The French rugby federation (FFR) medical commission president told *Midi Olympique* that what shocked him as much as the doctor's actions (or lack thereof) was the 'attitude of Guy Novès, who came looking for [Fritz] in the dressing room in order to get him back before the 15-minute time limit for blood injuries expired'. Another player explained to Australia's *Sydney Morning Herald* how 'Novès [had been] caught on camera apparently urging a player back into the fray who has since claimed to have been unconscious 15 minutes earlier'. Novès responded: 'I have been knocked out, played on and was fine; as you can see, I am still standing here.' *The Times* writer Daniel Schofield wrote that 'such a stone-age attitude demonstrates how far rugby has to go'. Novès was made national head coach the following year.

Novès seemed to improve his understanding of head injury protocols. During a Wales international in 2017 France appeared to have invoked the guidelines for tactical gain. Twenty minutes of overtime were played while the French pack camped on the Welsh line seeking the converted try that would bring them victory. While the French tried to push the scrum over the opposition try line, Rabah Slimani, the substituted French tight-head prop, started to warm up on the touchline. A conversation took place between a French medic and a coach who had strayed beyond his designated technical area. Then the medic came on to the pitch and spoke to Slimani's replacement, Uini Atonio. The referee asked Atonio about his health and was told he had a 'sore back'. The next scrum collapsed and the doctor returned to the pitch to take Atonio off. The superior scrummager, Slimani, returned while the doctor told the referee that Atonio required an HIA.

Television clearly showed the prop walking alone down the tunnel. Protocols stipulate that players removed for HIAs need to be supervised during that process. The French finally scored the seven points to gain victory. Novès said the 'medics told me he was injured, so I had to take my responsibilities as a coach'. A change in tone from three years earlier.

Owen Slot of *The Times* wrote that analysis of footage found no point at which Atonio had taken a head blow. Slot found it 'difficult not to conclude that France manipulated the protocols surrounding the HIA', adding that concussion was 'a situation that has to be handled with unstinting responsibility. Yet it is that very sensitive issue that France may have hijacked to try and win a game.'

Rob Howley, the vanquished Welsh coach, said, 'Integrity in our game is pretty important and player welfare is equally important … The evidence suggests that [the incident] is not in the integrity of the game.' Barry O'Driscoll, an ex-World Rugby medical adviser, said, 'It was inevitable that the system would be abused at some point … It's open to abuse from coaches putting pressure on doctors.'

Most doctors are an integral part of an organisation trying above all to win a game. This potential conflict was highlighted by Toni Belli, an experienced Birmingham neurosurgeon. After an interview with the *Daily Mail* in 2014, Belli's concerns were reported under the headline 'The Catch-22 of concussion: Top surgeon claims team doctors fear the sack … for trying to protect their players'.

After an investigation, the French were reprimanded for not following HIA protocols. However, the Untoward Incident Review Group of the Six Nations said there was 'no clear evidence of intent to obtain a competitive advantage'. Novès departed the international scene less than a year later – not due to any involvement in skulduggery but, more mundanely, because of poor results.

Were the French emboldened by the lack of teeth in the 2017 inquiry?

The next year, in a close encounter with Ireland, French fly-half debutant, Matthieu Jalibert, injured his knee. French management claimed he had an additional head injury as he left the field, giving them the option to bring on an HIA replacement. This gave the French longer to assess the injury; if the knee settled Jalibert could return, claiming to have passed his HIA. He stayed off. Near the end of the game, France were leading 13-12 and defending for all their worth. They had used all their substitutes when replacement scrum-half, Antoine Dupont, clearly injured his knee. Television footage showed no obvious evidence of head contact yet, you've guessed it, the French claimed an accessory head injury and Dupont limped down the tunnel pointing to his head. By activating the HIA, France could bring back on the already replaced scrum-half Maxime Machenaud. The knee injury alone to Dupont would have left them with 14 men. The Irish complained but referee

Nigel Owens said he had to follow medical advice. To paraphrase Oscar Wilde: 'To lose one half-back with a head injury is a misfortune; to lose two looks highly suspicious!'

The French later explained that it was the independent doctor (who was the FFR medical committee vice-president) who had added an HIA to the knee problems. *L'Equipe* reported that the linesman was also concerned about a head injury despite Dupont and the on-field French medical team telling everybody the player had a knee injury. The die was set for an HIA.

Was this a result of a mistaken linesman, extreme sensitivity that any injured player may be concussed, or Gallic quick-thinking? France finished the game with 15 men but lost to a late Johnny Sexton drop goal.

British brain drain?

Have rugby heads come out of the clouds in Britain?

In the last few seasons I have experienced a sea change in attitudes both on and off the pitch generally. Rugby authorities' actions, media attention, and player education at all levels have gone a long way towards expunging the macho intent of carrying on after a concussion. Players are more likely to admit to a blow to the head and, as importantly, team-mates appear ready to indicate to the touchline concerns about a colleague. Such a revolution in attitudes can only help prevent long-term damage. However, at the highest echelons, reported concussion rates remain at worryingly high levels.

The 2014–2015 Professional Rugby Injury Surveillance Project reported that one in six English Premiership players had been concussed that season. Concussion rates had risen fourfold in six years. Double-teaming tacklers and ever higher tackling positions must take responsibility for some of this increase. In 2017, Wasps rugby director Dai Young reported an extra 50 collisions per game for his side compared to just one year before. Concussions were accounting for over one in five of all injuries during games and, worryingly, it was also the most common training injury. Numbers fell slightly in 2018 but the average length of absence from a concussion rose.

Despite measures put in place by rugby authorities there is always more that can be done. One flaw in the system was highlighted in 2016.

George North suffered a head injury playing for Northampton Saints against Leicester Tigers. Retrospective video assessment suggested he may have lost consciousness but the evidence was not available pitchside.

It was North's fifth head injury in two years. The subsequent Concussion Management Review Group report concluded that video evidence and the player's history and risk stratification meant he should not have returned to play. It would have been a difficult call for the 'blinded' medical team, particularly with the player denying 'any loss of consciousness with immediate recall of events'. North suffered a sixth head injury in February 2020.

In April 2018, Welsh side Gwent Dragons announced that their third player in three years had been forced to retire following a head injury. Scanning evidence showed brain injury. This is a very worrying cluster of concussions for one club and for the game as a whole.

Research in New Zealand in 2015 found that 77 per cent of amateur and 85 per cent of professional rugby players had been concussed at least once and that retired rugby players performed worse on a range of mental reasoning tests than non-rugby players.

Where have the improvements been?

The early seeds of sense returning to the game are beginning to appear. Perhaps administrators' heads are clearing, giving players' brains a chance.

International and Premiership rugby union games have numerous clinical staff prowling the touchlines ready to sprint to the aid of a stricken player. Each has received arduous training in emergency pitchside response protocols, with the emphasis on teamwork. Other sports have followed suit and I can attest to the comprehensive and effectiveness of these actions. However, it is a sad reflection on rugby that these emergency drills have become depressingly familiar.

Independent doctors have been drafted in at elite level to be responsible for decisions over blood and concussion replacements, and HIA assessments. This process started in the Premier League in 2019 and follows the measures American football adopted.

Various rugby bodies are ploughing money into research and auditing such injuries, and evidence is accumulating. Risk factors such as neck strength have been recognised and acted upon and trials have taken place to test 'smart' mouthguards that could be used in rugby and boxing. The threshold for removing players from the action has been lowered – even below elite level. In 2019 I was the pitchside doctor at a representative match. In the second half, five players were removed from the game for HIAs. All stayed off. Thirty years ago, there would have been no pitchside medical support and all five players would have played on.

The tackle has become a primary focus. Nearly half of all match injuries occur during the tackle and it is the most common cause of head injuries. Over two-thirds of those concussed are the tackler.

As player power and size has increased there has been an inexorable shift to using sheer bulk to halt hookers in their tracks; the contact area has moved upstairs and audits of head injuries have highlighted the evil of the high tackle, which is what experienced clinicians have known for a long time. If the tackler contacts their opponent's head, the risk of a head injury is 20 times greater than if the tackle is around the upper thighs.

In the past, the player in possession had to release the ball immediately on hitting the deck and so the incentive was to take his legs away. The neatly executed 'waist and below' tackle depends hugely on timing and technique and correct head and body position were drilled into players in the amateur era with an emphasis on using the ball carrier's own momentum to bring him to ground. Now, the emphasis is on wrapping up the player and the ball. Inevitably this means moving your point of contact north.

The RFU announced in July 2018 a trial of no tackling above the armpit for the Championship (second tier) cup competition for the 2018/19 season. Within a month, the number of head and neck tackles had reduced by two-thirds. But concussions did not reduce and the initiative was abandoned mid-competition. The problem was that players were adopting low body positions and continuing to risk head clashes – the immense power of the modern rugby player remains a problem.

By the end of 2018, following the deaths of the four young French players, the FFR canvassed World Rugby to ban all tackles above the waist, two-man tackles and head-on-head tackles. Its president, Bernard Laporte, pleaded for rugby to change its emphasis from impact to movement. World Rugby announced trials in under-20 games to reduce the upper level of contact from the shoulders to the nipple line and penalise tacklers who remained upright. Some experts want similar guidelines applied to the professional game.

In a welcome change to their recent head injury history, French rugby has been quick to act. By early 2019, games encouraging below-waist tackling and penalties for running directly at tacklers and double-team tackling were trialled. In August 2019, World Rugby announced that these trials had been approved. If effective they could be adopted at elite international level by 2023.

The proposals have not met with unanimous support.

Ex-Scotland forward Jim Hamilton told the media of his concerns about outlawing double-teaming tackles. He recalled spending countless training hours perfecting the technique and felt that a narrower tackle zone on the player's body would leave insufficient room for two men to pulverise the ball carrier. In my opinion this double-teaming is a scourge on the game. It is the second man who is most likely to cause damage by hitting an already stalled player. Hamilton's argument was that the single remaining tackler would have to 'monster' the ball carrier even more. We just need tough refereeing.

Where I do agree with Hamilton and other ex-players is on the need to consider reducing exposure to head injury by reducing the number of matches played by individuals.

An ex-England forward, Ben Kay, pleaded that rugby's DNA should not be changed by trying to make the game safer. I agree. Homo sapiens' DNA can be traced back to East Africa. Rugby's DNA can be traced back to 'Big Side' on the Barby Road at Rugby School. DNA evolves through the generations. I doubt whether the Reverend William Ellis would recognise the game that he started by accident. However, I regard the changes that have developed around the tackle area since professionalism as a genetic mutation of the game. There is a generation of players who have grown up believing that the tackle to the upper torso and higher has always been an important part of the game.

World Rugby announced its determination to clamp down on neck-high tackles and shoulder-first charges on the eve of the Rugby World Cup in Japan in September 2019. As a result, a record eight players were sent off in that tournament compared to only 17 in the previous eight World Cups. Injury substitution rates dropped from 2.08 to 1.13 per match and concussion levels were reduced by 35 per cent compared to elite rugby games the year before.

As the 2019 World Cup started, David Denton, the talented Scottish back-row forward, announced his retirement. He should have been playing in Japan but instead had to admit defeat following an 11-month battle to recover from a head injury sustained against Northampton. 'I have woken up every morning with pressure in my head, visual disturbances and not really knowing what is going on,' he said.

Whither the back-up?

At junior level, rugby is struggling to provide equivalent care to its participants.

My own experience of pitchside medical duties below elite level is that players, parents, officials and clinical staff have a heightened awareness of head injuries. I get telephone calls from junior club officials and GPs seeking advice on how to correctly advise junior club players, including teenagers, following one or more concussions.

The NHS is simply not geared up to provide this advice in a timely and all-encompassing manner. In the absence of experienced support some GPs may take understandably defensive positions when asked to advise injured players that they should retire from the game. Alternatively, players will make decisions themselves and return too early. The stakes can be high. In Ireland a youngster received £2.29m for injuries sustained during a school rugby match in 2009. The judgement was jointly against his school and the treating medical team.

The RFU has not been passive. Players, parents, coaches and officials can undertake free online courses such as 'Don't be a headcase'. Junior clubs do have advice cards for concussion assessment and brochures like 'Rugby Aware' freely available. The RFU and other equivalent bodies need to establish a group of suitably qualified doctors able and willing to provide help to these young players. Private companies like Return2Play provide excellent advice and support but may not be within the financial reach of all clubs, youngsters and families.

Sharks in hot soup

Legal eagles have already landed on Planet Rugby with respect to concussion, and the English and French judicial systems are being tested.

In August 2016 ex-Sale scrum half Cillian Willis started legal action against his former club and their doctors. He alleged clinical negligence after a series of head injuries in a cup tie against Saracens in 2013 and was the first player to sue his club for medical negligence in such circumstances. Willis, an ex-Ireland under-21 international, claimed he had sustained two concussions in the first half of the game but was deemed fit to continue after assessment. He received two further blows early in the second half, was initially passed fit to continue but ongoing symptoms led to his withdrawal in the 47th minute. He never played rugby again. The player had just returned after three months recovering from concussions against Wasps and Worcester in December 2012. Additionally, he had fractured his eye socket three times during his career.

A month later, Sale Sharks coach Steve Diamond criticised rugby's position following another head injury to a player. He commented, 'All you need is a slap on the head to be taken off,' a statement criticised by ex-Ireland international Alan Quinlan as, 'horrendous, ill-informed and dangerous'.

And even while the Willis case remained *sub judice*, senior voices within the English Premiership expressed concerns in the media over the implications of the episode. Rob Baxter, the Exeter coach, told the BBC that 'it puts club medical staff and doctors in a very, very difficult situation. If a player can suddenly turn around and start suing a rugby club, at what stage will it stop?' He added, 'My big concern is, are we going to create – if we are not very careful – a scenario for our medical staff where they are almost having to drag players off the field just in case? That's the big worry for me.'

Saracens director of rugby, Mark McCall, agreed. 'If you put yourself in the shoes of the medic, it's almost an impossible job. Would they want to return someone to the field of play if they have been taken off for an assessment now?'

Wasps coach Dai Young said, 'The Willis case could set a dangerous precedent. Let's hope it doesn't go down that path. But we all have total trust in our medics.'

In 2018 it was announced that the case against the Sale Sharks had been discontinued without a compensation payment. However, the action proceeded against the club's medical staff and was heard behind closed doors in Manchester in 2019, six years after the game. The outcome is unknown as it is subject to a confidentiality agreement, although Willis told the *Irish Times* after the case, 'If someone is looking for accountability or some sort of closure, for me the judicial system is not a place where you will necessarily find natural justice. I think it is a place you can get lost.'

Head and neck injuries continued at Sale Sharks, as elsewhere in rugby. In September 2018 England flanker Tom Curry was stretchered off in a neck brace while inhaling oxygen. 'He got a knock to the head but nothing serious there. If you're out, and I think he was momentarily out, that's what they have to go through,' explained Sale director of rugby Steve Diamond. Three weeks later Tom's twin, Ben Curry, suffered a neck injury. *Independent* journalist Sam Peters wrote that Diamond was heard to say, as the player lay on the pitch, 'There's six minutes until half-time; he's staying on.' The player continued.

Meanwhile, in 2019, across the Channel, Canadian Jamie Cudmore took legal action against his club Clermont Ferrand. His medical expert claimed that more than once Cudmore was cleared to return to play by his club's doctor when he was unfit to do so because of concussion.

A true warrior

The 28-year-old Springbok international Pat Lambie announced his retirement from the game in 2019. He had sustained concussions in 2012, 2016, 2017 (twice) and 2018 and was left with persistent post-concussion symptoms from which he failed to recover. Another South African has also experienced the effects of a serious head injury – Gerrit-Jan van Velze, or GJ, a no-nonsense back-row forward from the high veldt.

At 6ft 5in GJ is intimidating on the pitch but a gentle giant off it. In 2012, after four successful years in Pretoria with the Blue Bulls, he moved to Northampton Saints and two years later transferred allegiances to Worcester Warriors. He is a good family friend.

A year before GJ's move, Jonathan Thomas, the Welsh international back-row forward, joined Worcester and was immediately made captain. But he sustained multiple head traumas leading to brain damage and the development of a form of epilepsy thought to be related to the injuries, and was forced to retire in 2015. GJ had taken over as captain. In September 2016, during the season's opening game, GJ was body-checked but not knocked out. Initially he felt whiplash-type symptoms and pains throughout his head. He went on to develop eye and inner ear problems.

For the first four months after the incident, he was virtually housebound and banned from watching television, using his phone or driving. His balance was severely affected and he struggled to remain upright at times. He was unable to use lifts or escalators. Some of the early opinions he received from non-clinical staff were less than supportive. As he recovered, he immersed himself in developing a bespoke shoewear business and breeding sheep.

GJ received exemplary care from the Worcester medical team and expert advice from neurologists, neurosurgeons, audio-vestibular specialists and neuroradiologists. As a competitive professional athlete he found it hard to accept the lengthy process of investigations, multiple specialist advice and the prolonged recovery process. Inevitably, advice can vary as to the safety of returning to rugby. Despite the seniority of the opinions he received, there is still, in certain areas, no definitive evidence to guide a player and his advisors. It is a matter of balancing risk.

As part of his rehabilitation, GJ went through a stringent neck-strengthening programme, increasing his already impressive collar size from 17.5in to 18.5in. Athletes are used to seeing team-mates rehabilitating from physical injuries and surgical interventions but in his darkest moments GJ feared his colleagues and coaching staff might doubt that his neurological problems were genuine, as there was little external evidence of his symptoms. For him, though, every new headache or bodily ache raised questions as to whether it was the signal of a relapse. Throughout all of this he had the unstinting support of his doctor wife, Menanta.

It took GJ nine months to pass the stringent return-to-play protocols. A whole season was lost, and he feared at times that his career was over. He was not the only concussion victim at Warriors that season. The Lions and England centre Ben Te'o missed games and the Scottish international fly-half Tom Heathcote only played one further game that season after being knocked out in November 2016.

GJ resumed playing and captaining duties in September 2017. After eight outstanding games he suffered another head knock but missed only two weeks of play. He returned to his previous blistering form and I was relieved and delighted to see him performing so well in the final game of that season against Northampton Saints. GJ is symptom-free now. However, he has vowed to remain vigilant throughout the rest of his rugby career with regular neurological and psychological testing.

Athletes involved in collision and combative sports put their bodies on the line every time they train and play. They know the risks involved and accept them. Equally, they have a reasonable expectation that the sporting authorities sufficiently understand those risks and attempt to reduce them. This is achieved by adjusting guidelines and laws that control each sport as fresh evidence emerges. Athlete safety and long-term health must remain paramount over and above financial and sporting successes.

Chapter 18

BLOODGATE AND
THE MIGHTY QUINS

'It will have blood. They say; blood will have blood.'

William Shakespeare, *Macbeth* **(1606)**

IN APRIL 2009 Harlequins welcomed Leinster to the Stoop Memorial Ground in west London for a rugby European Cup quarter-final. Before the game Quins 1st XV physiotherapist, Steph Brennan, bought false blood capsules from a joke shop.

Towards the end of the game the visitors led 6-5. Quins leading goal kicker, Nick Evans, had been substituted but the club's director of rugby, Dean Richards, schemed to return Evans to the field for the closing minutes by manipulating blood substitution rules. He hoped that a goal-kicking opportunity would arise to enable his team to claim victory. Winger Tom Williams was made the sacrificial lamb and was given a joke blood capsule, which he hid in his sock. After a tackle Williams tried to bite the capsule open but it fell out of his mouth, and in full view of the crowd and TV cameras he picked it up and bit it open. He was then caught on camera winking to team-mates as he was led from the pitch by Brennan – with the equivalent of rhesus +ve type O tomato ketchup seeping from his mouth.

The Leinster team doctor was Professor Arthur Tanner, director of surgery at the College of Surgeons in Dublin and a man well able to distinguish blood from Heinz 57 at ten metres. A felony was suspected and Leinster demanded to know whether the injury was bona fide. Williams was in the medical room being looked after by Quins doctor

Wendy Chapman, a casualty specialist, while a storm raged outside the locked door. Leinster's doctors wanted to examine Williams. The player persuaded Chapman to cut his lip to establish the presence of a 'real injury'.

The bloody assizes

The repercussions for the principle figures were huge. Williams was banned, at first for one year, but Richards, Brennan and Chapman were initially cleared of misconduct. Excruciatingly slowly the truth came out – mostly due to the revised testimony of Williams. (Quins had tried to persuade the player not to reveal the whole story and offered him significant compensation.) Richards received a three-year worldwide coaching ban and Harlequins were fined £237,000. Williams had his ban reduced to four months and went on to complete 17 years at the club. Ten years later he admitted living with the memories daily and reflected that he was 'a pawn in a bigger picture' and 'part of a coercive culture'.

Steph Brennan was banned from rugby for two years and the physiotherapy regulatory body struck his name from its register in 2010. He took his case to the High Court and was reinstated in 2011. Brennan reflected, 'I want the profession, and most importantly sports physiotherapists, to learn from my mistakes. Sports physiotherapy is a very different role for the physiotherapist than any other job in public or private health, but that should not mean we forget our standards of ethics and practice.'

Chapman was suspended by the General Medical Council (GMC) from practising as a doctor but allowed back after a warning in August 2010. It took 16 months to reach the final verdict, which affected Chapman's well-being. She admitted to being 'ashamed'. Tanner gave evidence to the GMC and stated that, 'A sports doctor was working in a dysfunctional environment and often had to withstand pressure from players and coaches.' He complained about 'the condescending and arrogant attitude' of Dean Richards towards the Leinster medical team.

The moral maze

Articles appeared in the press relating to the moral confusions within sport. Simon Barnes of *The Times* wrote in August 2010 that, 'More and more, with every passing day, race by race and game by game, sport looks more and more like reality,' adding, 'Time and again in sport, you find people losing perspective, forgetting that what they do is not actually real,' and, 'The madness of Bloodgate was entirely about the illusion that the results of a rugby match actually matters a tinker's fart.' In the same paper, Antonia Fraser wrote, 'Dr Chapman's mistake was not the lip-cutting but becoming embroiled in sports medicine. It is a field in which hypocrisy abounds. The line between performance optimisation and performance manipulation looks fine to an outsider. Yet we wrap the whole edifice of sport in its own peculiar morality.'

This boundary-blurring presents significant ethical issues to all involved in sport.

Shane Sutton, formerly UK Cycling and Team Sky's coach, discussed Bradley Wiggins' asthma treatment and use of therapeutic use exemptions (TUEs) to 'find the gains'. He said, 'If you've got an athlete that's 95 per cent ready, and that little 5 per cent injury or niggle that's troubling, if you get that TUE to get them to 100 per cent, yeah of course you would in those days.'

There is additional evidence from elsewhere in this book that some coaches and managers directly interfere with the clinical management, including drug prescribing, of sports people. The threats to doctors and physiotherapists' clinical independence and professional status is clear.

Before Chapman's final GMC hearing, Brian Moore, an ex-Harlequins and England player and a qualified solicitor, pleaded for leniency for the medic. Moore pointed out that Chapman was working as an unpaid volunteer and was wrongly charged by the European Cup authorities, who later admitted that they had no jurisdiction over her. Chapman had no prior knowledge of the deceit and only cut Williams at his behest and clear consent. The GMC agreed that she did not pose a threat to the public. As Moore said, 'Does her mistaken, yet isolated and instantaneous act, under inordinate and personal pressure created by others, outweigh her many previous years of competent and professional service, witnessed by thousands of patients she has treated?'

One rule for all?

I would not condone Chapman's actions, for which she professed sincere regrets, but I was struck by the almost parallel activities of footballer Andy Carroll.

In 2008 Carroll was arrested by Newcastle police and cautioned in relation to an assault on a woman. The following January he had a training ground fight with a team-mate. No disciplinary action was taken. In December of that year he was arrested again after smashing a glass into somebody's face at a nightclub and was fined £1,000. In March 2010 he allegedly 'broke the jaw' of a team-mate in another training ground incident, which the *Daily Mail* reported as an 'unwelcome distraction for his manager'. That October, Carroll was charged with assault involving an ex-girlfriend. Charges were later dropped because of lack of evidence.

Carroll missed no football as a result of his behaviour. In fact, in October 2010 he was rewarded with an improved five-year contract. Three months later he moved to Liverpool for £35m – the most expensive British transfer ever at the time – but was offloaded to West Ham after 18 months and, 36 hours before his signing-on medical, was reportedly partying in Las Vegas dressed as a giant chipmunk. His injuries and meagre scoring record meant that he netted £800,000 per goal over six years. In 2019 he was back on Tyneside claiming that his wild days were over.

Footballers are 'box office'. Clinicians are not. Different rules apply. I rest my case m'lud.

Surely not at Twickers?

Blood replacements were allowed under Law 3.10 of the IRB rules and had been since 1993 when rugby union followed the lead of rugby league which introduced blood substitutions in 1991. It allowed bleeding players to be removed to receive appropriate attention.

Manipulation of the guidelines had long been suspected at the time of 'Bloodgate' and Brennan's professional inquiry revealed four previous fake blood incidents involving Quins, dating back to 2005. An ex-Quins player, George Robson, revealed that he had been part of a scheme similar to that involving Williams. And at a confidential RFU meeting Dean Richards said the 'use of fake blood, cutting players, re-opening wounds, feigning injury in the front row, jabbing players with anaesthetic all occur regularly throughout the game'. He gave seven specific incidents including one allegedly involving the England team during their successful 2003 World Cup campaign.

I was involved in two incidents preceding 'Bloodgate' that indicated the degree of scepticism about the game.

In April 2001 I was the orthopaedic surgeon for England against France at Twickenham. England had a succession of injuries in the first half including to Jason Leonard, Phil Greening and Steve Borthwick (an international debutant), who received head cuts requiring suturing. As I completed one set of stitches and returned a player to the field another would run down the tunnel.

The next day, in the *Sunday Times*, Stephen Jones was concerned that England had been attempting to have a fourth player, Ben Cohen, removed to the blood bin. There was an implication that all was not above board. The referee, David McHugh, had said, 'There is no blood. You can treat him, but you can't put him in the blood bin.' Certainly the Northampton Saint did not come my way, and, to my knowledge, all injuries were managed strictly according to guidelines.

The war of Bracken's ear

Four years later I was honorary orthopaedic surgeon at a Northampton Saints' home Premiership game against Saracens.

Shortly before half-time, Saracens' scrum-half Kyran Bracken left the field holding his shoulder. Saracens claimed he had a blood injury to his ear. My colleague, the late Dr Jon Raphael, was sitting on the Saints' bench with me. We could see no blood and requested permission to examine Bracken to verify the injury. Raphael was an ex-Northampton skipper and, like Saracens coach, Steve Diamond, a former hooker. A fractious encounter ensued on the touchline between the two former No. 2s, who heatedly argued and jostled.

Paul Boulton covered the incident in the *Daily Telegraph* under the heading, 'Diamond so abrasive'. He recorded the uncompromising nature of Diamond and how he was 'likely to find himself the subject of an official complaint for manhandling Northampton's doctor, Jon Raphael'. He said, 'It all made for a thoroughly unpleasant afternoon,' adding that 'Diamond angrily refuted suggestions from the home camp that he had spat at Northampton's team manager, Dave Newman, though he admitted that he pushed Raphael, a former England reserve hooker, when the Northampton doctor encroached into Saracens' technical area in a row over an injury to Kyran Bracken.' Boulton explained that 'Saracens claimed that scrum-half Bracken suffered internal bleeding from a perforated eardrum. Northampton alleged Bracken had a different injury and that Saracens were manipulating the regulations on blood replacements to give him a breather.' Bracken was recalled by referee Steve Lander and was immediately involved in a 90-metre move from one end of the pitch to the other. Bracken's sense organs did not appear impaired. Continued niggling from both benches reflected the closeness of the encounter, won by Saracens 21-20 through an injury-time penalty.

Perforated eardrums are examined through an otoscope, which requires skills beyond the scope of a physiotherapist's practice and cannot be undertaken on the field of play.

Fourteen years later, Diamond (now with Sale Sharks) had to defend his methods and reputation after an altercation with a journalist in a post-match press conference. The journalist called Diamond 'a bully' and accused him of creating an intimidating atmosphere and ignoring medical advice on injuries. Diamond strenuously denied the accusations.

Does this all matter?

Prior to Bloodgate, experienced observers suspected that blood substitutions were being manipulated. Bill Shankly, the late Liverpool manager, said, 'If a player is not interfering with play or seeking to gain an advantage, then he should be.' While admiring Shankly's passion, sport must be believable to survive, as we have found with the various doping scandals in cycling and athletics.

Rugby coaches were using blood substitutions to gain an illegal advantage which, by their nature, involved medical staff (unwittingly or not). Many of the latter were working unpaid in an honorary capacity. However, they faced potentially more draconian professional sanctions than the original perpetrators. As the Carroll comparison confirms, they are judged by different standards.

Chapter 19

WHEN IS A BROKEN LEG NOT A BROKEN LEG?

'Healing is a matter of time, but it is sometimes also a matter of opportunity.'

Hippocrates, Greek physician

BROKEN BONES conjure up many visions: on the one hand, shattered bones and rows of patients strung up on traction for months such as in *Carry on Doctor*. On the other, stress injuries to many bones can cause minimal disability. Such distinctions are not often made. Consequently, elite athletes are imbued with healing powers denied to mere mortals.

A sequoia snaps a strut?

In July 2015, New Zealand rugby winger Waisake Naholo (108kg) was reported to have 'broken his leg' against Argentina. He had damaged his fibula (the thin bone on the outside of the shin), which threatened his participation in the England-hosted Rugby World Cup that autumn. His coach, Steve Hansen, was realistic, saying, 'I think it is a wee bit strong to say he broke his leg. He only really had a small stress crack in it.' The winger decided to fly home to Fiji, where he underwent traditional medical treatment applied by his uncle, Isei Naiova , who was a doctor. Kawakawa leaves were applied to Naholo's leg.

Ten weeks later Naholo played against Georgia in the World Cup. The herbs were declared a 'miracle cure' and described by his uncle as a 'gift from God'. The great news was relayed around the world by the media.

Healthy scepticism surfaced. Wellington-based surgeon Nigel Willis felt Naholo's recovery time was as expected but that the leaves may have helped relieve pain. 'All cultures have their own natural healing methods, but whether that's making a difference, or whether it's all about a belief system and managing pain – it would be hard to sort of tell the difference,' he said. Hansen was blunter: 'There has been a lot of talk about a miracle cure, but he has come back when we expected him to.'

People worldwide believe in the medicinal powers of witch doctors. The travels of rugby player Manu Tuilagi, when he sought treatment from his Samoan witch doctor to rid him of his catalogue of injuries, have been chronicled in this book. Criticism of traditional herbal treatments is unfair. The kawakawa has been used by Maori healers for many problems, ranging from rheumatism to gonorrhoea. However, Naholo's return to play was very much as anticipated and Willis and Hansen were right.

There is an epitaph to this story. Naholo re-fractured the same bone less than five months after the first injury. His Highlanders' team doctor, Greg MacLeod, said the player would not be returning to Fiji for similar treatment this time. Naholo returned to play ten weeks later.

'And all Ernie had to offer was a pint of milk a day.'

Benny Hill, 'Ernie (The Fastest Milkman in the West)' (1971)

What about the recuperative powers of gold top milk for fibula stress fractures?

If Naholo's reappearance after ten weeks was declared 'a miracle', what about Joe Mahler's return to international rugby only five weeks after a similar problem? The Harlequins prop (116kg) announced he had broken his fibula playing against Worcester in January 2017. The injury was only diagnosed after Mahler tried to play a game one week later. His club said, 'Joe will undergo a period of rehabilitation and is expected to be fit to play again in four to five weeks.' Mahler duly appeared in February 2017 for England against France.

The media was in raptures and back pages were filled with the news that a diet including two pints of milk per day had majorly contributed to his 'remarkable recovery'. Reminding us of the importance of calcium for healthy bones was helpful but it could have played no more than a marginal role in his recovery: the timescale was too short. Good nutrition may have helped but only because of foundations laid down over years.

It is the long-term good nutrition of elite athletes which is critical to optimising recovery.

Supermen appear at the Super Bowl

Mahler's sensational return to play was trumped less than one day later when Alex Mack appeared at the 51st Super Bowl. Mack (141kg) was a starting offensive centre for the Atlanta Falcons. A fortnight before the event he had sustained a hairline crack of his fibula. He had fractured the same bone in 2014 requiring a plate to be inserted.

Bravely, Mack eschewed the use of South Pacific herbal vegetation and the contents of bottles left by the early morning milkman and was named in the team's line-up. His coach, Dan Quinn, was unsympathetic. Mack was 'going to hurt, but a lot of guys are playing through stuff'. Using local anaesthetic injections, Mack played in the game. He joined two previous owners of fibula fractures who had played in the Super Bowl – Jack Youngblood (1979) and Terrell Owens (2005). All three finished on the losing side.

Wiggins' woes on ice

One week after Mahler and Mack, another superstar succumbed to the curse of a fibula stress injury. Sir Bradley Wiggins was injured practising for Channel 4's alpine spectacular, *The Jump!* Wiggins favoured the Mack approach – ignore it and carry on. However, wiser counsels prevailed and Wiggins reassured fans, 'Seen a specialist, I have a small leg fracture and need to rest for three to six weeks. Good news, no surgery or cast required.' Wiggins saw no need to double his weekly milk bill or fly off to a tropical island.

Nature and nurture

Sensational headlines about wonder leaves and full cream milk sell newspapers but they detract from the hard work of the clinicians and the skills of the S&C teams maintaining an athlete's fitness. This is what allows sportspeople to return with minimal delay once their fracture is comfortable. Far from exhibiting supernormal recuperative powers, Naholo and Mahler appear relatively sluggish in North American terms. Perhaps the only unscientific observation that can be made from these case studies is that the heavier you are the quicker you appear to heal.

Chapter 20

THE FIELDS ARE GREEN, THE SKIES ARE BLUE ...

'The fields are green, the skies are blue ...'

Northamptonshire CCC victory song

NORTHAMPTONSHIRE ARE not a glamour county cricket club.

With Somerset and Gloucestershire, they are one of only three counties never to have won the County Championship. If Somerset, with Botham and Richards in tandem, and Gloucestershire, with W.G. Grace dissecting the bowling, could not triumph, what hope the 'Wantage Road Irregulars'? They didn't win a trophy until 1976 – the 60-over NatWest Cup.

Despite the club's modest success their cricket has inspired local journalists, so much so that Andrew Radd and former *Wisden Cricketers' Almanack* editor Matthew Engel wrote a definitive club history. My father introduced me to Northamptonshire cricket in the late 1950s. The old press box where I sat survives still, in dilapidated splendour. It housed a variety of hacks from local and visiting rags. Fred Speakman was one of them and had been covering local sport since the war. He held court while devouring his lunchbox. Speakman never missed a home cricket day in 30 years and knew most of the gossip around the ground. His successor reported that 'his pockets usually contained a piece of toast, a bundle of cheques and fourpence for the telephone'.

Later, I ventured further afield. In 1968 Surrey played Australia at the Oval. Dad's friend John Morris was my host. Surrey featured the England opener, John Edrich, and Australia such luminaries as Bill

Lawry, Dougie Walters and Graham McKenzie. As I edged into the press box an Australian beckoned me to sit next to him. It was the great Jack Fingleton, a distinguished Test cricketer between the world wars. He played in the 1932–33 Bodyline series but was dropped after the 3rd Adelaide Test for revealing details of an altercation between his captain, Bill Woodfull, and the England manager, Plum Warner. Woodfull had said, 'There are two sides out there. One is trying to play cricket and the other is not!' Disclosing a private conversation between two gentlemen was simply not cricket in the 1930s. To pour further oil on the flames Fingleton and Sir Don Bradman had a series of disagreements that festered before and after the Second World War. I sat for several hours listening to Fingleton, who mixed observations of the present game with reminiscences of days of yore. It was an unforgettable meeting with someone described by E.W. Swanton as, 'surely, as cricket writer and broadcaster, the best his country has'.

Building unbreakable bonds

As a child I spent summers at the County Ground with my ten shilling junior season ticket. It kept my friends and I out of trouble. We saw our heroes close up – swashbuckling Colin Milburn, England wicketkeeper Keith Andrew, and later the bespectacled David Steele. In 1975 Steele became the most unlikely recipient of the BBC *SPOTY* award.

The paucity of success for your club needs to be borne and should never become a barrier to forming an unbreakable bond with your local team. Support should never be determined by media exposure or trophy success, but by the accident of geography of your personal birthing unit or, exceptionally, that of a parent. Most fans spend 95 per cent of their time suffering, but it is a communal affliction and makes any rare victory treasured.

However, times change. So many local youngsters appear in my clinic with a red cast on their arm that matches their Manchester United shirt. When I ask, 'Why don't you support Northampton?' they reply, 'Because they are rubbish, mate.' My riposte of 'rubbish or not, they are still your team' falls on deaf ears.

In 1995 the class and sheer determination of the Springbok-turned-Englishman Allan Lamb came closest to delivering the County Championship Holy Grail. He was 41 and in the last year of his captaincy and his career. It was the summer in which I decided to abandon London and return home after 23 years. That August I made the pilgrimage back to Wantage Road to witness 'Lamby finally bringing home the bacon'. Sadly, it didn't transpire. After leading by 43 points at the end of June we lost out painfully to Warwickshire and finished third.

An opening partnership

The following year was inevitably a case of 'after the Lord Mayor's show' and coincided with my first season of professional involvement at the club. We dropped vertiginously from third from top to third from bottom. I hoped my presence was just coincidental.

Over the next two decades I established an excellent relationship with the club's clinical team, led in turn by physiotherapists Kirk Russell (who went on to work with the national team), Andy Roberts and Barry Goudriaan.

My work with Northamptonshire led to requests from other counties to look after their players and my specific surgical interests meant that the usual patients were fast bowlers. Over the years I formed a view on the relative kindness of different grounds for fast bowlers' ankles and feet. Old Trafford, Trent Bridge and the County Ground, Derby, figured prominently for being unkind; Northampton seemed benign in comparison

A trickle of international cricketers found their way to my clinic. It was a privilege to work with these players and the famous 2005 Ashes series was the pinnacle of my England team experiences. Close working relationships with a side involved in such a momentous series that gripped and galvanised the nation is special. It felt at the time that you were a very small part of a massive machine working collectively to place the best XI on the pitch to realise the dream of winning the Ashes.

Call to alms

Before 2012 my association with Northants had been purely as an orthopaedic surgeon. Daily medical concerns were dealt with by the chief medical officer (CMO), who was a local GP. In 2012 the club's finances were parlous, however, and officials decided that they couldn't afford a very part-time CMO.

After 15 years' unstinting service the doctor departed. This caused problems. The ECB requires each county to have an appointed CMO and there were no volunteers. I was approached by chief executive David Smith, who was always direct.

'Would you be our CMO? We haven't got any money, though.'

It was a difficult decision. The club was in my blood but I was unhappy about the circumstances which had bought about the offer. I accepted, nevertheless, and received excellent support from Barry Goudriaan, who had been the club's lead physiotherapist since 2004. My CMO's duties were different from the more tangential contact I had had with the team as their surgeon. I would be consulted about problems ranging from worrisome moles to the abdominal problems of a player's grandmother.

In 2013, my first full season, the club won promotion to the Championship first division. The team produced scintillating displays, not least from our Aussie fast bowler Trent Copeland. He ran through the opposition in the first two months of the season, giving us a mighty points cushion that would see us through to September. The following year we were relegated without registering a single victory for the first time in 76 years. The increased intensity of the cricket could be judged by medical factors. Of the 20 registered players we had eight with finger fractures, double our historical annual average.

The 2013 T20 competition produced unexpected riches. By May, Northants were in a one-day-game slump having lost 32 of their previous 37 white-ball matches. But from then on, they went on the march and reached only their second finals day three months later. Edgbaston finals day is a special occasion, with the four top T20 teams taking part and their supporters in fine song for a three-game shoot-out to crown the champions.

The splendour of the recently refurbished Edgbaston ground and the team and support staff facilities were a pleasant change from those of our ground. We were fourth favourites with Essex, Hampshire and Surrey blocking our way. As Chapter 3 recalls, we made it to the final against Surrey, but playing two high-pressure games in a single day took its toll and one of our batsmen was withdrawn from the final with a wrist injury, to everybody's disappointment.

Persistent rain delayed the scheduled 6pm start to the final and it was almost postponed to the following morning. The relationship between the sides was testy, particularly between David Willey and Surrey's Jade Dernbach. Cameron White anchored our innings and, as in the semi-final, kept his wicket intact until the end. I sat in the dugout next to our head coach, David Ripley, as Surrey replied. We pinched ourselves in disbelief as Surrey got further and further behind and Willey finished them off with a hat-trick at the death.

The Northants side invited the support staff to join in celebrating our first cup for 21 years. We mounted the victory dais as champagne corks popped and fireworks went off behind. As we bounced up and down I spotted my wife in the stands in front of me making unmistakeable gestures indicating that I needed to get off and act my age. We were hours late for a family social engagement and arrived after midnight. I was in the doghouse but still wagging my tail. The team awarded me one of the T20 medals as a 'thank you' for my season's work. It was better than any financial remuneration and almost worth incurring my wife's wrath for. The year finished with an open-top bus ride and reception at the town hall for players and staff.

We reached another T20 final in 2015, only to be defeated by Lancashire. In 2016, we won again against Durham, who had proven superstars in Ben Stokes, Paul Collingwood and Mark Wood. The county got home in the last over in heavy rain after a match-winning innings from Josh Cobb.

Because of financial constraints, Northants went through 2016 with a squad of 18 players – one of the smallest in the country. Such small numbers leave little room for injuries and put considerable importance on balancing play with adequate rest. We needed luck and got it: there were no hand fractures all season. By 2017 our squad had grown by one player but injuries reduced coach Ripley's options. A helmet strike to a batsman left the player with significant concussion and unable to play for eight weeks – one of the most prolonged recoveries nationally in recent seasons. However, we kept our championship promotion aspirations going until the season's last day, when we lost out by five points having had five points controversially deducted for slow play. Promotion was achieved at the end of 2019, although the coronavirus pandemic meant that the truncated 2020 season was re-engineered.

In ten seasons Northants sustained more than 40 finger fractures. Effectively, the side can expect to be one player short at any time during the season from this injury. Add in the ubiquitous sore backs, shin splints and tight 'hammies', and playing resources get thinly spread.

Most cricketers' salaries are relatively modest, and historically many needed to supplement their incomes during the off-season. Some worked locally in non-sport-related occupations or studied for further qualifications and others followed the swallows south. Younger players have opportunities to gain experience and maturity. Others may go on organised tours and training camps and some may pick up lucrative overseas T20 contracts.

These winter trips can be a headache for the medical team, particularly when players secure weekend-grade cricket contracts in the southern hemisphere. Medical support may be lacking there and players can nurse injuries without proper treatment. The worst scenario is a player returning for pre-season with a chronic injury that leaves them unfit for weeks. Most players start pre-season training in the new year, while others appear in dribs and drabs in the following months. Overseas players may be tied into contracts at home that overlap with the English season. International players may come back late from tours and others will come in for white-ball cricket only. Jose Mourinho would really have something to complain about if his key centre-back was injured moonlighting in Melbourne or if squad members didn't turn up until September, having accepted better offers elsewhere.

Parachuting in foreign recruits can have its problems – not just in cricket. In the 1990s, Northampton Saints played at Saracens in an early season rugby match. How would our new Antipodean forward shape up? All was well until deep into the second half when he started crawling around the middle of the pitch while the game continued around him. Physio Phil Pask and I ran on and enquired after his health. He replied, 'I've lost my contact lens.' We urged him to re-join the fray and use his other eye but he told us that he was blind in that eye. No one had had time to examine him and discover this between his leaving the plane at Heathrow and starting his first match.

Beyond the wealthiest sports clubs, medical teams are rarely involved in decisions over signings – especially those of overseas players. It is cloak and dagger stuff until the media release is issued. I try to do some research on our new star batsman/striker/prop-forward. How many games did they play last season? What injuries have they sustained? It is depressing when the latest team saviour makes one of their first priorities a visit to the physiotherapists to sort out their chronic back problem aggravated by a long flight. Professional players should provide evidence of satisfactory health and screening, such as for heart checks. Trying to trace their home country MRI scans, operation records or echocardiograms (heart scans for abnormalities) can be testing and some sporting medical departments I've been part of have been served up a few challenges.

Seasons in the sun

Soccer games last 90 minutes – whatever the competition – and football's league structure has changed little in over 60 years. The FA Cup has its own traditional rhythm – set times for rounds and a Wembley final each May.

The cricket season is shorter, has a timetable that is tweaked annually, and has three principal competitions – the four-day red-ball County Championship, the one-day white-ball 50-over Royal London Cup, and the T20 white-ball format introduced in 2003. Each competition places different emphasis on the skills and stamina of its participants. The Championship was split into two divisions in 2000. Before 1988, games were played over three days but, bizarrely, from 1988 to 1992, some games were played over three days and others over four. Now all are played over four days. Test matches are usually played over five days with occasional variations including 'timeless Tests'. Some people would prefer four-day Tests. In my youth, Tests started on Thursdays and finished on Tuesdays with the Sunday as a rest day. Tom Graveney used the Sunday of a 1969 West Indies Test to play in his own testimonial game at Luton. He did not play for England again. From 1969 to 2009 the Sunday league could interrupt the Championship game that straddled it.

The number of balls per over was not finally agreed until 40 years ago. In the 1880s, four-ball overs were common. The southern hemisphere experimented with up to eight balls at various times until 1979. Now we have compromised on six. Over the last 50 years, the game has toyed with 20-, 40-, 45-, 50-, 55- and 60-over one-day formats. From 2021, we will have the 100-ball competition with ten balls per over delivered by one or two bowlers. The English season's structure is resembling shifting sands in a storm and the Championship is increasingly bookending the season. The 100-ball format will force further change.

From 1962 the denouement of the season was traditionally the Lord's one-day final. This disappeared as various formats were tried and discarded. Now the riotous Edgbaston T20 finals day is the flagship event in the one-day calendar.

Would football ever make so many fundamental changes to its configuration and playing times? Have all these changes succeeded in increasing playing and spectating participation in an ever-congested sporting market? Sport England's Active People 2016 survey reported that cricket lost 19 per cent of its players at all levels in the previous decade. This covered a period when T20 competitions were being introduced. Many other sports lost numbers during the decade that covered a home Olympiad. Boxing overtook our national summer sport in terms of fitness choices.

Lord's is cricket's cathedral and the game can be likened to the Church of England. Faced with falling congregations, it forlornly looks for the right form of service to present to the masses. However, changes have alienated traditionalists while failing to arrest the fall in numbers coming into the game.

All involved must adapt and predict how these alterations will affect performance, playing staff requirements and participants' health. The medical care of the professional cricketer has evolved enormously over the last 20 years and the ECB has established an inspiring centre at Loughborough University which supports professional players at all levels. The central support supplied to county doctors has been equally impressive.

Local sporting family dynasties

Like lower league football players, some good cricketers move on. Northamptonshire is not traditionally the first port of call for national selectors and cricketers based at Northampton and selected for England do so despite rather than because of their club allegiance.

It is always sad when locally born lads seek pastures new – especially when you have witnessed their early development. David Willey to Yorkshire and Graeme Swann to Nottinghamshire are prime examples. Their international careers flourished after their moves.

David Willey's father, Peter, was an established international cricketer and umpire and is remembered for the oft-mentioned quote, 'The bowler's Holding, the batsman's Willey,' during the 1976 Oval Test match. The quote is attributed to the broadcaster Brian Johnston but is probably apocryphal. The Willey family remain strong supporters of Northants cricket and I even persuaded Peter to act as a celebrity croupier for a charity casino evening.

Graeme Swann's father, Ray, taught PE locally and was an outstanding all-rounder for my local junior club. In later years we played veterans rugby together. He was a natural at that, too. With those genes, it was not unexpected that his two sons, Alec and Graeme, would become fine first-class cricketers. Both started at Northants the year I returned to Northampton. Three years later, Graeme toured South Africa with England at the age of 20. His infectious personality is as genuine in person as it is in the media and on *Strictly Come Dancing*.

The 1999–2000 winter tour was led by coach Duncan Fletcher, a no-nonsense Zimbabwean. Despite Swanny making his debut in a one-day international he did not endear himself to management. Famously, he overslept and missed the team bus, twice. Another seven years passed before Swanny got his chance again; he went on to became one of the greatest English spin bowlers since the war.

The years 2000 to 2007 were Swanny's wilderness years. My village pub is three miles from the County Ground and became the unofficial watering hole of some players. There, I was able to keep up with the bacchanalian tendencies of certain team members. One overseas player had to be extricated out of a 'convenience cubicle' looking very green.

Swanny was a village regular and New Year's Eve fancy dress parties were his forte. He became great friends with my offspring. One night I got home from the hospital to find Swanny sprawled on the sofa with a vice-like grip on the TV remote control.

For years the county cricketers would participate in our village six-a-side competition – five has-beens or never-will-bes plus a professional. Swanny played a big part in making sure these annual events prospered, one year joining my mix of mediocre medics and opening the batting with me. I had to face the menacing South African fast bowler Andre Nel – albeit bowling off three paces. The day before, Nel had appeared at Lord's against England in the NatWest series final and taken Michael Vaughan's wicket. I glimpsed the first ball as it left his hand, heard a swoosh and took up a cowardly defensive pose with my bat held high. Matters got worse. Later, I had to bowl to Michael Hussey, the Australian Test batsman. My donkey drops and daisy cutters were despatched disdainfully to the boundary. I avoided the ignominy of conceding 36 runs in an over – but it was a close-run thing. Another time, one seasoned pro deposited my full toss over the sight screen and said, 'That's for the injection you gave me last month.' It was certainly a new angle on sledging.

In 2004 Swanny moved to Trent Bridge during a fractious period in Northants' history. His autobiography, *The Breaks Are Off*, chronicled his altercations with the county's coach. He was particularly annoyed at the banning of the club's traditional victory song, commenting that the club 'was in danger of losing its identity as the county's cricket club, unless there is a conscious effort to rebuild the sense of pride and kinship for the town and people'.

I feel that this has been achieved. Since I became CMO in 2012 I have been helped enormously by David Ripley and his team. All are rooted in Northamptonshire cricket; I have known many of them since their own playing days. The club has returned to its roots. It is a modest and honest club still capable of turning over the big boys in various cricketing formats. The performance management team understand and respect the efforts of the medical team. It certainly makes our lives easier.

Chapter 21

THE SKIES ARE GREY?

IN 2017 Northamptonshire were pushing for Championship promotion but daily attendance for their seven home games averaged just 500.

Low attendance is why many of the 18 county cricket clubs are not financially sustainable as independent entities. Gate money revenues will not buy new tractors for the groundsmen or repaint the pavilion, let alone pay the employees. No number of rock concerts performed at your ground will balance the books. Clubs are dependent on central funding.

Television revenues, live attendances for international cricket and T20 games, and merchandising are the currency. English cricket needed a successful 2019 World Cup and the 2020 100-ball competition to bolster income streams and promote participation by youngsters. These are county cricket's saviours. In return, county cricket needs to identify and nurture future England stars. Sadly, these dreams turned into a nightmare when the COVID-19 pandemic decimated the 2020 summer season. As a pragmatist I appreciate that Northamptonshire, Derbyshire, Leicestershire and Gloucestershire might be first in the firing line if the 18-team structure was reduced. As a traditionalist I think such a move would be a great shame.

However, central power might help preserve and promote the game in the face of so much competition; while stifling individualism, it allows decisions to be made for the greater good of all. At no time was this better demonstrated than in the summer of 2020 as will be explained later in Chapter 32.

More than football and rugby, individual cricket clubs are beholden to their masters. In 2000, elite male England players were awarded central contracts, allowing better control of their cricketing workload. The sport remains decades ahead of English men's rugby in this respect. Senior soccer clubs would never accede to more centralised power.

Belatedly, women's cricket received support with central contracts offered to leading players in 2014. This ushered in a fully professional era for the women. England women's rugby was five years behind, offering contracts to players in 2019. Better promotion of female participation in cricket is afoot, including closer alignment with the men's game. In 2009, *Wisden* made Claire Taylor one of its five cricketers of the year and in 2014 created a separate section for women's cricket. Four years later its front cover depicted Anya Shrubsole, and three females were included in its famous five.

The ECB has turned its thoughts increasingly to cricket's governance, with policies and regulations designed to improve player welfare at all levels. As the ECB holds the purse-strings, these changes can have real teeth compared to soccer. As explained in Chapter 17, in the 2018 World Cup, FIFA admitted it couldn't enforce its own regulations on head injury assessment when Morocco resorted to face slapping as part of concussion management.

Cricket has changed quickly and medical teams have had to react. County players may have one-day or four-day duties only. Overseas players fly in for T20 games and then leave for similar competitions elsewhere in the world. Clinicians and S&C teams need to be ready for these fluxes, predict when pinch points will arise and prepare and treat players accordingly. It is understood that athletes perform better and are healthier when not over- or under-worked. Sudden uplifts in activity followed by downtime can play havoc with spines, muscles and tendons. This is why, pre-season, it is so important to reintroduce 'sporting bodies' to incremental workloads and keep them below breaking point throughout the season.

Americans might have got it wrong this time

How athletic is cricket? The Americans have come up with an interesting assessment.

In 2005, American heart specialists provided guidelines for people with cardiac complaints. They classified sporting pursuits to aid the prescription of suitable exercise regimes for compromised patients. It was known as the Mitchell Classification and was endorsed by doctors in Europe. It is still in use and updated.

Sports were analysed in three ways. The first was 'impact risk', such as concussion exposure. Cricket was awarded 'impact not expected' alongside riflery and archery. Clearly, the Americans had not seen the 1976 footage of 38-year-old Brian Close, bareheaded and without chest protector or arm guards, facing 97mph deliveries from Michael Holding. The hard, red 'cherry' hit him repeatedly on his torso leaving him black and blue afterwards but unbowed.

Sports were then graded according to their perceived 'dynamic and static components'. The former gauged heart stress and the latter a sport's effect on blood pressure. Cricket was placed in the lowest category for each, alongside yoga and curling. Synchronised swimming and softball were placed in more strenuous categories. Americans believe cricket should be the preserve of octogenarians on blood thinners and fitted with pacemakers. We still have a lot of educating to do stateside.

So where might these surprising conclusions have come from? Traditionally, many cricketers did not look athletic and a few were clearly overweight; sports science and cricket were not a match made in heaven. I recall arranging for a professional cricketer to rehabilitate with a professional rugby team following knee ligament reconstruction, because of rugby's greater experience of such injuries. The player was horrified at the torture he was subjected to.

The length of the game and periods sitting in the pavilion did not help preconceived prejudices; cricket was more about skill, honed technique and what players possessed between their ears. Research in the 1950s concluded that energy expenditure during a Test match only slightly outflanked the effort required to spectate at the game – although the study did include player time spent watching from the balcony. Over 50 years later similar conclusions were being drawn by some observers. However, other research had changed views. A South African study in 2000 demonstrated that cricketers possessed similar strength and short-sprint speed to rugby players.

Cricket in all its formats has become increasingly demanding physiologically and the one-day game has improved fielding standards and athleticism. Placing a ball in the top tier of the balcony is no longer the preserve of the top order. Tail-enders come in and flay the ball to cow corner with aplomb. During a 50-over one-day international, cricketers might engage in 200 sprints with distances covered potentially greater than those of a Premier League footballer in a single game. Furthermore, recent research suggests that batting can involve three to four times higher energy expenditure than the 1950s calculations. During one-day batting, average heart rates frequently reach 75 per cent of maximum – around 150 beats per minute. Bowling spells reveal similarly high cardiac demands.

Estimates of injury rates vary, but the greater risk occurs in one-day formats. Using daily overs bowled per day (40 for T20; 100 for 50 overs; 96 for red-ball games), I calculated that injuries in T20 were between two and three times higher than in 50-over games and four times higher than the longest format. Players need to train and prepare for different challenges, to reduce injury and improve split-second decision-making while working under considerable physiological stresses.

Apologies to our American cousins, but cricket is not a game for the faint-hearted. It never was.

'Anyone who had a heart'
Dionne Warwick, 'Anyone Who Had a Heart' (1963)

Medical screening is used to identify early the presence of diseases such as cancer or congenital (from birth) disease.

While compassion should be at the heart of all medicine, health economics need to be applied to such programmes. Is screening the best use of limited resources? Who should be tested, what is the cost and how many lives will be saved? These arguments came to the fore during the 2020 coronavirus pandemic. Enter the debate over cardiac screening in the young (particularly sports people) for which cardiologists worldwide cannot agree the merits.

One recent frightening image was Fabrice Muamba's resuscitation at White Hart Lane in 2012. He suffered a cardiac arrest while playing for Bolton Wanderers against Tottenham in the FA Cup. His heart stopped for 78 minutes but he survived thanks to the efforts of a spectating cardiologist, the clubs' medical teams and the emergency services. Others have not been so lucky. Since 1945 at least 83 professional footballers worldwide have died from cardiac causes during games. In the lower reaches of the sport, many more have perished.

Cricket has been luckier with three recorded sudden cardiac deaths (SCD) directly related to playing the game. Most high-profile was suffered by Wilf Slack, the England and Middlesex player, who died in 1989 aged 34. He had been investigated for blackouts, before collapsing and dying while playing in The Gambia.

SCD is the most common cause of death of young athletes during sport. Only 20 per cent have any history suggesting such an impending tragedy. It devastates families, friends and communities and may impact on other youngsters becoming involved in the activity. It can be caused by peculiar electrical activity and structural heart changes. What argument can there be for not offering all young sports people cardiac screening? Since 2008, the ECB has offered screening for all players involved in county cricket.

In America, an average of 150 youngsters die annually on the sports field from SCD. However, 14,000 youngsters die in accidents each year, 8,000 suffer a non-sports-related sudden death, 4,100 are murdered and 2,200 commit suicide. Should scarce resources be targeted more at teenage mental health, road safety and crime prevention? Is it ethical to just target sports-minded youngsters? Youngsters participating in sport may have a two to five times increased risk of SCD compared to a sedentary friend. However, 65 per cent of American youngsters dying from SCD are high school students. Should screening take place in senior schools rather than in professional sports organisations, as 40 per cent of SCD in youngsters occurs away from sport, including 13 per cent during sleep?

SCD is variably reported to occur in between 1 and 3/100,000 young athletes, but 1 in 300 youngsters may harbour a cardiac condition that may lead to SCD. Screening can wrongly indicate that a problem is present (false positives). The results of strenuous training can alter the appearance of electrocardiograms (ECGs, which check the heart's rhythm and electrical activity) in young athletes, causing concern and prompting additional investigations. It requires an experienced physician to provide safe advice. The effects of restricting youngsters' sport and saddling parents and sporting organisations with extra medical bills must be considered.

America restricts screening to a medical history and examination but some affected youngsters can be missed. ECGs and echocardiograms – scans that look at the heart and nearby blood vessels – are more expensive but are favoured by many European countries. In Italy, everybody taking part in organised sport must undergo heart screening. In the UK, the charity CRY (Cardiac Risk in the Young) offers awareness, education and mobile screening to schools and sporting organisations.

Such programmes will not eliminate all SCDs. Current UK government policy is that there is insufficient evidence to warrant widespread screening of our youth. Sports such as cricket do screen, however, and have identified unsuspected heart problems in seemingly fit teenagers and young adults. In 2016, at the age of 26, the England batsman James Taylor was diagnosed with a rare heart condition. He retired immediately and had a defibrillator implanted. Intense exercise can lead to life-threatening heart irregularities. Chest trauma from a strongly hit cricket ball can cause death from a cardiac arrest in previously healthy individuals. Peter Bruckner, the ex-Australian team doctor, identified 13 such cricket deaths in Australia alone.

All major sports have improved their standards of urgent medical care at grounds. Team clinicians regularly attend refresher courses, and umpires, coaches and other staff are encouraged to become familiar with resuscitation techniques. It is all about the immediate assembly of a team singing from the same hymn sheet.

The debate over who, how and when youngsters' hearts should be screened will go on. Cricket has pinned its colours to the mast and instituted a comprehensive programme for its sport.

'You can leave your hat on'
Randy Newman, 'You Can Leave Your Hat On' (1972)

Ever since the first village blacksmith held a cricket ball in his hand there have been concerns about head injuries.

In 1870 George Summers died several days after being struck on the head at Lord's while batting for Nottinghamshire. The next batsman arrived at the crease with his head wrapped in a towel for protection.

The first prototype safety helmet is credited to the wife of Middlesex and England batsman 'Patsy' Hendren in 1933. Concern over serious head injuries had reached a peak the winter before during the infamous Bodyline series in Australia, when Harold Larwood and Bill Voce had terrorised Aussie batsmen by bowling into their bodies and Australian wicketkeeper Bertie Oldfield had fractured his skull while top-edging a Larwood delivery. The English skipper Douglas Jardine was demonised and angry exchanges reached government level.

The good Mrs Hendren produced a rubber cricket cap embellished with side flaps of the same material to protect her husband against beamers from the likes of Learie (later Lord) Constantine. It made Hendren look like a sporting Sherlock Holmes. It was not a good look and the cap did not catch on. However, the battery of fast and short bowling from Australian and Caribbean quickies in the 1970s prompted permanent change.

Even England fast bowlers delivered balls that whistled around your ears. In 1975, debutant and batting rabbit Ewan Chatfield was holding up the English bowlers trying to finish off the New Zealand innings. He had contributed to a last wicket stand of 44 when he received a John Lever bouncer, which fractured his skull and caused him to swallow his tongue. The quick-thinking England physio, Bernard Thomas, administered cardiac resuscitation to save his life. Chatfield played 42 more Tests for the Kiwis.

In 1977, Dennis Amiss, the England opener, played while wearing a helmet during the Australian pirate World Series. He was booed by the crowd and must have felt like a Christian facing the lions in the Colosseum. The fibreglass headpiece had been made by a motorcycle helmet manufacturer and had a visor that 'could withstand a shotgun blast at 10 yards'. It later retailed at £29.

How quickly did it catch on? I investigated by reading my collection of *Wisden*. The magazine awards five people the accolade of cricketer of the year and a photograph accompanies each honouree's write-up. From 1979 to 1982 the 11 batsmen-winners appeared bareheaded or in traditional headgear. Only in 1982 was Allan Border depicted with skull side protectants.

In *Wisden*'s editor comments on topical cricketing issues between 1979 and 1982 helmets failed to escape attention. In 1979 a *Wisden* article titled 'The Ugly Helmet' noted that the Test and County Cricket Board, which preceded the ECB, had ruled that helmet wearing gave fielders an unfair advantage – despite Derbyshire's Philip Russell fracturing his cheekbone when the ball lodged inside his helmet visor when fielding. A year later, the Marylebone Cricket Club (MCC) were minded to outlaw helmets, especially for fielders. They retreated after considering the repercussions of an injured player being denied their use. Fear of the law is not a new sporting phenomenon. In 1981, in an article titled 'Donning the Helmet', then editor John Woodcock acknowledged the changes on safety grounds but remained unhappy. He believed that protectants encouraged 'bumpers' – very fast, short-pitched deliveries designed to make the batsman duck – which he felt had wrought the helmet revolution and rendered the cricketer underneath anonymous. It was 'sartorially and aesthetically an objectional trend', he said. The following year Woodcock claimed that helmets had increased the number of 'bouncers', particularly the number aimed at lower-order batsmen. Ex-England skipper Tony Greig and the great West Indian batsman Viv Richards agreed. The latter regarded helmets as cowardly and did not wear one through to his retirement in 1991.

Those arguments mirrored the simultaneous debate over car seatbelts, which were made compulsory in 1983. We then quickly felt exposed without our safety devices. For similar reasons most cricketers became wedded to their helmets. However, debate continues as to whether helmets have encouraged intimidatory bowling. Are umpires less quick to step in and warn bowlers of such tactics? Ex-England skipper Alastair Cook and others have raised concerns over whether certain helmets might slow reflexes and become distracting.

Helmets are here to stay but do not prevent head injuries completely. In 1986 England batsman Mike Gatting suffered a nasty facial injury while trying to hook Malcolm Marshall in a one-day international in Jamaica. Such was the impact that fragments of his nose were embedded in the ball. My cycling buddy, Allan Lamb, replaced Gatting with some trepidation. Lamby remembers that he 'walked off a nick' from Marshall even though the umpire didn't give him out – for the first time in his career. Up next was another Northampton friend, Peter Willey, who was caught off Marshall's bowling.

In 2014, two terrible incidents affected the thinking on player protection. In July of that year England wicketkeeper Craig Kieswetter sustained awful facial injuries playing for Somerset at Northampton. A delivery from Peter Willey's son David squeezed between grill and helmet peak as the batsman tried to hook a bouncer. It was my second year as Northants club CMO. Despite facial reconstructive surgery, Kieswetter was left with visual disturbances and retired the next year.

In the following November Phillip Hughes's death shocked the sporting world. He was hit behind the ear attempting to hook a bouncer from Sean Abbott while playing at the Sydney Cricket Ground. The injury split a major artery to his brain and he died two days later without regaining consciousness. It took two years for the coronial inquest to begin. It concluded that Hughes had suffered a dreadful accident for which no one was to blame.

Various new helmet designs were introduced, including those with neck guards, and in 2016 the ECB required all batsmen, wicketkeepers and close fielders to cover up. Recommendations were made about the grill design and the gap between grill and helmet.

Batsmen's improved strength and technique coupled with increasing bat weight is worrisome, however, particularly in T20 cricket. Bowlers and umpires must feel like sitting ducks in a fairground shooting gallery. In 2018 I tended an injured square-leg umpire who was hit 30 yards from the action.

The ECB has put considerable resources into researching helmet strike events and concussion. Every ball bowled in county and Test cricket is recorded and every head injury analysed. This provides details of ball speed, point of impact and where the ball finished. Helmet damage can be analysed and lessons learnt, leading to safer helmet design and knowledge of which type of impacts cause most damage.

Like other contact sports, cricket has detailed guidelines for assessing concussion victims. Before every season, players undergo baseline tests to assess their normal neuropsychological state. The answers to carefully designed questions and the results of tests after concussive episodes are recorded and return-to-play criteria are mapped out, mirroring measures adopted in other sports.

In 2018, English cricket followed Australia by introducing concussion substitutes. This allows clinicians time to fully assess injured players and reduces the pressure to return them to the game. In June of that year Lancashire's Danny Lamb became the first concussion substitute, replacing Joe Mennie in a game against Worcestershire. The next day, Max Waller subbed in for Jack Leach for Somerset against Surrey. Concussion rates are low compared to other sports such as rugby and horse racing but research by John Orchard showed that concussion numbers reported in Australian cricket doubled in the season of Phillip Hughes's death. The English experience is similar, with reported head injuries quadrupling in the summer after the tragedy. Cricket had to take this issue very seriously. Undoubtedly some of this is greater awareness and players being willing to admit they have symptoms, and it mirrors the reporting trends in other sports, particularly rugby. Most counties will experience at least one concussive episode annually.

Within the general population between 20 per cent and 30 per cent experience long-term persistent post-concussion symptoms so why should cricketers be immune? There is anecdotal evidence that the effect of a concussive episode on a batsman can have repercussions long after they return to play, by adversely affecting performance.

Cricket and rugby are involved in research to assess the use of saliva testing in head injury diagnosis. This follows evidence that road traffic accident patients have altered levels of small particles known as microRNAs, which help predict brain injury severity. If proven, this will help eliminate some of the dilemmas in decision-making concerning concussed sporting athletes.

We cannot prevent another concussion in cricket. However, the measures being taken on many fronts – helmet design, helmet strike analysis, concussion protocols, player education, concussion substitutes and innovative research – are combining to make it a safer environment for the short- and long-term welfare of the player.

White rabbits, anyone?

> *'One pill makes you larger*
> *And one pill makes you small*
> *And the ones that mother gives you*
> *Don't do anything at all.'*

Jefferson Airplane, 'White Rabbit' (1969)

Professional cricketers have all the strengths and weaknesses of their peers.

A 2013 government survey revealed that 15 per cent of 16–59-year-olds had used class A drugs, such as cocaine or ecstasy. Some cricketers joined their ranks. Lord Ian Botham was banned for two months in 1986 for smoking cannabis and Ed Giddins was banned for 18 months for cocaine use in 1996.

The death of Surrey's Tom Maynard in 2012 shook the entire cricketing community from any complacency. The 23-year-old was electrocuted on a railway line fleeing from police. He was four times over the alcohol limit and had taken cocaine and ecstasy.

Now the ECB has a comprehensive illicit drugs policy (IDP). Education, support, monitoring and appropriate rehabilitation are its central tenets. The IDP uses out-of-competition testing on hair samples to identify the use of substances such as stimulants, narcotics and cannabinoids. A small length of scalp hair can detect cannabis use in the previous three months. Other sports and industry have similar policies.

A first violation is confidential and a welfare issue. The player is counselled and a programme of rehabilitation and monitoring agreed. A second violation is more serious and results in bigger fines, stricter treatment regimens and the wider involvement of the player's senior management team. A third violation means a year-long ban and prompts questions about the player's future cricketing career. This range of actions is continually being reviewed by the ECB. It adds to my potential portfolio of responsibilities and is markedly different to my normal day-to-day activities in the operating theatre. The difficulties of dealing with recreational drug abuse as a confidential welfare issue was brought into the spotlight when England batsman Alex Hales was outed for a second offence and lost his place in the English World Cup-winning team of 2019.

A drinking culture has traditionally been part of many sports and, in recent times, has led to ugly incidents appearing on social media sites such as YouTube. The use of illegal drugs is in another league, however. In the past it would have seemed absurd that players would take performance-enhancing substances. The game's evolution, in terms of formats and financial rewards, has changed that.

Incidents in American baseball should be a warning to all. The home-run hitting feats of big 'sluggers' such as Barry Bonds and Mark McGwire have been tarnished by admissions of anabolic steroid abuse. Mark McGwire's 1998 confession caused the sales of his preferred poison to increase by 1,000 per cent, such was other players' desire to copy the miscreant. In 2001, 8 per cent of male US high school athletes admitted trying steroids.

In 2003, baseball's random and anonymous testing revealed that between 5 per cent and 7 per cent of players were using steroids and from 2004 players were tested annually. The first offence penalty was a ten-day suspension. A consequence of this 'get tough' policy was players swopping to human growth hormone (HGH). The 2007 Mitchell Report detailed widespread use of steroids and HGH, naming and shaming 89 Major League Baseball players. Testing was made biannual but pre-season HGH testing was not agreed until 2012. Now, a first-time offender is suspended for 80 games. Mitchell emphasised that the whole baseball community was responsible for eradicating drug abuse.

The T20 format has affected many aspects of cricket. Bat technology has altered, for example, with size, shape, weight distribution and materials all being investigated to create a weapon capable of producing a six-run hitting feast. Technique, good reflexes and strength are essential, too, and are the result of years of practice and conditioning. Even Test cricket scoring rates have increased in recent years. Spectators must believe in what they are seeing, which requires a robust testing programme for illegal drug use. It has taken time.

WADA was established in 1999 to control drug-taking in sport and produces lists of prohibited drugs. Cricket signed up in 2006. Every pre-season, cricketers attend educational meetings and are provided with a 'kit bag card' for reference. Advice is readily accessible.

The first cricketer banned for performance-enhancing drug use was one of *Wisden*'s five cricketers of the 20th century, Shane Warne. In 2003 the Aussie 'leggie' took a diuretic that he claimed his mother had produced to help him lose fluid and improve his appearance. One wag produced a banner at a match: 'Warnie, it's been worth the weight'.

Supplements can catch players out. Vitamins and trace elements are frequently advised but their origin needs consideration. Players should use sources that have been batch-tested for the inclusion of banned substances. This reduces but does not eliminate risk.

WADA's 'whereabouts rule' has caused controversy. It was introduced in 2004 and required athletes to specify their location for one hour daily to enable random drug testing. Certain Indian cricketers, backed by the Board of Control for Cricket in India, objected and cited concerns over security and privacy and, until compromise was reached in 2011, India risked being listed as WADA non-compliant. FIFA and UEFA have expressed similar concerns over infringements of footballers' personal rights.

Over the last decade or so the holes in cricket's drug-testing net have become smaller. Both small and big fry have been caught. In 2006 the Pakistan fast bowlers Shoaib Akhtar and Mohammed Asif tested positive for the anabolic steroid nandrolone. Both were banned but had their cases overturned on appeal. Asif cited a lack of awareness in Asia of the dangers of contaminated supplements. In 2011 Sri Lankan batsman Upul Tharanga tested positive for the steroids prednisolone and prednisone. He claimed they were in a herbal remedy but was banned for three months. The same year West Indian batswoman Treymane Smartt was banned for five months for diuretic abuse. And in 2014 Pakistani all-rounder Kashif Siddiq was banned for two years for testing positive for an undisclosed drug.

The present ECB anti-doping policy is a weighty document that underlines the determination of sporting authorities to root out any performance-enhancing drug-taking culture. The unannounced appearance of a drug-testing team is common in UK sport. They arrive, identify a safe centre of operations and inform players on the selected list. It is a necessary inconvenience that is part of modern professional sporting life. For cricket, it prevents a baseball-like scandal and maintains an even playing square for all.

Back to black

'And I tread a troubled track
My odds are stacked
I'll go back to black'

Amy Winehouse, 'Back to Black' (2006)

Cricket has a problem with the mental well-being of some active and retired players.

Many sports have athletes who experience mental health concerns. This reflects society's struggles. Danny Rose, the Tottenham and England footballer, was very candid about his depression during the 2018 World Cup build-up. Likewise, later, the Manchester United player Michael Carrick. Snooker heroes such as Ronnie O'Sullivan, Willie Thorne and Mark Allen have openly discussed their fights with the demons. Every sport has similar tales.

Early talent identification can take its toll. From 2010 to 2017 the number of teenage suicides nationally increased by 67 per cent. In 2018, 18-year-old snowboarder Ellie Soutter took her life. Her father felt that elite performance pressures may have contributed, saying, 'Mental health awareness needs to be really looked at and made more public,' in young athletes. He felt that five head injuries, including a bad concussion three months before her death, may have been a factor.

I saw a young injured sportsperson requiring surgery. The patient was mature and engaging and became an Olympic gold medallist at 21. The injury was a major setback, but, with a healthy attitude to its management the athlete came back firing on all cylinders. I wondered how it must feel to reach such a goal so young. Most of us work hard and progressively achieve experience, knowledge and skills through most of our adult lives. This is different. This athlete had an excellent personal and sporting support network to add to their own natural equanimity. Others are not so lucky. Different athletes handle early success differently but what happens when the buzz of training and competing has gone, when requests for interviews stop? Those remaining in sport via coaching, mentoring or the media may find it easier. Phenomenal early success needs as much careful handling as the more common sporting rejection.

The increasing segmentation of cricket's different formats can increase pressure on its participants. A contract only for one-day competition leaves players twiddling their thumbs for the early months of the season. Half the sides will not advance to the competitions' quarter-finals and it is all over in less than six weeks. A smack on that untwiddled thumb during fielding practice in late June may signal no T20 action until next year. It can be devastating.

In the four-day format, a batsman could collect a 'golden pair' (out first ball both innings) even though his side goes on to win. Despite joyous celebrations around him, he knows he hasn't contributed to the triumph. In football and rugby, there is usually time to atone for one or two mistakes. Cricket remains an individual game played within a team setting.

A run of poor performances can leave players fearful of their place in the side and this can happen at any time in players' careers – the youngster trying to establish himself and gain a new contract; the veteran fighting slowing reflexes and aching joints – Winston Churchill's 'black dog days'.

Long international tours can have their victims. Media attention intensifies when form disappears and the player is relegated to bringing on the interval drinks. England batsmen such as Michael Trescothick and Jonathan Trott have been open about the difficulties and anxieties leading to their decisions to quit overseas trips and curtail their international careers.

External pressures can affect performance. Relatives' health concerns or coping with unhappy spouses struggling in new environments can adversely impact on-field performances. Overseas signings and players moving from other counties might have to leave settled families at home. Homesickness can affect players of any seniority.

Early September is the saddest time of the cricket season. Who will be retained and who will be released? Reviews are scheduled and the news (good or bad) presented. Seeing team-mates leave after seasons of unstinting club service is painful, although like taxes and death it comes to everyone. Some will choose when to retire, some will be forced by injury to retire and others will be ushered through the door. Some will find employment with another team but for many it means exploring the wider world. Ben Stokes admitted, 'I'm not a person to think about the future. I very much live in the present, only dealing with what's on my plate. Life after cricket can be planned nearer the time.' Encouragement and support to attain non-cricketing qualifications, coaching badges and experience media training is available and supported by the Professional Cricketers' Association (PCA).

The women's game is becoming more popular, professional and subject to increased media attention, and strains are beginning to show. In 2016 two English players required 'time-out' due to anxiety and depressive episodes. Both returned to the game but one, Sarah Taylor, retired two years later citing chronic anxiety.

Perhaps the major worry is the post-cricket years. Retired elite cricketers are reported to be four times more likely to admit to anxiety and twice as likely to suffer from depression than non-sporting counterparts. Phil Hopley of psychiatric specialists Cognacity reported in 2013 that one-third of professional athletes felt out of control in the immediate two years after retirement. Others suffered from anxiety, lack of self-esteem, despair and depression.

David Frith's 2001 book *Silence of the Heart* assessed the suicides of more than 100 cricketers. He calculated that British ex-cricketers were 75 per cent more likely to commit suicide than their peers. The suicide rate for British former cricketers was 1.8 per cent, in Australia it was 2.7 per cent, the rate in New Zealand was 3.9 per cent and in South Africa it was 4.1 per cent. In the book, Mike Brearley, ex-England Test captain and psychoanalyst, wrote, 'The uncertainty of cricket is not always glorious or exciting; it can be disillusioning and anxiety-creating.' Frith pondered whether cricket turned susceptible personalities into 'brooding, insecure and ultimately self-destructive men'. Later, following Ben Stokes's acquittal for affray in 2018, the *Sunday Times* writer Simon Barnes asked, 'Is cricket irresistibly attractive to odd types, to extreme personalities … or does cricket make them that way?'

The fifth decade of life is the most common time for a crisis. David Bairstow, the Yorkshire and England wicketkeeper, committed suicide aged 46 in 1998. Thankfully, his son, Jonny, has been able to overcome this loss to forge his own magnificent international career.

Virtually every player at some time needs a safety net but who provides it? It starts in the dressing room where camaraderie should be strong enough to support team-mates when their form is poor, when they have personal concerns or are making forced exits. Management, captains and senior players set the tone. New players (and their families) must feel fully supported on arrival. It makes no sense to pay megabucks but not allow your star signing to hit their straps immediately. Away from the sport there are houses and schools to be found. Belatedly, sport has recognised the need to provide welfare services. A huge salary doesn't mean that the player and family know where to register with a GP.

Team physiotherapists do more than lay on healing hands. They become the player's sounding board and confidante, particularly during injury rehabilitation when doubts can set in. They perform a valuable pastoral role. At Northants, we supplement this with the considerable skills of our club chaplain, David Chawner.

Most sporting organisations employ experienced sports psychologists to help players during troubled times. They are usually one step removed from day-to-day game pressures. Likewise, the UK has psychiatrists steeped in managing the mental health of sportspeople. Professionals such as Dr Steve Peters, who has worked in cycling, football, athletics and taekwondo, and Hopley, an ex-professional rugby player himself.

Unusually in medicine, 95 per cent of team doctors' interactions with player-patients are when they are well and engaged in their sport. This is different to other medical disciplines when you only see the ill or injured. These times can be used positively and help when the 'proverbial hits the fan' for the athlete.

The role of the PCA cannot be overemphasised. In 1975 it canvassed for a standard county cricket contract and minimum wage. In 2000, the PCA Benevolent Fund was created to support past and present players during times of hardship. Like the PFA in soccer, the PCA provides a point of contact and practical support. Its local representatives are known to all players; they support professional cricketers transitioning to civvy street. The PCA liaises closely with the ECB on policy and advice and support on such issues as drug abuse and medical screening. My friend Tim Munton, the ex-Warwickshire and England fast bowler, was a director of the PCA from 2002 to 2005. I can attest to the hard work and care taken by the association.

I have been working with local professional sports teams in Northampton for a quarter of a century. Many of their athletes settle nearby after retirement and many are patients. I see others at social events or shopping with their families. Those youngsters from the 1990s are in their fifties now. The pleasure of seeing them and hearing of their post-game personal and professional successes never diminishes.

Cricket has worked hard to support players' mental well-being. This will not stop another tragedy but networks are available during and after their careers. Hopefully they will be used.

'Here comes the sun, and I say
It's all right'

The Beatles, 'Here Comes the Sun' (1969)

I travelled to New Zealand for the first time in 2015. Within hours of arriving the intense sun made the top of my head feel as if it was being drilled. On my first day friends took me to the Canterbury Agricultural and Pastoral Association Show near Christchurch on the South Island. I marvelled at how a sheep could be separated from its fleece in a few minutes and watched in awe as male and female competitors chopped felled tree trunks with axes. It was November and late spring under the Southern Cross. It was not particularly hot but the sun's rays were burning my scalp.

Auckland is on the North Island and is the melanoma capital of the world. Kiwis have the highest death rate from skin cancer globally. Ultraviolet (UV) radiation intensities are 40 per cent greater there than in comparable European latitudes. The hole in the Antarctic ozone layer lies just to the south. I put my hat on.

Australia fares no better. Two-thirds of Australians are diagnosed with some form of skin cancer by the age of 70. Annually, 2,000 Aussies die from skin cancer. In Victoria state, the mortality rate is 150 per cent higher than from road accidents. What does this have to do with cricket? Richie Benaud, for a start.

The great Aussie cricketer and broadcaster died from skin cancer in 2015. It started on his forehead and scalp. He blamed the problem on not wearing a hat while playing. He was not alone. Ex-Australian fast bowler Max Walker died in 2016 aged 68 from malignant melanoma, and former Australia captain Michael Clarke has had three facial skin cancers removed.

It is not just an Antipodean problem. In 2010 the former England coach and Zimbabwean batsman-wicketkeeper Andy Flower had a facial melanoma removed when aged 42. Another former England coach and spinner, John Emburey, had a forehead cancer removed in 2014. The *Daily Mail*'s headline was 'Cricket gave me skin cancer'. Emburey blamed the disease on not wearing sun cream and a hat.

Skin cancers appear years after sun exposure; there is no room for complacency. UK melanoma rates have soared by 128 per cent in the last 30 years. Outdoor summer professions, including sport, are clearly at risk. Cricketing authorities had to act and had to be seen to be taking reasonable steps to avoid harm during players' careers. In 2009 the PCA launched its Skin Awareness Campaign and stated 'that it takes the disease very seriously and is working to raise awareness of the dangers, screening players and umpires to ensure that any signs are detected and treated early'. All professional cricketers are offered screening and onward dermatology referral for suspicious lesions. This is why so many cricketers plaster their faces with creams and use caps and floppy hats.

From a CMO's viewpoint such assessments are important. At-risk skin types need identifying. Those with fair skin and freckles and red or fair hair are many times more likely to develop skin cancer. I am most concerned about two groups: English cricketers wintering abroad and Australasian and southern African players joining us in our summers. All need monitoring.

Our understandable warnings about protection from UV light can come at a price – low vitamin D levels. The main source of vitamin D is our skin and the problems of under-manufacture of vitamin D were detailed earlier. It is recommended that our professional cricketers are regularly screened for vitamin D deficiency to help reduce stress fracture rates and aid healing.

Many sports are monitoring this problem. In 2019 it was announced that low vitamin D levels contributed to the three arm breaks suffered by England rugby No. 8 Billy Vunipola. Pills containing vitamin D need to be stringently batch-tested to exclude WADA-banned additives, however; they're alright for Joe Public but not for professional athletes – it's another minefield for our sports people to navigate.

Drawing stumps

Over my many years of involvement, cricket has developed hugely in terms of player care and has pulled ahead of other sports in some respects. The game was slow to accept the input of sports science and medicine but could now be regarded as a leader in this area and beacon of best practice. It will never have the perfect answers to all problems but it is pushing hard in the right directions.

Chapter 22

BIG HEARTS AND BIG BOTTOMS

'To be a great fast bowler, you need a
big heart and a big bottom.'

Fred Trueman (1931–2006), Yorkshire
and England fast bowler

HOW DOES sportspeople's resilience compare between eras?

Coping with injury, workload and setbacks is an impossible task to compare precisely across the ages. But cricket's bowlers have statistics on appearances and overs bowled and are a good place to start. For an unscientific piece of research, I compared Fred Trueman's English summer of 1965 with Stuart Broad's equivalent 50 years later.

Today's cricketers have access to physiotherapists, masseurs, S&C coaches, sports physicians, fast bowling coaches, sports scientists, analysts, podiatrists and nutritionists. Bowling workload is monitored and the cream come under the ECB umbrella at Loughborough University. A king's ransom is spent at elite level providing medical and scientific support. Do these contributions have a significant impact? Would present injury levels be higher but for our analyses, prehabilitation regimens, conditioning, access to expensive scans, and improved physiotherapy and surgical interventions?

The swingin' sixties and Yorkshire's finest

Why Trueman and why 1965?

'Fiery Fred' was a hero for many people of a certain vintage. He was the first cricketer to take 300 Test wickets; he played his last Test series in 1965. Trueman was the subject of discussion and concern: the BBC commentator Brian Johnston once announced that an elderly female listener had sent in money for Fred to get his hair cut because of his unkempt appearance.

By then, Trueman was 34 and on the wane. He had been dropped for England's four-month South African winter tour of 1964–1965, so after having his feet up started the season for Yorkshire on 28 April at Lord's against the MCC. Each county team played 28 Championship matches of three days' duration – 84 days' play in total. The 60-over, one-day Gillette Cup was in its third year. Counties would also play the MCC, tourists and universities, when strong sides were expected to be selected. Trueman never shirked his responsibilities to his county.

The wickets were certainly different, with debate on covering squares still in flux in 1965. Wickets could be covered only before the match and on Sundays. *Wisden* commented, 'A rain affected pitch and the consequent interesting cricket it might produce still remained a part of the game.'

The Almanack also reported that Trueman had 'had a mixed season'. He bowled 568 Championship overs at a wonderful average of 11.36 runs/wicket and played all four victorious games for Yorkshire in the Gillette Cup, bowling a total of 40.2 overs. Overall, he bowled 754 overs in first-class cricket. Was this extraordinarily onerous? *Wisden* reveals that 31 bowlers were busier of whom eight delivered over 1,000 overs. Indeed, 1965 was a relatively sluggish year for Trueman. From 1959 to 1962 he bowled on average more than 1,100 overs annually.

What did Trueman's 'quiet' summer look like? The season finished on 14 September – it was 140 days long. He had 49 days off in that time – one every three days. Sundays accounted for 14 days, games finishing early for another four, and he missed three days having been disciplined by Yorkshire for writing a newspaper article. There were no days off for injury, tiredness or because the opposition weren't worthy of him.

In one memorable spell he played a Test against New Zealand at Edgbaston – five days' play split by a Sunday of rest. The next morning he began a three-day game at Bradford, also against New Zealand. The game ended on a Friday and he appeared on the Saturday at Old Trafford for a three-day game (with Sunday off) against Lancashire. On the Tuesday night he drove to Swansea for a three-day match against Glamorgan. Mercifully, the game finished a day early allowing a day off before his three-day game against Nottingham at Sheffield. After one day's rest he played for England against New Zealand in the Lord's 2nd Test. The following day he played for Yorkshire against

Somerset in Taunton in a 60-over one-day game: 28 days with six days off.

It is exhausting recounting his toil and travel arrangements; he must have been on his knees. He was dropped for the next Test on his home ground, Headingley, and never chosen for England again. Is it any wonder?

> '... *the very model of a modern Major-General'*.

Gilbert and Sullivan, *The Pirates of Penzance* **(1879)**

Why Stuart Broad?

I needed a fast bowler of similar stature 50 years on. Broad is a gifted and hard-working international sportsman and stayed fit for the period of analysis. In 2015 he was 29 – five years younger than Trueman was in 1965.

In 2015, England played 101 days of international cricket. The schedule comprised 14 Tests against five countries, 26 50-over matches and five T20 games. Not a month elapsed in 2015 when England were not playing cricket somewhere on the planet.

In 1965, international one-day cricket was still six years away. England played nine Tests – three away and three at home against South Africa and three at home against New Zealand – totalling 45 days' play.

Broad bowled 271 first-class cricket overs in the 2015 summer. Only eight England-based bowlers delivered more than 500 overs. Durham's Chris Rushworth topped the workload with 641 overs – 113 short of Trueman.

Broad played County Championship cricket twice in 2015, bowling a total of 51.3 overs. Both games were in the middle of lengthy downtimes between Tests – 26 and 50 days respectively. He played in only one Nottinghamshire one-day game, bowling ten overs. Broad and Jimmy Anderson were regarded as our main Test bowlers and were to be protected from burnout or serious injury. Broad played for 84 days that season of which all but nine were for his country – seven days less than Trueman.

Broad's total bowling stint in 2015 was 601.4 overs spread across 350 days. In 1965, Trueman bowled 794.2 overs in 140 days. With higher over rates and less one-day cricket in 1965, Trueman bowled on average 21 per cent more balls per game-day.

Were cricketers of earlier years capable of greater workloads than the modern cricketer? Were the 'Truemans' made of sterner stuff? Broad was centrally contracted and his playing schedule was planned and monitored by the ECB. Intense cricketing activity was interleaved with rest, review and recovery. Modern cricketers have access to ice baths, cryotherapy chambers and sports massage, and work in the nets and gym to iron out flaws revealed by hours of technical analysis.

Broad and his colleagues must be men for all seasons and continents, adapting to conditions in Birmingham, Brisbane or Bangladesh. Modern travel is quicker and more comfortable, but cricketers must criss-cross countries, for example, during World Cups.

Fred's fast bowling fraternity

The three bowlers taken in preference to Trueman for the marathon 1964–65 four-month tour to southern Africa didn't let up on returning to Blighty.

Tom Cartwright (aged 30) bowled 735 overs in the 1965 summer despite breaking a metatarsal on tour. He was injured again in early summer and then broke his thumb during the second New Zealand Test. Like Trueman, his reward was never to play for England again. Ian Thomson (36) bowled 797 overs that summer. Only John Price (28) had a modest summer workload. Injury limited his season and he bowled only 322 overs.

Modern cricketers are more athletic in the field and catching standards and run-saving feats are quite astonishing. Bats are heavier and require considerable strength to use to full effect. Test match scoring rates have increased putting extra pressures on batsmen and fielders.

In contrast, the white, leather ankle boots players wore in the 1960s lacked the finesse of today's modern materials, design and manufacturing standards. Over rates have fallen significantly in the last half-century, leading to fewer balls being bowled per hour, day or game.

In the 1960s, many cricketers believed that 'to get fit for cricket you needed to play cricket'. Such views are still held by some sportspeople. In 2017, footballer Wayne Rooney said, 'I know I am at my best when I play. Everyone is different. I've played with lots of players who will miss two days' training and then they will train one day before the game because it is better for their bodies. I know I need to keep training and keep playing. That's when I know you will get the best out of me.'

In the 1950s and 1960s recovery tools following a day in the outfield might include a hot bath, lighting a fag and downing a pint of ale. To be fair, I still see first-class cricketers sitting on the balcony and smoking during a game.

The cricketers of my youth were born during times of real austerity in the inter-war and Second World War years. The 1930–1950s were times of shortage, true hardship and poor health. Food rationing did not stop until the year of my birth, 1954. In contrast, modern cricketers were raised in times of plenty and receive excellent advice about nutrition to aid health, strength and how to maximise recovery. The increase in the size of adults since the 1950s might be playing a part in causing increased physical stresses and strains. Apart from the obesity crisis, there are other signs that our nutritional status is not all that it might be. Trueman was no willow, though – he was 5ft 10in tall and weighed 13st. He had hip and chest circumferences of 46in; no shrinking specimen of Yorkshire manhood there.

But, surely, modern fast bowlers put more effort into their deliveries than our heroes of yesteryear. Who were the fastest bowlers of all time? Jeff Thompson and Michael Holding from the 1970s or Shoaib Akhtar and Brett Lee from more recent years? There are many others to add to the list and 1950s and 1960s fast bowlers would have to be included.

Frank 'Typhoon' Tyson died in 2015. Many believed he was the fastest bowler of all time and arguably capable of delivering the 100mph delivery. He was the toast of Northampton in my childhood and I was given a book by my dad containing a panoramic photograph of him preparing to bowl at our county ground. Tyson started his run-up 200ft from his wicketkeeper who was often stationed closer to the boundary than the batsman. Trueman had also been quick and had rapid accomplices, particularly the Lancastrian Brian Statham.

Did aspiring young players and established professional cricketers have as many injuries 50 years ago as today? It is likely that cricketers' injuries were less reported in the media and that many went unnoticed. Furthermore, players in the 50s and 60s were more likely to play through injury than their modern counterparts. An insight into 1960s attitudes towards injury and treatment was found in the 2017 *Times* obituary of Brian Taylor, Essex cricket captain from 1967 to 1973. Ex-colleagues described him as being 'very Victorian' and said he 'never believed in cricketers being injured or in physiotherapy', about which he was quoted as saying, 'Good players don't need it; bad players aren't worth it.'

Whistle. While you work

The cry many years ago was that when England needed another fast bowler somebody whistled down a coal mine. Preferably in Nottinghamshire.

Strong backs, biceps and buttocks, the ability to toil all day and a phlegmatic approach to life were strong attributes for a quickie. The little mining village of Nuncargate in Nottinghamshire produced five England cricketers, including Harold Larwood and Bill Voce, who shared the new ball in the Bodyline Australian series of 1932–33. Youngsters of the 1930s and 1940s probably underwent a form of unrecognised progressive conditioning as a result of their more physical lifestyle, preparing them for the vigours of professional cricket. Many finished education at 15, took up manual employment and played weekend cricket before being spotted by their local county.

Wisden recounts how the England cricket team were imprisoned on a ship en route to the 1961 Ashes Tour. They were press-ganged into fitness work by the great Gordon Pirie, double 5,000m Olympic medallist and 1955 *SPOTY* winner, who was a fellow passenger. Pirie told Trueman, 'It's your leg muscles that want strengthening.' Fiery Fred replied, 'Well, let me tell you they've held me for over 1,000 overs and more this year already. And they've never let me down when I've been performing for England. It's a lot more than a lot of sportsmen can say.'

Modern sport funnels talented youngsters into academies to acquire sport-specific skills and, for many teenagers, impromptu cricket and football games on the local Rec have been replaced by solitary indoor computer games. In 2010 it was reported by the *Daily Telegraph* that only a third of children were given the opportunity to play school cricket. In the same year, the charity A Chance to Shine claimed that less than 10 per cent of children in state education played 'meaningful cricket'. Fewer school playing fields, fewer qualified and willing teaching staff, and the scheduling of exams before the May half-term break have combined to erode school cricket's position.

England's potential strong seam of cricketing talent from less affluent areas is not being identified. In 2013 an *Economist* article entitled 'Class and cricket. A lower-order collapse' calculated that from 1945 to 2000, 60 per cent of England cricketers were state educated. That figure was halved over the next decade. There are a huge number of sports vying for youngsters' attention, particularly football, whose spectre haunts other pastimes and hoovers up so many talented young athletes.

A similar lament can be made for ethnic minorities' representation in English cricket. One of my most wondrous sporting sights was the great West Indian fast bowler Michael Holding in action: loose limbed, economy of effort, sheer athleticism; beautiful biomechanics; born to bowl. In the late 1970s and early 1980s 'Whispering Death' and his mates terrorised batsmen around the world. Every Afro-Caribbean young cricketer wanted to emulate them. By the 1980s, around 30 black players were in the English county set-up and five players of Caribbean descent represented England in 1991. Many more followed in the next decade. Then the change started. West Indian cricketing dominance declined and British ex-Caribbean generations lengthened, increasing youngsters' cultural distance from their roots and historic heroes. Alternative sports and other attractions beckoned. By 2018, only eight black or mixed-race cricketers qualified to play for England played in the County Championship.

After 1945 a male teenager had two main choices for a professional career in sport: football or cricket, unless they lived in a rugby league northern citadel. Even the successful would probably not become wealthy. The average national weekly wage in the 1950s was about £2 per week; in 1951, an English professional footballer's maximum weekly wage was £14. Fast forward 20 years when Kevin Keegan signed for Liverpool on a basic weekly wage of £50.

The post-war national football team were not exactly world beaters and in their first World Cup in 1950 they lost to the USA. In 1953 the 'Magical Magyars' of Hungary humiliated England 6-3 at Wembley. Our team contained greats such as Stanley Matthews, Alf Ramsey and Stan Mortensen but Hungary were playing a game from another planet and the shock to British soccer was profound. My father gave me an illustrated brochure of 'The Wembley Game' so that I could study the genius of Ferenc Puskás and his mates.

Therefore, in the 1950s, relatively more youngsters would dream of being the next England Test player. There were plenty of role models, including Tyson, Jim Laker, Tony Locke and Peter May. Dennis Compton was the swashbuckling batsman of his day. He was known as 'The Brylcreem Boy' for endorsing hair cream. He won FA Cup and league titles with Arsenal.

International English footballers' origins are the converse of cricket, according to one analysis, and most come from working-class backgrounds. The greater ease with which football can be practised and the lower cost of equipment are among many factors. Both cricket and football are the poorer for ignoring talent from large swathes of the potential playing pool, and both would benefit from merging personalities and ideas from all corners of our multicultural society.

Comparing conkers with conkers?

Were the likes of Fred Trueman examples of survival of the fittest?

Were Trueman, Statham and Tyson simply rare combinations of perfection? Did they have an unblemished anatomy, physiology and psychology and the appropriate opportunity at a critical time? With less medical support, were many more talented youngsters in the 1950s not fulfilling their potential because of sheer bad luck or faulty mechanics causing a cricket-finishing injury?

Conversely, does the present availability of sports medicine and science at sporting academies do some a disservice? Many athletes in earlier times would have been lost because of the absence of such support. But by patching up youngsters, does it deliver into adult professional sport individuals who have subtle biomechanical flaws that make them more prone to overuse injury compared to the seemingly indestructible Truemans of former years?

The Broads of today are more akin to track and field athletes. Their sporting calendar is mapped out ahead so that they peak at certain times. For Trueman and his mates, seasons were mostly short, brutish and unrelenting. Even the thoroughbreds resembled carthorses by the end of them.

Are short bursts of intense cricket followed by recovery and rehabilitation preferable to more prosaic, continuous cricket? Are cricketers more or less injury prone as a result? This question is particularly pertinent as white-ball formats become increasingly dominant. As in Rooney's comments on footballers, I suspect there are individual variations. The art and science of our work is to recognise who would benefit from different programmes.

In 2017, Jimmy Anderson recorded his 500th Test wicket at the age of 35. In the *Sunday Times* Ed Smith suggested that Anderson's 39 summer Test wickets were aided by his seven-month break from international cricket. He felt that Anderson's key was maintaining a 'lean and athletic' body, advising, 'Work with your natural body shape rather than against it … In the late 1990s, too many bowlers made the opposite mistake, bulking up in the gym with mindless weights training. Even when they gained a yard, they often lost years from their careers.' In 2018, Smith became chief national cricket selector.

We now understand better the pattern and predictability of injuries to modern fast bowlers. These whirling dervishes certainly represent an endangered species if their injury rates are an indication. Sports science has tried to identify how to ping balls at 80–90 mph around a batsman's ears. Not unsurprisingly, a fast run-up helps. Additionally, delaying bringing the delivery arm over like a sling shot, increasing trunk forward bending to harness power, and delivering the ball with a straight front leg all help raise the numbers on the radar speed gun.

Broad and Trueman absorbed forces up to eight times their body mass during ball delivery. They covered greater distances (20–80 per cent) per playing day than other team members and recorded between two and seven times more sprints (in run-ups) with 35 per cent less recovery time. Their injury rates are multiples of those experienced by spinners, wicketkeepers and batsmen.

In 2003, John Orchard suggested that both over- and under-bowling increased injury risks. A gap between bowling sessions of three to four days minimised injury risk. The ideal number of deliveries per week was between 123 and 188. By 2004–2005, evidence suggested that juniors who bowled with less than 3.5 days between sessions were significantly more at risk of injury. Back injuries have been a major concern. Many youngsters play school cricket during the week and back-to-back club cricket at weekends.

We understand better the timing of injuries to fast bowlers. In red-ball cricket, quickies bowling more than 50 overs per match have a significantly increased injury risk. If they bowl more than 30 overs in the second innings their risk increases by up to 22 per cent. However, the onset of injuries may be delayed for up to four weeks.

This is what cricketers and coaches have known for ages: fast bowlers need systematic incremental workloads pre-season or after injury. It prepares them for sudden surges in games and reduces problems such as stress fractures of the lower spine.

Going back to the summer of 1965, how can we explain how Trueman and his mates managed their workloads? Only once did Trueman exceed 51 overs in a game – in the first New Zealand Test at Edgbaston. He built his fitness from late April with hors d'oeuvres against the MCC and Cambridge University. By the late-May Kiwi Test he had played in seven three-day games, bowling an average of 18 overs per game. He was match hardened without being played out.

What is more difficult to explain is what happened after the Edgbaston Test, which finished on 1 June. His merciless schedule was described earlier but he was never injured. However, England dropped him at the end of that period and never selected him again.

Clearly, the programme affected his performance even if he was injury-free.

Arguments will continue about whether today's elite sportspeople are more or less resilient than their counterparts in days gone by. Whatever our views, present-day clinicians and scientists should not feel we have a monopoly on knowledge and skills. There is a lot to learn from our sporting past, and merging forgotten practices with modern theories may help the care of athletes in our charge. Every athlete is different – all have individual needs and considerations. There is no *Mrs Beeton's Book of Household Management* with recipes that suit all.

Chapter 23

SCHUMI AND I
11 July 1999

'Well I'm not braggin' babe so don't put me down
But I've got the fastest set of wheels in town'

Beach Boys, 'Little Deuce Coupe' (1963)

THE FORMULA 1 caravan moves to Silverstone in the southern corner of rural Northamptonshire every July.

In 1999, Michael Schumacher was hoping to deliver the World Championship to the 'prancing horse' for the first time in 20 years. He had won world titles with Benetton in 1994 and 1995 but the championship had eluded him in his first three seasons with Ferrari. Schumacher's early lead in 1999 had been eroded by the Finn, Mika Häkkinen, who led the German by eight points at the halfway mark in the F1 series.

On the first lap at Silverstone, Schumacher tried to pass his team-mate Eddie Irvine at Stowe Corner but disaster struck. His car's rear brake failed and the vehicle was catapulted into a wall at 200mph. The car absorbed most of the impact but Schumacher suffered a broken leg. The manoeuvre may have been unnecessary because the race had been stopped following a stall by Italian Alex Zanardi.

That weekend I was the on-call orthopaedic consultant at Northampton General Hospital and we'd seen the usual numbers of broken hips, wrists and ankles. I'd worked most of the weekend and was looking forward to some respite and watching the Grand Prix on TV at home.

'Lazy Sunday afternoon
I've got no mind to worry ...'

Small Faces, 'Lazy Sunday' (1968)

Silverstone weekend is always a busy time for local medics; it is the equivalent of a small town moving into the hospital's catchment area. About 60,000 people watch qualifying on the Friday and Saturday and double that number turn up for the race itself. Silverstone's medical facilities are excellent for drivers and the crowd and are staffed by a talented multidisciplinary team. At the time of Schumacher's crash, Professor Sid Watkins, who died in 2012, organised global medical care for the sport and did much to transform the safety of grand prix circuits. He was a neurosurgeon and chronicled his career in two books, *Life at the Limit* and *Beyond the Limit*.

After the crash the emergency car was deployed with ex-F1 driver Alex Ribeiro at the wheel, accompanied by Dr Phil Rayner. They were with Schumacher 86 seconds after impact. Initially it was reported that Schumacher had sustained a head injury, which was tragically ironic in view of his devastating skiing injury of 2013. He was able to wave and acknowledge the crowd from his cockpit, however, and I realised my services as the local orthopaedic surgeon might be required. The arrangements were that head injuries at Silverstone went to Oxford and everything else to Northampton.

I drove to the hospital less than two miles away ready to receive the stricken driver while listening to Radio 5 Live. Schumacher was in a helicopter and the BBC reassured listeners that he was en route to one of the country's premier trauma units. Nottingham was mentioned but not my small market town. The helicopter landed across the road from the hospital on the local school playing fields.

Schumacher was stable and communicative and was taken straight to a resuscitation room where the leg of his red Ferrari jumpsuit was removed with scissors. Careful examination confirmed a closed fracture of his tibia and fibula (shin) with no evidence of complicating factors.

All was calm initially but our semblance of peace disappeared with the arrival of the Ferrari team who had followed by road. Among them was Jean Todt, sporting director of Ferrari and later president of the Fédération Internationale de l'Automobile (FIA). In the background I heard plans being hatched to transfer Schumacher by air to Paris for treatment.

I explained that Schumacher had been involved in a high-speed accident and required stability, investigation and observation, and that placing him in an aircraft so soon after his accident carried risks. Ferrari then said they would fly in a French surgeon. I explained that overseas surgeons could not operate in the UK without the necessary licences and insurance.

There was a temporary impasse before it was agreed that I would consult with a French surgeon by telephone. That surgeon asked in a lovely Gallic accent whether I had examined the patient and if his toes were pink. They were. 'Good,' the surgeon said, 'carry on,' and he was gone. Watkins phoned shortly after and I outlined the injury, Ferrari's wishes and the brief, unusual conversation with my Parisian colleague. He asked me to do the necessary.

The hospital rapidly filled with press and interested locals. I accompanied Michael to X-ray, and passers-by in the corridors offered words of support and advice such as 'put his leg on backwards to slow him down'. The Ferrari circus was asked to stay in casualty giving me a single opportunity to discuss the situation alone with my patient. We scrutinised the X-rays together in the imaging room and I described the advantages and disadvantages of various treatment options and recommended surgery to insert a nail across the fracture.

Schumacher remained calm and absorbed the information quickly – abilities that had made him such an outstanding driver. He assumed control when we returned to casualty and quietly informed the Ferrari management that he wanted surgery as quickly as possible and for me to carry it out.

A media scrum would be difficult to control so we decided to take him to the sanctuary of the recovery area in the operating complex, where I became aware of the hospital's chief executive, the very personable David Wilson. It was rare to see any hospital CEO on an early Sunday evening, let alone in the operating complex. Wilson looked concerned and, looking me straight in the eye, pleaded, 'For goodness sake, Bill, don't cock this up or you'll bankrupt the hospital.'

With that ringing endorsement I was next assailed by Todt, who had somehow managed to get into the operating complex. He poked me in the chest and said, 'Michael is my best friend and I pay him $16m per year to drive for me. I tell you for him to have surgery in your hospital is a big responsibility for me, but I tell you it is an even bigger responsibility for you!' Wilson, standing behind him, paled even more. I wondered whether my successful attempt to dissuade Ferrari from putting him in a private jet to the European mainland was a mistake.

The surgery was relatively routine orthopaedic trauma work but I remember thinking that of all the operations I would undertake I would probably be remembered for this one. I felt strongly that we should be able to deal with this leg injury irrespective of who it was attached to. Within five hours of the accident Schumacher's leg was moving as one again.

After the operation I was 'invited' to the CEO's office where Schumacher's wife, Corinna, brother and fellow driver, Ralf, friend Jean Alesi and Todt joined us. A press release for issue the next morning would say that surgery had gone well and that Michael was comfortable and had enjoyed his breakfast. The latter was removed after Ralf Schumacher said it was impossible for anybody to enjoy an English breakfast.

Michael remained in the hospital for 48 hours after surgery to allow swelling to abate and for monitoring. He was on an NHS ward and under the care of the hospital's senior ward sister Denise Sweeney. His treatment was free, as it was for all EU nationals involved in a motor vehicle accident.

The next year, 2000, another German driver was admitted on to the same ward following an accident at Silverstone. He complained about being housed on the ward and our ward sister told him that it had been good enough for his compatriot. He refused to believe that Schumacher had been there, claiming that he would never have had surgery in Northampton.

Fast forward to December 2013 and the coverage of Schumacher's terrible head injury suffered while skiing. The *Daily Mail* credited at different times the Parisian doctor with undertaking Schumacher's 1999 surgery and overseeing his subsequent care.

'Oh Monday mornin' you gave me no warnin'
of what was to be ...'
The Mamas and the Papas, 'Monday, Monday' (1966)

With the permission of Schumacher and his family I was wheeled out on the Monday morning following the driver's surgery to face the international media, accompanied by Wilson and Todt. The press conference was held in the small staff car park outside casualty. Back in 1999, without internet and social media, we relied on TV and newspapers for information, and friends across the world told me of their surprise at seeing me in front of the cameras.

I then continued with normal operating lists and clinics, with meetings with members of Schumacher's team in between, including his excellent media manager Sabine Kehm and dedicated personal physiotherapist Balbir Singh. Throughout, the family were extremely friendly and tolerant of the surrounding maelstrom.

'All we hear is Radio Ga Ga'

Queen, 'Radio Ga Ga' (1984)

The hospital informed me that Nicky Campbell from Radio 5 Live wished to interview me the next morning. Both hospital and patient gave permission and at about 8am on the Tuesday morning I was ushered into a BBC outside broadcast van in the hospital car park for the interview.

I explained to the producer that I could not give detailed surgical information. 'All understood,' came the comforting reply. Cue and countdown followed. The next voice I heard was that of Campbell who was informing listeners that he was going live to speak to Michael Schumacher's surgeon. My heart rate increased like a sports car going from 0–60mph. Campbell's opening gambit was short and to the point.

'Well, Bill, tell us all about the operation.'

I stalled. I gulped. I thought I had an agreement about the scope of the interview – at least with the producer. After a second that seemed like an hour I replied that I couldn't give precise surgical details because of patient confidentiality. A disappointed Campbell retorted, 'Oh come on, Bill. A leg's a leg.'

'And a patient is a patient and I am not going to tell you,' I replied.

The interview picked up after that with an unspoken understanding that we would stick to generalities, and concluded with a discussion about shin fractures and likely timescales for recovery. Family and friends who have listened to the broadcast told me they had laughed and laughed at my obvious discomfiture.

'If you leave me now, you'll take away the biggest part of me'

Chicago, 'If You Leave Me Now' (1976)

Schumacher was to be discharged the same day and another car park press conference was planned as an elaborate ruse: he would be taken from the back of the hospital while reporters were trained on Messrs Wilson, Todt and Ribbans. Within minutes of the start, however, a bright spark at the back shouted that Schumacher was being smuggled out via another exit, and within seconds we were left staring at an empty car park.

It was a great relief to me that the whole race team entourage disappeared as quickly as it had arrived, on Schumacher's private jet back to Switzerland. The surgeon who supervised his aftercare kept me updated on his progress. For 48 hours I had been party to the circus that surrounded him for most of his career. I was astonished that they all managed to maintain their equanimity.

Recoveries and reunions

I came to the view that Schumacher was the consummate sporting professional and expected anybody who came within his orbit to deliver their own skill set as a matter of course. His recovery from the injury was nothing short of miraculous. Average bone healing time is three to four months, but it can take over double that time to rehabilitate fully. Having been written off for the rest of the Formula 1 season, rumours circulated that Schumacher might compete in the last couple of races and, astonishingly, he returned for the penultimate race in Malaysia on 17 October – 14 weeks after the accident.

Media requests restarted for me in the build-up to that race, including from BBC Radio Northampton and Radio 5 Live. We kept to generalities – vibrations in Formula 1 cars, comfort levels and mobility so soon after such fractures. The hospital was approached by a best-selling car magazine which wanted to feature me – and take my picture while gowned up in the operating theatre holding a tibial nail.

Schumacher won pole position and shepherded his team-mate, the Irishman Eddie Irvine, to a Ferrari 1–2, leaving the latter leading the championship with one race to go. In a thrilling denouement in Japan, Schumacher again claimed pole but Häkkinen won ahead of Schumacher and Irvine in third. The Finn beat Irvine to the championship by two points. However, Ferrari, with the help of Schumacher, claimed their first constructors' title since 1983, by four points.

The 2000 British Grand Prix, when the second German driver was hurt, was switched to Easter Sunday – a controversial change by the FIA that only lasted a year. Dreadful weather caused misery for the thousands of attending fans. Ferrari invited me to the weekend as their guest and asked my wife and I to their motorhome. It was a lovely end to an interesting professional episode, in the season in which Schumacher finally won the championship for Ferrari. It was the first of his five consecutive seasons of domination with the 'red machine'.

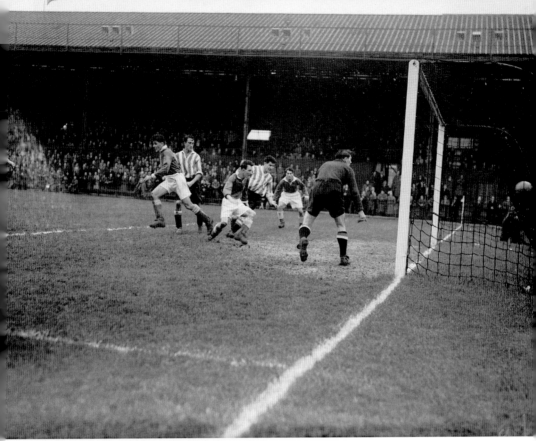

Figure 1. 27 November 1954. Griffin Park. Brentford 1-3 Northampton Town FC. The author's father was reporting the game while his mother was in 'labour'.

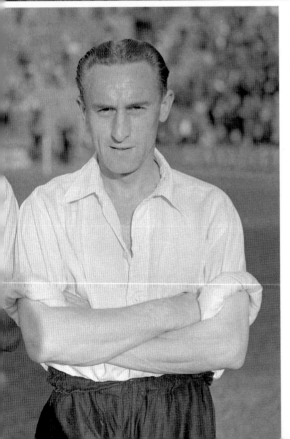

Figure 2. A Flash of Genius. Tommy 'Flash' Fowler. Northampton Town FC footballer of the 20th century.

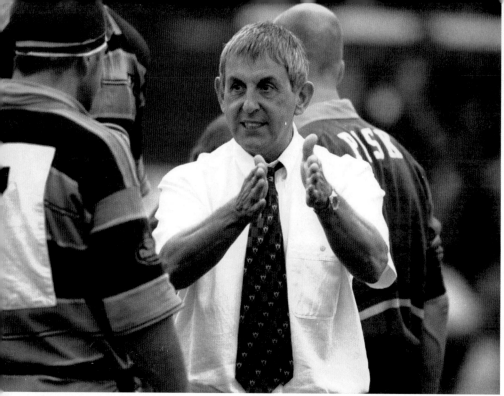

Figure 3. *Sir Ian McGeechan. Northampton Saints, Scotland and British Lions coach talks to Budge Pountney with Phil Pask behind at Franklin's Gardens, Northampton. 1998.*

Figure 4. *22 April 1992. Wembley Arena. Frank Bruno knocks out the Cuban, José Ribalta.*

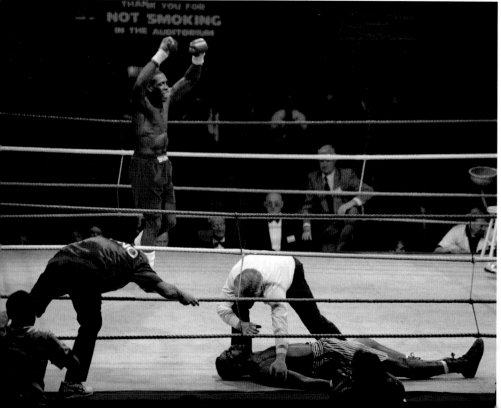

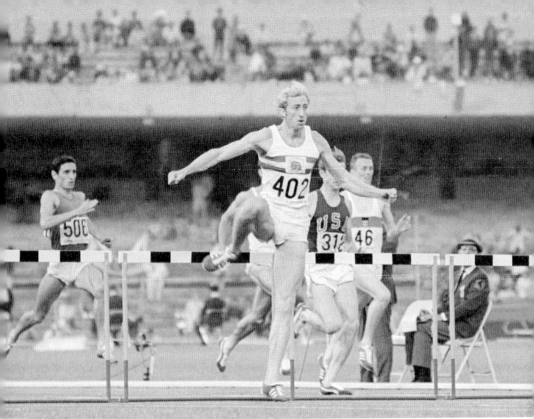

Figure 5. *12 October 1968. Mexico City. David Hemery wins the Olympic 400m hurdles in a world record time of 48.12 seconds.*

Figure 6. *20 October 1968. Mexico City. Lilian Board right) is beaten by Colette Besson in the final of the women's 400m by 9/100ths of a second.*

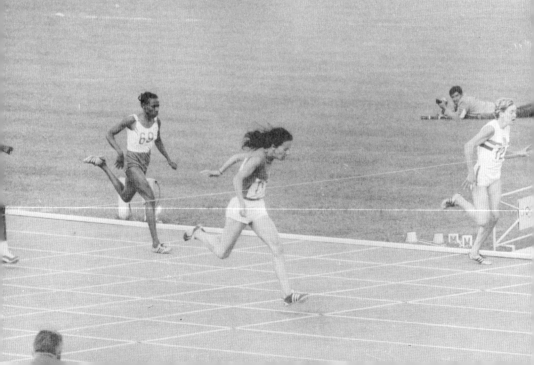

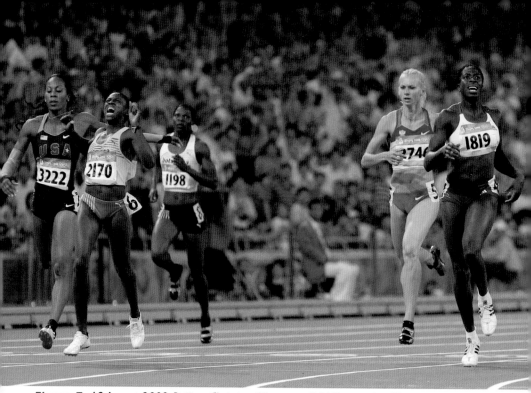

Figure 7. *19 August 2008. Beijing. Christine Ohuruogu (1819) wins the Olympic women's 400m gold medal to add to her world championship title.*

Figure 8. *4 August 2012. London. Greg Rutherford leaps to Olympic men's gold on the incredible evening of British success with Jessica Ennis and Mo Farah.*

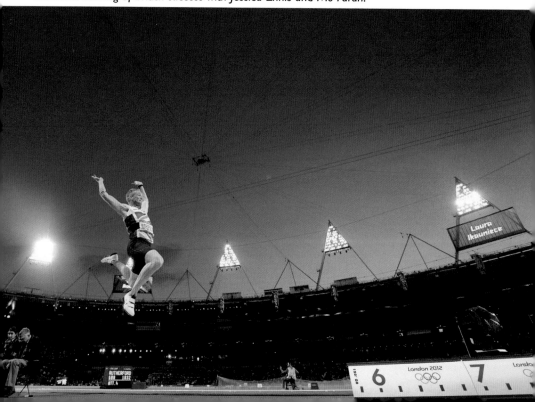

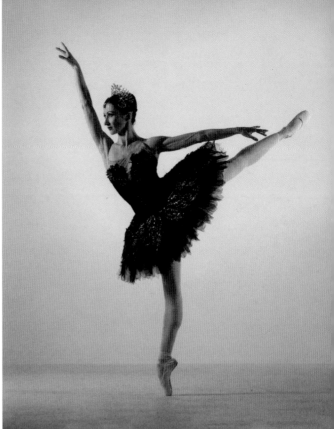

Figure 9. The grace and poise of prima ballerina, Daria Klimentova. Photographer Hugo Glendinnig

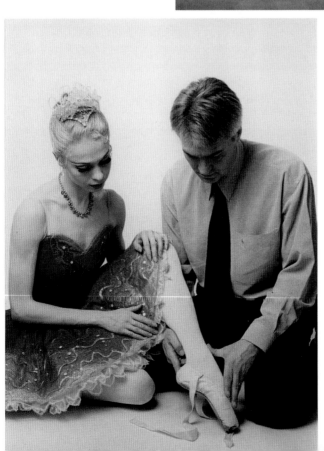

Figure 10. The author with the Sugar Plum Fairy, prima ballerina Agnes Oakes. The Daily Telegraph. Christmas 2009.

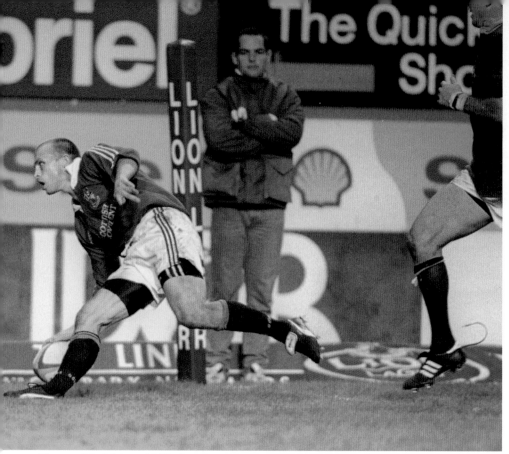

Figure 11. 21 June 1997. Cape Town. South Africa vs British Lions 1st Test. Matt Dawson scores a try in the corner after an outrageous dummy on Springbok captain, Gary Teichmann.

Figure 12. 27 May 2000. Twickenham. Northampton Saints beat Munster 9-8 to win the Heineken European Cup.

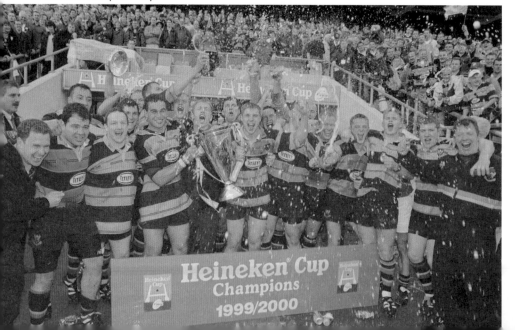

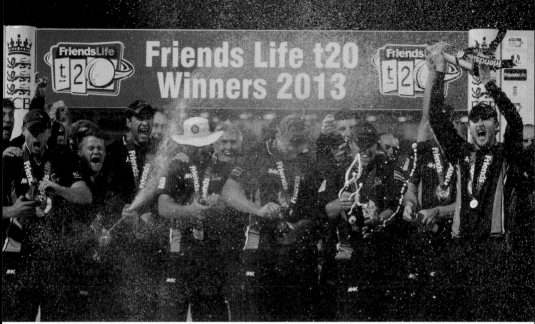

Figure 13. 17 August 2013. Edgbaston. Northants CCC celebrate winning their first T20 final against Surrey. The author is to be found to the right of the white hat – much to his wife's displeasure.

Figure 14. 11 July 1999. Silverstone British Grand Prix. Michael Schumacher's Ferrari crashes at Stowe Corner on the first lap. [Motorsport Images]

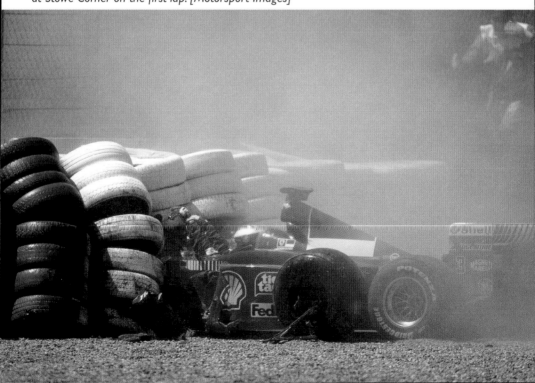

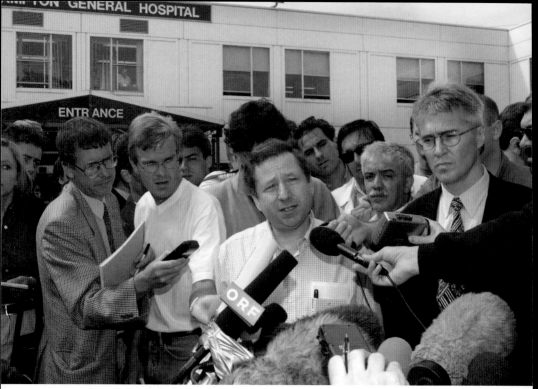

Figure 15. *12 July 1999. Northampton General Hospital. Jean Todt, sporting director of Ferrari, and the author are interrogated by the media.*

Figure 16. *Easter weekend 2000. Silverstone. Michael Schumacher and the author. WJR's own collection.*

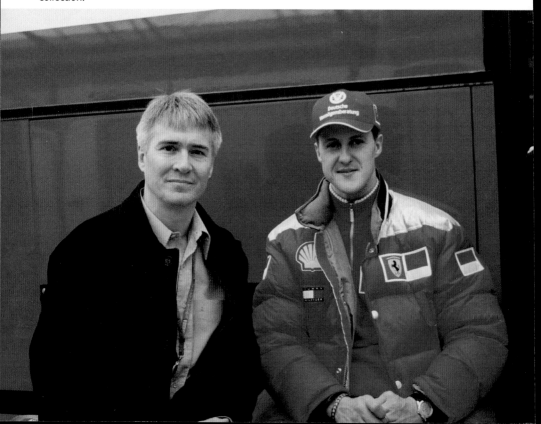

Chapter 24

BEST FOOT FORWARD –
A DANCE ODYSSEY

'Dance, then, wherever you may be,
I am the Lord of the dance, said he'

Sydney Carter, 'Lord of the Dance' (1963)

I HAVE long been fascinated by the role of dance in our society and its health benefits.

Every civilisation has embraced dance; it has fulfilled many functions. It has been a courtship ritual or been used to pass on stories; it has been part of thanksgiving celebrations, an invocation to the gods, a welcome to guests and part of battle preparations. People also dance to let their hair down.

Our forebears flocked to the cinemas to watch matinee idols such as Fred Astaire, Ginger Rogers and Gene Kelly dance. We have been entertained more recently by such dance blockbusters as *Saturday Night Fever*, *Grease* and *Dirty Dancing*. Television has its own dance-themed programmes such as *Strictly Come Dancing* and *Fame*. All provide escapism and promote participation. Dance is accessible to all ages, from pre-school ballet to jive, to ballroom and ceroc classes for adults. There are tea dances and there is line dancing for the even younger at heart.

The health benefits of dance should be self-evident. It provides cardiovascular and respiratory exercise and improves coordination and balance – protecting against falls in the elderly. The calories consumed help any diet. Less easily measured benefits include the feeling of well-being that accompanies regular exercise. Dance also helps improve social skills in the young and helps offset feelings of isolation in the elderly.

Ballet bound

'Congratulations on getting your Royal Free consultant post, my boy. Do you want to join me in Harley Street?'

The voice on the telephone belonged to my mentor, Justin Howse. His invitation opened a new world for me; he was the doyen of dance medicine and surgery. In 1980 he established the Remedial Dance Clinic in Harley Street with the talented physiotherapist Shirley Hancock. Together they wrote the definitive textbook *Dance Technique and Injury Prevention*. His 2013 obituaries in the broadsheets attested to his influence. I had been Howse's senior registrar at the Central Middlesex hospital in the late 1980s. He introduced me to the management of a host of subtle dance injuries which even now go undiagnosed by many clinicians.

I joined the Howse Empire in January 1991. I hadn't the slightest idea what my fees should be or how to organise a diary or secretariat and my hand was led gently through the mechanics of establishing myself. Early patients included dancers from all disciplines – ballet, ballroom and various musicals. Since then I've seen thousands of amateurs and professionals from dance and drama schools, ballet companies, *Strictly Come Dancing* sets and musical productions.

Howse was honorary orthopaedic surgeon for The Royal Ballet School at White Lodge in Richmond Park. The venue had been King George II's hunting lodge but in 1955 became the educational establishment for the next Fonteyns and Nureyevs. When Howse was elsewhere I was despatched to south-west London. I felt the disappointment of the teachers, physiotherapists and dancers when the lad appeared instead of the master. I was permitted to slip quietly into the back of lessons and observe the expert tuition – the cream of young British dance talent being put through their steps under the watchful eye of former Royal Ballet luminaries such as Dame Merle Park.

I attended assessments for ballet school applications, which took place in one of the large stately rooms. Assembled was a panel of ballet teachers, educational assessors, admissions staff, physiotherapists ... and myself. We sat on one side of a long boardroom table and the young applicants stood in front. My role was to identify physical problems or possible future concerns that could affect a dancer's ability to reach their full potential. The 2000 film *Billy Elliot* beautifully captured the assessment scene and the terrors it engendered in applicants. The assessment was less scientific than it is today but identified most orthopaedic concerns. Hopefully my input was positive for the school and dancer.

My knowledge of the dance world increased exponentially and I developed an enormous respect for the dance profession. The dancers were an interesting counterpoise to the huge rugby players attending my other clinics. I came to view them as being 'as tough as old boots'. They performed with injuries that would sideline others. In the 1990s I operated on a prima ballerina's foot. Inevitably she was press-ganged back into service ahead of the pre-operatively agreed schedule, to appear on the opening night of a classic production. She had learnt to adapt by changing her weight transmission through her *pointe* shoe and toe block to offload the surgical area. All was well until halfway through the performance when an audible crack signalled a metatarsal breaking.

She tried to carry on – her understudy was not there because she was jetlagged from a recent trip abroad – but eventually had to bow to the inevitable, and the audience, and exit stage right. I read of the drama in *The Times* the next morning while eating my corn flakes. She made a swift and full recovery.

Another dancer recalled how once she pushed back into place her dislocated kneecap on stage with the help of another ballerina and on another occasion experienced the crack of a breaking metatarsal while performing a solo. She carried on through the pain.

A very English company?

It was my fortune to become honorary orthopaedic surgeon to the English National Ballet (ENB) in the early 1990s. The ENB clinical team comprised physiotherapists, masseurs and a general practitioner supported by Pilates instructors, remedial coaches, podiatrists, psychologists, nutritionists and sports scientists. For most of my ENB tenure, I worked closely with the highly knowledgeable physiotherapist Jackie Pelly. Major dance companies should have preventative health measures in place, including regular formal fitness assessments, Pilates reviews, technical correction sessions, bone density scans and general medical reviews.

The ENB employs dancers from all over the world, which can mean language barriers and limited access to past medical notes for clinical staff. Cultural differences are inevitable and a suspicion of all things foreign is not confined to the British. As with sportspeople, dancers may prefer home physicians or want to try alternative therapies. Homesickness for young dancers can lie barely hidden below the surface.

'All the world's a stage,
And all men and women merely players;
They have their exits and entrances;
And one man in his time plays many parts'

William Shakespeare *As You Like It* (1599)

For the ENB I provided telephone advice, saw dancers in my clinic and carried out surgery. I visited ENB headquarters for rehearsals and provided injury advice before performances and during intervals. I became familiar with the stage doors of many West End and regional theatres. The dancers were fulsome with their time after productions, even allowing my young daughters to don tutus and glissade across an empty stage. Prospective sons-in-law have had their mettle tested by being asked to sit through a production of *Giselle*.

The orthopaedic surgeon must support the company physiotherapist and physician, and not being involved in day-to-day activities can be advantageous, particularly at times of critical decision-making. The surgeon needs to be aware that, despite having less frequent involvement, their role is more than 'just putting in the knife' and must watch, listen, learn and communicate as a team player in a multidisciplinary setting. Surgeons need an awareness of the technical aspects of various dance disciplines and to be knowledgeable about an individual dancer's past achievements and forthcoming events.

The relationship between the dance company and the dancer is no different to other professional sports. One must be aware of the difficulties that arise through the natural inquisitiveness of coaches, trainers, artistic directors and the media in relation to patient confidentiality.

Surgeons can become the dancers' advocate when medical decisions are coloured by contract requirements and career crossroads. Even senior dancers can find their contract suspended following an injury, only for it to be renewed once the dancer has fully recovered. Dancers move abroad to find work with foreign companies and a new and vibrant European city has its attractions until the first major injury. The young dancer may then find access to medical care hard to source and even more difficult to fund. Emails and calls from abroad for advice have been frequent over the years.

The psychological aspects integral to any changing room are found equally in a dance dressing room. Inevitably, travelling, training and performing together as a company creates strong bonds, tensions and protectionist sympathies. There is tremendous support for each other within dance companies and the independence honed by dancers having travelled widely as youngsters is impressive.

'You're a very fine swan indeed!'

'The Ugly Duckling' from the film
***Hans Christian Andersen* (1952)**

What does the ugly duckling have to go through to become the beautiful swan?

Dance is still beset with problems that have been overcome elsewhere by sports that are better planned and financed. With no overarching umbrella structure, such as national federations or the Premier League football machinery, there is no common strategy or accountability to enable the promotion of optimal employee health.

Major companies receive Arts Council and other charitable grants but dance is not an industry awash with money. Medical support has traditionally been poor. Even nowadays, some elite dancers are shorn of the clinical care taken for granted by many sporting organisations. Dancers need help when they are injured and advice on how to prevent further injury.

Most dancers perform with chronic injuries – often from a young age – and most suffer acute injuries every year, requiring time off from rehearsal and performance. Only a tiny percentage dance professionally beyond 35. Lower limb injuries predominate, especially to the foot and ankle.

The Birmingham Royal Ballet research group, led by physiotherapist Nick Allen and to which I have contributed, has calculated a rate of 4.4 injuries per 1,000 hours of dance. The figures equate to five significant injuries each week in a company of 40 dancers. Amateur dancers suffer fewer injuries than professionals, although they are still significant. Overuse injuries predominate in all dance forms.

Shakespeare's Melancholy Jaques described the seven ages of man in *As You Like It* but in dancers I believe there to be five orthopaedic dance ages: infant to young teenager; the teenage years; the young adult; the mature dancer; the retired dancer.

#1. The cygnets

Young dancers start at local academies and perform at festivals. Like any child they are susceptible to specific, numerous paediatric injuries caused by acute damage or chronic overuse. Poor teaching in dance schools may embed technical faults, subsequently leading to injury. The child's changing body shape puts altering demands on their musculoskeletal system.

#2. Pubertal plumage

By their teens, aspiring dancers are usually enrolled at a dance college or a ballet company school. Classes become more frequent and the associated physical demands can cause overuse injuries. Subtle biomechanical and technical weaknesses become more obvious.

Young female dancers look forward to starting *en pointe* work but too early a debut in *pointe* shoes can lead to injury and setbacks. The timing is not simply a matter of chronological age, but more the duration of training and competency of the dancer combined with adequate strength and control. Specific assessments such as the 'airplane', 'sauté' and 'topple' tests have been developed to test youngsters' readiness.

Young dancers develop muscle strength, speed, balance and coordination to such an extent that their poise and performance eventually appears effortless. Long rehearsal hours develop the muscle memory that enables performance at elite levels. Some classic dance positions, such as turn-out, place unanatomical stresses on young bodies and dancers should be sufficiently fit for these and must learn to harness their skills economically. They must develop a steel psychological core so that they can tolerate rehearsal, discomfiture and the inevitable rejections.

It is recognised that activities such as dance, which emphasise thinness or muscularity, are associated with a high degree of body uneasiness and inappropriate eating attitudes and behaviours. Weight concerns and nutrition are a problem in our society for a significant minority of teenage females. As with many sportspeople, such as those involved in horse racing and gymnastics, young dancers need a diet that minimises injury susceptibility and rehabilitation problems.

It can be difficult for young dancers living away from home for the first time to find the right calorie balance. There is a fine line between being too thin and too heavy and they must cope with evolving body shapes and replenishing energy burnt during rehearsals and performance. Dancers' diets are reported to be poorly balanced compared to other athletes, particularly with respect to carbohydrates, vitamins and trace elements. This can manifest medically in many ways, including reduced immunity and more viral infections, wound-healing problems and reactions to the soft tissue injections required for injuries. Ballerinas have been found to have almost double the rate of eating disorders compared to matched groups in the general population. Dancers develop strategies to control weight, which often lead to amenorrhea – the cessation of periods. Many require professional support and major companies engage nutritionists to advise on home cuisine and eating on their travels.

As has been previously discussed, the tyro dancer risks developing the female athlete triad – disordered eating and disturbed menstrual patterns leading to a reduction in the amount of circulating female hormones such as oestrogen. The result is osteoporosis or weakened bone. The condition was described in the 1980s and recognised by the IOC in 2005. It has since been renamed Relative Energy Deficiency in Sport (RED-S). Sufferers, female or male, are unable or unwilling to replenish their high energy expenditure by diet. The condition also affects other systems such as immunity and cardiovascular health. Like many sports, dancers are prone to burnout when subjected to a remorseless schedule of training and performing. They need proper rest to recover mentally and physically from the inevitable fatigue that occurs. An energy deficiency was found in three-quarters of dancers examined from a single professional company.

Young female dancers risk delaying the start of their periods – for several reasons including their weight, exercise schedule and the psychological effects of training – a time known as the menarche. A delay beyond 14 years old is considered late but occurs in many dancers. Increased dance training intensity prior to the expected menarche appears to increase the risks of delay. Both teenage and adult female dancers have an increased tendency to irregular periods and many have long episodes with no periods at all, causing chronic problems with fertility and bone health.

A child's bone density increases with age. However, the peak female accumulation of bone strength occurs following the menarche. The bone accumulation rate levels off after 16 years old irrespective of the age at which periods began. Peak bone mass is attained in early adult life; after that it is all downhill until we become jelly.

Squeezing the time for maximum bone accumulation during teenage years because of delayed periods risks low final peak bone mass. This stores up trouble for later in the shape of fragility fractures to wrists, hips and spines.

What about the positive influences of regular exercise on bone strength? Research from around the world suggests that dance increases strength in lower limb bones but is not so effective in the arms or spine. Consequently, osteoporosis in ballet dancers remains a concern. A 2013 American study of over 113,000 dance-related injuries in the under-20s showed increased problems as training became more intense. One American dance school reported that three-quarters of their teenagers were injured every year.

Who would be a teacher of young dancers? There is an enormous burden on those charged with young dancers' development. In this modern world, when even polite and gentle questioning of a young girl's gynaecological status may be deemed intrusive and suspicious, a coach must have the innate wisdom of Solomon to ensure safe progression of their charges. Increased emphasis must be placed on the education and support of the youngster and their parents.

The last year of dance school is vital for aspiring Darcy Bussells seeking to win professional contracts. Final year performances are watched by agents and employers and an untimely injury that forces withdrawal from such productions can have a devastating impact on career progression. Many students have chosen to dance through an injury and delay treatment, including surgery, until they have displayed their skills to the waiting world.

#3. Swans on tour

There is another incremental step in workload, skill level and fitness once a dancer joins a professional company. Frequent travel at home and abroad and learning to adapt to different performing venues pose extra challenges.

At any one time, adult ballerinas are six times more likely not to have periods than non-dancer females of a similar profile – nearly one-quarter of professional dancers. Female dancers whose periods have stopped risk losing bone density, and the longer the time without periods the greater the risk of stress fractures. A 1992 American study revealed that 31 per cent of dancers had had stress fractures, of which one-third reported multiple fractures and two-thirds had suffered stress fractures of the foot. Risk factors included the duration of training and dancing each day and menstrual irregularities. In the same year, a study of New York ballerinas found that those with stress fractures were more likely to suffer eating disorders and weighed less than control groups.

Historically, when speed, power and strength have been tested, dancers generally have fared poorly in comparison to other elite athletic groups. Female dancers lack strength and have lower body weights, factors associated with a greater incidence of back and lower limb injuries. Further, the average dancer has been found historically to have aerobic fitness, measured by VO2 max, only just above that of sedentary controls. Traditional barre and floorwork are not sufficient to improve aerobic fitness. Overwork and traditional training methods may be at fault. Modern understanding of sports science and medicine is helping to rectify these issues.

The ENB travels the globe and performs in many different venues at which performance surfaces can be less than optimal – wooden sprung floors are ideal. A male dancer returned from a tour of the Far East where performance floors were frequently hard and unsuitable. He experienced pain in his shin bone but refused to stop for fear of letting down his friends. His tibia looked like a tiger's torso – the tell-tale X-ray stripes revealed multiple stress fractures. Dancers develop a tolerance of pain higher than the ordinary mortal. Pain is part of daily class and the dancer is programmed to perform through aches and pains. Consequently, dancers may not respond appropriately when a 'new pain' warns of something more serious. Impending and established stress fractures are but one example.

Dancers have mostly a healthy attitude towards surgery – it is to be avoided at all costs. Inevitably there are times when surgery is the only way forward, however. I have lost count of the times when dancers have delayed the inevitable to complete a tour or series of performances. It is that feeling of not letting the company down.

#4. Elevation to the officers' mess

Senior and talented ballet dancers will be asked eventually to take on more demanding roles. The busy scheduling of these prime company positions makes it more difficult to time surgery, but management utilising repeated injections to manage chronic issues involves risk. A prima ballerina required surgical intervention to the back of her ankle, but the after-effects of previous, repeated steroid jabs had left her skin resembling tissue paper by the time I met her and I feared for her ability to heal.

Prima ballerinas and principal male dancers are in demand for short-term contracts all over the world. Elite dancers' earnings are dwarfed by footballers and those of other sportspeople, and these contracts are a chance for stars to save for the future. However, travel, rehearsing with unfamiliar dance companies and performing at peak power takes its toll.

I have caught up with dance patients in far-flung places such as Cape Town while there to participate in conferences.

For some dancers, changes in positions within the company can be explored – character roles, for example, offer a means of extending careers and continuing to perform without the excessive demands on body and soul. The character Baron von Rothbart, for example, the evil sorcerer in *Swan Lake*, is a delicious role for the older male dancer.

#5. Post-P45

A dancer forced to finish their career early needs tact and understanding and the value of a team approach, including the orthopaedic surgeon, cannot be over-emphasised. The decision to stop often involves parents, teachers, spouses and partners and the reaction of dancers themselves can be surprising. More than once I have seen a young dancer relieved that the decision has been taken out of their hands. Often, they have feared letting down family or teachers.

At the end of a dance career other issues arise and dancers can face the same difficulties experienced by professional sportspeople. The loss of bonds developed with other dancers within the company can have a profound effect. Dancers must find new sources of income and new professional directions, and cope with the increasing aches from decades of performance and the physical and psychological impacts of altered fitness and body shape.

'Dem bones, dem bones, dem dancin' bones'!

Spiritual song by James Weldon Johnson and J. Rosamund Johnson (1928)

The extreme positions required of an ankle and foot in classical ballet positions such as *plié*, *pointe* and *demi-pointe* put enormous strains on joints and soft tissues. The dancers' feet are the equivalent of the hands of most manual professions.

A number of problems can develop: bunions and big toe arthritis are common; lesser toes develop hammer and mallet toes and dislocate; swollen, painful nerves; stress fractures, ankle sprains and tendon tears; bone spurs in front and behind the ankle (and the heel), which cause disability and limit movement.

Male dancers place massive strains on their Achilles tendons, which become prone to swelling, pain and can even rupture. I looked after a wonderfully athletic male dancer for over 15 years and he nursed a swollen Achilles for most of that time. Finally it ruptured while he was performing at a Boxing Day gala in Tokyo. Cue frantic phone call and my advice to get on a plane home. He was in his mid-thirties and I counselled him that this might be the end of elite performing. His tendon contained more calcium than most people's molars and I doubted whether my surgery would be sufficient. Would it allow him to reach the heights he had previously attained? Male dancers require enormous power to hang effortlessly in mid-air during jumps – as if time has been suspended. Moreover, they need to support their female partner without a discernible muscle quiver.

The dancer would not entertain my fears and rehabilitated like a Trojan, and nine months later, at the quaint Theatre Royal in Bath, I watched in trepidation as if watching *Dr Who* in my childhood from behind the sofa. I should not have worried. The dancer's determination combined with the excellence of his rehabilitation delivered him back to his incomparable best. The hang-time of his leaps belied his time away. He never looked back. Relief. It is situations like that when a surgeon's skills are laid bare for public approbation.

The wider corps de ballet

Both young and established dancers require the same clinical input that has become de rigeur in professional sport. Dancers, parents and coaches need to be educated about the importance of nutrition and body shape. A change in attitude and openness about periods and puberty in young female trainees should be encouraged. Workload and recovery for all dancers needs foresight and execution, and consideration must be given to encouraging the inclusion of other forms of exercise that work the arms, core and spine, to improve bone and muscle strength. The evidence clearly shows that dancers' injuries can be significantly reduced if professional dance companies have ready access to multidisciplinary clinical teams. This access should be entrenched in all serious dance companies out of a duty of care to the dancers and, from an economic front for cash-strapped organisations, to maximise the availability of their most precious resources – the dancers.

Curtain call

Galen, a Greek doctor sometimes called the Father of Anatomy, said over 2,000 years ago that the 'best exercises are those that train the body and delight the mind'. Dance fits both these criteria and gives pleasure to millions of people every year. However, the strains on professional performers are enormous. Dancers must maintain healthy bodies and minds to enjoy a long, successful and comfortable career, and to be able to enjoy their post-performance life in optimal health. This can only be enabled by expert input from the many clinically related disciplines.

Chapter 25

GOLDEN GIRLS
AND LEAPING LORDS

Golden numbers: 48.12, 3.59.4 and 4,801

In October 1968 I was transfixed by the TV coverage of the Olympic men's 400m hurdles final beamed from Mexico City.

David Hemery streaked home to gold in a world record time of 48.12s. He was voted sports review personality of the year and became one of the most recognisable people in British sport. A signed photograph of him negotiating the last hurdle has pride of place in my clinic even now.

Four months after that race my PE teacher, Dennis Whitby, was looking for a hurdler for the school team. At mediocre height I was not the most obvious choice but Whitby felt I was worth persevering with. The following July I found myself at the English schools' athletics finals, the breeding ground of future Olympians. The same year, Marilyn Neufville won the championships' 150yds female sprint – the furthest a 16-year-old girl could race. A year later, she broke the senior 400m world record in taking Commonwealth gold in Edinburgh. My achievements were nowhere near as stellar but I managed a fourth in my final. The highlight of the experience was being presented on the podium to David Hemery.

In 1972 at the Munich Olympiastadion I watched Hemery defend his title. Despite leading through the final bend, he was overtaken by the amazing Ugandan John Akii-Bua, who became the first man to dip under 48 seconds. Hemery faded to third but his stature in my mind remained undiminished. Ironically, his defeat was planned by another Brit, Malcolm Arnold, who trained the new Olympic champion in East Africa. After returning to the UK Arnold guided Colin Jackson and others, such as Andy Pozzi, to Continental and global hurdles titles. Nearly 40 years after Akii-Bua's success Arnold and I spoke at a sports conference in Bath. His lecture on training methods was far more riveting than my contribution on the genetics of tendon injuries.

Hemery retired from athletics after Munich and began teaching at Millfield School in Somerset. A year later my school rugby side travelled to Millfield and played on the pitch that had produced such luminaries as Gareth Edwards. On the wing I found myself only inches away from Hemery, who was delivering instructions to the opposition from the touchline. To my disappointment I did not set the game alight and Northampton went down to a clear defeat.

Twenty years after Hemery's Olympic triumph I was on my American Harvard fellowship in Boston. This was where Hemery had studied and prepared for the 1968 Olympics. As I ran beside the Charles River I wondered if a previous Englishman abroad had pounded the same streets – albeit at a much faster pace!

In the mid-1980s I worked at St Mary's Hospital in London, where Sir Roger Bannister was a senior consultant. Six months before my birth in 1954, Bannister had broken the four-minute-mile barrier in Oxford, running the distance in 3m 59.4s. Along with England's 1966 World Cup triumph and David Hemery's 1968 Olympic gold, his achievement was one of the sentinel sporting feats from which I took inspiration.

Bannister became an eminent neurologist and edited the textbook *Brain's Clinical Neurology*, which became my undergraduate bible on the subject. Like Hemery, Bannister had made Boston his temporary home while at Harvard in 1962.

Whenever medical duties allowed, I ran around London's royal parks at lunchtimes. The hospital changing room was in the medical school basement. On several occasions the great man was to be found on a similar health mission. Bannister still retained an enthusiasm for fitness in his mid-fifties, although a road traffic accident had badly injured his ankle. Respect and shyness prevented me from making more than a fleeting salutation. However, being in the presence of sporting and medical nobility, even if he was only tying up his shoelaces, was a spur to my endeavours as I circled the Serpentine lake minutes later.

Bannister's achievements as a doctor, researcher, administrator and athlete seem barely credible. I had the privilege to be at his memorial meeting at the Royal College of Physicians in 2018. How the man had time to sleep? He was a brilliant neurologist, pioneering researcher, evangelical educator and publisher, chairman of the Sports Council's research and planning committee, and advisor and supporter of umpteen sports medicine-related societies, associations and faculties. However, what came over most was his inherent kindness, love and care for patients, colleagues, fellow athletes, family and friends. For me, Bannister and Hemery represented the epitome of cerebral sporting Hercules, whom Britain specialised in producing in the pre-professional athletics arena.

Mary Peters was the British darling of the 1972 Olympiad. Alongside hundreds of cheering Brits I saw the Ulsterwoman triumph over the German favourite, Heide Rosendahl, in breaking the world pentathlon record by just ten points with a score of 4,801.

At the 1996 Atlanta Olympics 24 years later I was standing in a queue with my daughters to buy tickets for the rowing. Immediately in front and patiently waiting was Lady Mary herself, alongside Lord Jeffrey Archer. It was a surreal experience a quarter of a century on since my last Olympic experience. That morning, Redgrave and Pinsent won the men's coxless pairs (the fourth of Redgrave's five triumphs). It was Britain's only gold medal of the entire Games – so different to 2012 and 2016.

I regard track and field as the purest of sports and the one that I have most consistently enjoyed being medically involved with. It is clean, decisive and, at times, brutal and has no allowance for subjectivity. Rarely are there histrionics in the stands from coaches and, unlike many sports, athletics remains a sport for all body shapes and sizes. Endomorph, mesomorph and ectomorph body type all have a place in one of athletics' disciplines.

What people accomplish with the body they inherited never ceases to amaze me. One example is flat feet, which can occasionally be painful but cause no problems in most. An athlete consulted me about an injury and while examining him I couldn't ignore the enormous pancakes at the bottom of his legs. They were some of the flattest feet I had ever seen. He had never had any problems, was one of the fastest humans on the planet and had a World Athletics Championships' gold medal. A photograph of him in action adorns my clinic wall. It is a reminder not to judge a book by its cover or a foot by its shoe or insole prescription.

We all stand together

The National Lottery became a game-changer for Olympic sport in 1994; from 15 Olympic medals in 1996 to 67 medals 20 years later is a fine track record. Athletics has been one of the main beneficiaries.

The funds have allowed athletics to become more organised, provide better training and coaching facilities and improve its sports science and medical support. My own involvement with UK Athletics has straddled this transformation, which has allowed many talented and dedicated sports physicians and physiotherapists to become involved. They include doctors such as Bryan English, Bruce Hamilton, John Rogers, Paul Dijkstra, Noel Pollock and James Brown, and physiotherapists such as Mark Buckingham, Alison Rose and Neil Black. The latter became UK Athletics performance director in 2012.

The success of British athletics means that other sports and countries have come looking for the sources of the sport's marginal gains. Clinicians have disappeared abroad, to Qatar in the Middle East for example. Others get poached by that great white shark of British sport, football. However, this has allowed well-trained young doctors to come forward and take their places.

When an elite athlete requires surgery, with their permission I welcome the presence of the sports doctor or physiotherapist in the operating theatre. It fosters a multidisciplinary approach to the problem from the outset. Seeing the torn tendon or ligament carefully reconstructed or the broken bone nailed, screwed or plated gives everybody perspective on what the athlete must overcome to be at their best again. It helps with the naturally curious athlete's concerns in the weeks that follow. It certainly makes my job easier.

I want to be free

For all the central funding and administration, athletics remains an individual sport and this is reflected in training locations. Loughborough and London remain the main hub – both, fortunately, one hour from Northampton.

However, British athletes are often scattered across the globe – winter camps in Potchefstroom and Stellenbosch in South Africa, European pre-games holding camps in Portugal, and altitude bases in East Africa and New Mexico have been favourites. Long jumper Greg Rutherford preferred American warm-weather locations.

This can cause logistical problems for medical teams trying to co-ordinate care. One Saturday evening I looked at MRI scans on my laptop while Paula Radcliffe simultaneously looked at the same images in New Mexico. It is much easier looking after a Premier League football team when the squad spend most of the season close to base.

Conversely, the individualism of athletics and the itinerant nature of training and competition fosters a maturity and independence in its participants not always seen in major team sports. Athletes are more likely to research their own injuries and arrive for consultations armed with relevant questions. Radcliffe was always formidably well-informed and exuded a persona of calm and authority. She was delightful and respectful of my views but was always clear about what she wanted from her injury management based upon painstaking pre-meeting research and thought.

'When you wish upon a star
Makes no difference who you are'

'When You Wish Upon a Star', from the film
***Pinocchio* (1940)**

For the elite athlete there are just six major championships each four years – one Olympics, one Commonwealth Games and two World and European Championships. The cream strive to peak for these events.

I try to conjure a mental map of the specific four-year cycle of the athlete sitting in front of me, including qualifying events and factors such as age and retirement plans. How many more games do they have in them? This is influenced by the athlete's physical state and their continued ability to cope with punishing training schedules. Many elite athletes only have one shot at an Olympiad. Even when young, one can never be sure whether that opportunity will come again. To lose the chance of competing at an Olympics is devastating and the postponement of the 2020 Tokyo Games will have shattered many dreams. Competitive outings can be few and far between for some disciplines – marathon runners, decathletes and heptathletes may only leave their training camps two or three times each year.

The build-up to an Olympics feels special, even from my distant medical clinic. Emails and telephone messages requesting sports doctors' and physiotherapists' input become increasingly strident. The threshold for scanning gets lower. A serious injury weeks before a major games is a personal disaster for the athlete. However, the decision-making about the injury is more straightforward. Do what is necessary, move on and plan for the next major championships. This, though, can leave the athlete scarred physically and mentally.

Injuries four to six months before a major games can be more difficult. Does the athlete have enough time to recover, train and find enough form to compete following my surgery? This is where multi-team decision-making comes into its own. From a surgeon's point of view it is important to be honest about recovery timescales based on previous experience. Realism is as important as surgical skill.

Many Olympic sports have similar concerns relating to the primacy of the Games. In late 2018 I was already being asked whether surgery for niggling injuries would 'guarantee' a free run-up to 2020 Games' qualifying competition. Conversely, athletes who had lost their chance of appearing at Tokyo 2020 because of injury glimpsed hope in the rescheduled date.

Track and field athletes appear to spend more time injured than other professional sportspeople, but not because they are less tough. The difference between winning a 2016 Olympic 100m medal and finishing sixth was 0.5 per cent for men and 1.8 per cent for women; elite athletes cannot carry injuries that reduce performance by 2–3 per cent.

In some team sports, an individual might still contribute despite carrying an injury, but in athletics there is no hiding place in lane eight. Reaching your full potential during the narrow windows of significant competition available requires the gods to smile on you. This was alluded to in Chapter 7 in my Swiss cheese analogy.

Injuries beset the mind and the body. Greg Rutherford remarked that 'when the body constantly breaks down – a strain here, a tear there – it takes a lot out of you, not just physically but mentally'.

Kelly Holmes has been open about the toll injuries have taken on her. This supremely gifted runner won the 1994 Commonwealth Games 1500m aged 24. She then suffered multiple injuries that would have broken most and admitted that she had contemplated suicide before being treated for depression; she had resorted to physical self-harm in despair. Ten years later, physically and psychologically healthy, she unleashed her true talent and became only the third woman to claim the Olympic 800m and 1500m crowns in the same Games. It would have been a calamity if she had been robbed of that opportunity. She reminded me recently that only 13 one-hundredths of a second separated the first four in the 800m final – so fine are the margins.

Doping, diaries and doubts

Athletics is haunted by the spectre of drugs. Its victims come in different guises and include athletes who lose out to drug cheats and those unknowingly implicated in institutionalised doping. There have been other issues, too.

In 1991 I operated on a major games gold medallist. On the evening after surgery the ward sister told me that the patient had been urged out of bed by 'persons unknown' – the athlete had been selected for drug testing despite being full of anaesthetic gases and painkilling drugs. Without requesting permission from staff, the testers had persuaded my patient to swing their legs out of bed and stand on the operated foot to provide a urine sample. Goodness knows what pharmaceutical cocktail of legitimate drugs the subsequent analysis revealed. My long list of safety, confidentiality and common-sense concerns were relayed to the drug-testing authorities. Predictably, I never received a reply.

Over the last 30 years I have looked after several athletes who have fallen foul of drug testing. Two were victims of faulty laboratory processing and others were guilty of taking contaminated supplements and were cleared of knowingly cheating. Another seemed guilty primarily of poor diary keeping.

While declaring my full support for WADA and United Kingdom Anti-Doping the collateral damage to athletes caught up in the fight against the real cheats is significant. Some of my patients put their ordeals behind them but none come out unscathed mentally. The stresses extend to athletes' families and coaches. Time taken to clear their names might include their potential 'golden years'. One athlete bankrupted themselves in attempting to do this through the courts – which was finally successful.

Stress fractures

A running theme in this book has been the menace of stress fractures to athletes in all sports. Why do they fill up our sports clinics?

Bones are capable of fatigue and failure like any structure in nature. They will fracture if the imposed stresses from exercise are repeatedly beyond the bone's endurance limit. Workload management in sport is designed to keep our skeletons below that breaking limit – whether it be marathon training or fast bowling.

Everybody has different bone endurance limits. We need strong bone by our early twenties, good nutrition, genes and health, combined with carefully graduated training programmes to improve bone strength and resistance to injury. No bone is immune, and each can be broken if subjected to enough force.

Stress fractures cause enough damage to break a bone but not enough to make it splinter into two or more parts. They are sustained by athletes of all shapes, sizes and abilities and occur frequently after sportspeople try to pick up training following a period of injury or indolence. In the 2020 months following COVID-19 lockdown, my clinics were swelled by runners with stress fractures. Many had gone from nought to silly miles in a couple of weeks as they embraced the freedom of working from home.

Different sports have different 'pinch points' and it often takes time for athletes to realise that their problem is more than a transient ache. Frequently, the athlete tries to carry on training in the hope of 'running it off'.

Runners' stress fractures are usually located below the knee and involve shins, ankles, heels and feet. Other areas are not immune, though. Longer-distance runners can fracture their upper femurs (thigh bones) just below the hip joint. The London Marathon throws up these injuries frequently but they're not limited to runners: I looked after an international rugby fly-half who fractured his pelvis as a result of assiduous kicking practice, which placed enormous stresses on his dominant side.

The foot absorbs huge forces during the running required in many sports. One specific bone at risk is the navicular (so called because of its likeness to a boat). Fractures of this bone can take an eternity to diagnose and heal. The high hurdler Andy Pozzi lost several years of his early career to such fractures in both feet. Surgery enabled them to heal and allowed him to take European and world indoor high hurdles titles.

I see cricket fast bowlers with lower back stress fractures which are often related to surges in overs delivered, poor bone strength and accelerated pre-season or post-injury rehabilitation programmes. Other vital parts of the bowling action can break down, such as Jofra Archer's elbow and Jimmy Anderson's rib stress fractures of early 2020. Less hostile sports such as golf have their own recognised patterns of overuse injuries from the peculiarities of the golf swing, and fractures of the tibia have laid low such giants as Tiger Woods. Watching crowds have heard the pistol shot of a splintering shin as the golfer completes their tee shot. Gripping your club handle too tightly can fracture small bones in your wrist and practice that is too vigorous can break your ribs.

Sportspeople with heel fractures arrive predictably in my clinics in the early months of the year, as athletes increase their mileage preparing for spring challenges. They were first recognised during the Second World War when sympathy from the medical profession was not always in abundant supply. They were 'found for the most part in older soldiers who are inadequate physically and structurally, and who frequently have inadequate personalities'. It is interesting to speculate whether any publication nowadays would allow doctors to make such scurrilous assertions about the mental capacities of their patients based on a foot injury.

The metatarsals join your midfoot to your toes. Second and third metatarsal fractures were initially recorded in 1855 by the Prussian military physician Breithaupt, who described what is known as a march fracture. Traditionally, callow squaddies lined up outside the platoon medical officer's door the morning after their first major trek across the moors. A mass mutiny was suspected until X-rays a week later confirmed the damage. In more modern times, these injuries have been hijacked by footballers such as David Beckham.

Other footballers, such as Wayne Rooney, Michael Owen and Steven Gerrard, and All Black rugby legend Richie McCaw, have broken their fifth metatarsal, which is on the outer border of the foot. The first recorded example of this injury was sustained by Sir Robert Jones while dancing round a military maypole in 1902. He rose to the rank of major general during the First World War and saved thousands of servicemen's lives through the organisation of their care following battleground injury. He became one of the forefathers of British orthopaedic surgery.

Sports field midfoot dislocations are seen in rugby and American football but their recognition dates to the Napoleonic wars. Jacques Lisfranc de St Martin was a gynaecologist and one of the Emperor's military surgeons. He noted the devastating injuries sustained by cavalrymen thrown from their saddles and dragged along the ground with their feet trapped in the stirrup. Nowadays, similar damage is caused by a 300lb prop-forward landing on your outstretched foot.

They can be heroes for more than one day

'I, I will be king
And you, you will be queen'

David Bowie, 'Heroes' (1977)

Queen of the quarter

When Christine Ohuoruogu won bronze with her team-mates in the 4x400m women's relay in the 2005 Beijing World Championships nobody could have predicted that that achievement would be the start of a streak encompassing nine successive global championships (Olympic and World), from 2005 to 2016, during which she would win at least one medal at each – three golds, two silvers and seven bronzes – a record she shares with two Jamaicans, Merlene Ottey and Usain Bolt.

It is even more amazing to remember that this run nearly hit the buffers when Ohuruogu was hardly out of the blocks. Between October 2005 and July 2006 she fell foul of the 'whereabouts' rule for drug-testing availability on three occasions. The final violation occurred when she changed her training venue because of a clash with a school sports day. She passed drugs tests nine days before and three days after the missed knock on the door and numerous other tests during that ten-month period. She was banned for one year, although an independent investigation recorded, 'There is no suggestion, nor any grounds for suspicion, that the offence may have been deliberate in order to prevent testing.' She accepted the penalty with her trademark grace.

It would have been a very difficult situation for any 22-year-old to cope with but Ohuruogu and her coach Lloyd Cowan looked for a silver lining to the disaster, deciding to sort out Christine's painful Achilles, which had limited her training despite numerous attempts to get it to settle. Six weeks after the ban was confirmed, Ohuruogu underwent Achilles surgery to both legs. Within 24 days of her ban finishing she won Britain's only gold medal at the Osaka World Championships. I interrupted my morning clinic to find a television so that I could scream at the screen in support. The rest is history – Olympic, world and Commonwealth champion.

The Tadpole

Part of any doctor's life is helping patients come to terms with disappointments resulting from illness or injury. For athletes, the setback is magnified when it entails withdrawal from an important sporting event – one they have focused on for months or years.

In May 2008 Jessica Ennis was 22 years old and the rising star of heptathlon. She was vying with Kelly Sotherton for number-one status in the UK and had already won a Commonwealth Games bronze medal. Sotherton referred to her younger rival as 'Tadpole' because of her small stature. The Beijing Olympics were intended to be the springboard which would establish Ennis within the pantheon of top-class heptathletes.

Then disaster struck. A niggle in her right foot developed into three midfoot stress fractures.

In her autobiography, *Unbelievable*, Ennis described the ordeal of missing the 2008 Olympiad and my involvement. 'He was caring and brilliant and got the timeframe right.' Like Ohuruogu, she was incredibly mature in dealing with adversity and received strong support from her coach Toni Minichiello. They analysed the problems and decided to change Ennis's long jump take-off foot to reduce future risk. Quite a feat. In 2009 she won the World Championship heptathlon and three years later claimed gold under the extreme pressure of being the poster girl for her home Olympics.

I was fortunate to be at the Olympic stadium for Ennis's opening day events and Greg Rutherford's long jump qualifying session in 2012. The next day, on that wonderful August Saturday evening, Ennis, Rutherford and Mo Farah produced their astonishing performances.

Happy as a sandboy

Jumpers are unlikely to enjoy an injury-free career.

The speed and power required to jump at elite level places the most immense stresses on the body, especially the legs and back.

Over several decades I have seen the damage around the ankles sustained by many of our international jumpers. The impact at take-off to the back of the ankle can squeeze an existing bone spur like a Brazil nut pincered in a pair of crackers. The British jumps squad have endured a minor epidemic of this. The greatest British long jumper and ultimate competitor of his generation has been Rutherford. He has himself catalogued the range of injuries that peppered his career.

I first met Rutherford in 2005 shortly after he won the European Junior Championship long jump. He was 18 years old but already the toll on his ankle was causing problems. 'I couldn't really bend the ankle properly at all,' he recalled in his autobiography, *Unexpected*. He had nut-crackered himself once too often. A year after surgery he won his first senior medal, a silver in the Europeans. However, new injuries to the same foot appeared and 17 months later more running repairs were required.

It was another four years before he won a second senior medal – silver again, in the New Delhi Commonwealths. The Radio 5 Live presenter Nicky Campbell debated the importance of the Games in India and used Rutherford as an example. He asked if anybody but his mother knew who he was. Within two years, the whole world would know.

Even while leaping to Olympic gold, Rutherford's right take-off foot had new problems. 'I needed surgery on the foot issue that I'd been dealing with for a few years.' Ten weeks after that golden night, he underwent further surgery but managed to take his first World Championship title the next season.

He always remained extremely grounded for a jumper and opened our new clinic in 2013. On another occasion he arrived for a consultation without the means of getting home. He patiently waited until the end of my clinic when I gave him a lift back to Woburn Sands – the appropriately named home of one of our most prolific athletes.

The finishing tape

Elite athletes really are the Ferrari of the sporting world. When finely tuned, their engines simply purr. However, the electronics that control the machine are complex and prone to overload and the constituent parts prone to wear and tear. To be allowed to peer under the bonnet and effect the necessary repairs has been a privilege.

Chapter 26

THE HISTORY OF SPORTS MEDICINE IN BRITAIN AND BEYOND

'History will be kind to me for I intend to write it.'
Winston Churchill (1874–1965)

HOW HAS medicine responded to the increasing prominence of athletes, the wealth of its major stars and the organisations controlling sport?

While a student in the 1970s and junior doctor in the 1980s care for injured athletes appeared haphazard. Despite good intentions, Britain lagged behind the advances in sports medicine abroad.

In 1983 the late Professor John King started a sports medicine course at the Royal London Hospital. He recalled the daunting task of programme setting, telling me that 'as no one knew what sports medicine was, this was a challenge'.

First stirrings from abroad

In ancient times, emphasis was placed on fitness and health in the young. In the 5th century BC, Herodicus, a Tracian physician, understood the benefits of exercise for health and recovery from illness. Around 700 years later Galen was appointed as physician to the Roman gladiators. Was he the first team doctor?

Modern interest in sport and exercise medicine dates back more than a century. Before the First World War it was recognised as an area that would promote well-being. The Germans and French were among the leading exponents; congresses were organised. In 1915 Dr Arthur Mallwitz, a German doctor, became probably the first full-time sports physician of modern times. In 1928 doctors from 11 countries met in St Moritz to form the Association Internationale Médico-Sportive. It survives today as the International Federation of Sports Medicine (FIMS).

Home front foundations

Education in sports medicine and organising care for athletes in Britain was slower to develop. The British Association of Sport and Medicine was established in 1952 and continues as the British Association of Sport and Exercise Medicine (BASEM). It achieved full membership of FIMS in 1961. These pioneer clinicians worked to create an understanding of athletes' problems and optimal methods of treating them.

Junior doctor J.G.P. Williams published *Sports Medicine* in 1962. It dealt with injuries and contained sections on basic sciences. It explained the extraordinary physiology of the athlete and emphasised the importance of understanding the technical aspects of specific sports being treated. A later version of the book was jointly edited by Williams and Peter Sperryn and published in 1976. It became a much-thumbed tome during my student years and in my early professional work. The work of Williams, Sperryn and colleagues to establish sports medicine as a recognised speciality was long and arduous. Other visionaries followed, including physicians and surgeons such as Donald MacLeod, John King and Charles Galasko, who worked tirelessly in its cause.

In 1979, my final student year, I was seconded to Farnham Park Rehabilitation Centre, which was run by Williams. This stately house in leafy Buckinghamshire opened for medical services in 1947 and its magnificent grounds served as open-air settings for treating many patients. It had a large group of talented physiotherapists, remedial gymnasts and occupational therapists.

Its old-fashioned decor and regulations gave the house the air of a 1930s boarding school. Most patients were resident and had strict timetables extending beyond normal working hours – including lights-out time. During my stay, a number absconded at night to the local pub. I know, because I joined them.

The multidisciplinary working atmosphere produced excellent results for the patients. Williams oversaw operations like a slightly austere autocrat. Small procedures were undertaken at the house itself.

An epidural was administered to relieve back pain on a table in the former kitchen. Surgery took place at nearby Wexham Park Hospital and Williams ran the operating lists with a rod of iron. I recall dodging as instruments were despatched to the four corners of the theatre to catch the attention of staff whose minds might be wandering.

Take-off overseas

Britain was not alone in arriving late to sports medicine and progress was similarly slow stateside. The American College of Sports Medicine was established in 1954 and the American Orthopaedic Society for Sports Medicine in 1972.

While at Harvard in the 1980s I attended American football, ice hockey, basketball and baseball games. There was a huge difference in the variety and numbers of medical personnel in attendance. I spent part of my time working for sports surgeons such as Bert Zarins and Arthur Boland. Both made important contributions to surgery on the injured athlete.

Australia and South Africa have enviable records of producing outstanding sports doctors. When the UK was training insufficient doctors of its own, numerous southern hemisphere physicians came here to staff clinics and work with various sports. Sports Medicine Australia was founded in 1963 and the Australian Institute of Sport in 1981. The latter acted as a training hub for many sports; its establishment was a piece of innovative thinking and delivery and brought together experts in many fields of sports science and medicine. The historic ability of Australia to punch above its weight in so many sports is due in no small part to the vision of the AIS. Aussie physicians such as Peter Bruckner have made telling contributions in their homeland and abroad, including at Liverpool FC.

The South African Sports Medicine Association was formed in 1985. Of many excellent physicians from that country, Tim Noakes stands out. He was a giant of the discipline and made enormous educational and research contributions and was tireless in his questioning of accepted normal practice. His autobiography, *Challenging Beliefs*, would be of equal interest to clinicians, athletes and keen sports fans. It outlines the difficulties he faced in overcoming prejudices, self-interest and politics. I have met Noakes only briefly, on several occasions, but have been proud to work closely with his research team at the National Institute of Sports Medicine in Cape Town since 2007.

Even so-called 'smaller nations' have been more proactive than Britain in establishing centres of sporting excellence. Norway established their own Olympic training centre in Oslo in 1985. I visited in 2014 when it was a hive of activity, including in carrying out education and research to support the country's many world-class facilities and coaches. Norway's small population (5.2 million) may have meant it was easier to establish such a facility, where national sports teams can train and access medical facilities. At the time it was one of only nine sites recognised worldwide by the IOC as a leading centre for sports medicine research. America had none.

It is no coincidence that Norway has been one of the most successful Winter Olympics countries. In 2018 Norway topped the medal table at the Pyeonchang Games, a feat achieved on a Games budget of £13.7m – less than half the budget of Britain, which spent £28.35m.

Norway's success is not limited to snow. *Soccernomics* by Simon Kuper and Stefan Szymanski analysed the world's most successful nations across a range of sports. Weightings depended on popularity and degree of global participation, methodology the authors admitted was not without flaws. Not surprisingly the USA came top. However, when the successes were divided by national population Norway was the world's best per capita nation. Its sporting successes were calculated to be greater than all of Africa and Asia combined.

The present-day, self-professed jewel in the crown of sports medicine is the Aspetar hospital in Qatar. Since 2007 it has spared no expense in the facilities built and personnel recruited from across the globe. It claims to be the 'world's leading specialised orthopaedic and sports medicine hospital'. This tiny Middle Eastern peninsula state of 2.5 million people hosts the FIFA World Cup in 2022. Aspetar claims to provide support for its 20,000 registered athletes and has embarked on comprehensive research and educational programmes. As it is based in a country that has the highest per capita income in the world, Aspetar's aspiration to be regarded as the global leader in sports medicine does not seem fanciful.

> *'Rub–a–dub–dub,*
> *Three men in a tub*
> *And who do you think they were?'*

Traditional nursery rhyme

In the 1980s Britain's sports doctors were drawn predominantly from three areas of medicine: orthopaedic surgeons who operated on athletes, general practitioners who brought wide medical knowledge to the table, and consultants in rheumatology and rehabilitation who had excellent knowledge of joint and soft tissue assessment and greater experience of medication and injection techniques.

These doctors worked at a time when today's sophisticated imaging and investigations were not available. MRI was in its infancy and had restricted access. Other techniques, such as ultrasound, were more basic than they are today. It can be argued that tools such as MRI have been a mixed blessing. They make clinicians more reliant on secondary methods of diagnosis and less competent in traditional clinical examination.

Cutting one's teeth

In 1981 I was working as a junior in casualty and orthopaedics at Luton and Dunstable Hospital. The hospital is next to the M1, close to the A5 and near busy factories. It was pre-seat belt days. On my first day I was instructed on how to use the amputation saw in tight spaces to extract drivers from crumpled cars. I spent the rest of my time there terrified that I would be called on to brandish it. Fortunately the call never came.

I asked if I might start a Monday evening sports injuries clinic in my free time. Amazingly, it was agreed; in today's NHS it would never be approved – it would have to be consultant-led, equipped, funded and have protocols established. I started with a lot of enthusiasm and little knowledge but was ably helped by one of the senior physiotherapists, who provided the expertise.

Injured athletes were diagnosed, provided with home treatment information, referred for physiotherapy or given an orthopaedic appointment. I learnt rapidly; so did the local sports people. We were a self-referral clinic and became inundated, and attracted vitriol from local clinics who complained that our free service was threatening their livelihoods.

The scope of problems we saw rapidly extended from fresh weekend injuries to chronic problems, sometimes years in their genesis and mostly suffered by middle-aged athletes who thought they were still 18. We soldiered on. When I left, the clinic became part of the casualty department offering and was taken on by a senior colleague.

Later in the 1980s I worked as a senior registrar at the Middlesex Hospital in central London. It had one of the few NHS sports injury clinics and possibly one of the oldest. It had masqueraded as the 'athletic clinic' in the 1950s and in 1958 reported the first series of stress fractures of the tibia in runners – an injury commonly seen nowadays and known to all sports clinicians. The clinic accepted difficult cases for second opinions and provided invaluable experience but, like Luton, was mostly populated by chronic problems that were not always soluble.

Handicaps and hurdles

Everywhere cottage industries were springing up. At Northampton General Hospital rheumatologist Tim Beer and the excellent GP colleague, Frank Newton, provided a weekly NHS sports injuries clinic. Like every hospital, Northampton struggled with resources and waiting lists, which prevented prompt access for newly injured athletes.

In the mid to late 1990s Northamptonshire health services looked after over 600,000 people. They had one MRI scanner. In my clinics, patients could take a year to return with their MRI results. Subsequent surgery might wait a further two years.

In 1991 there were 862 orthopaedic surgeons in England and Wales – an average of 125,000 legs or arms for each surgeon to look after. This ratio of surgeons to potential patients was three and a quarter times greater than elsewhere in Europe. We were firefighting and it was difficult for surgeons to develop expertise in areas such as sports surgery.

In the NHS I felt that sports-related injuries were regarded, sometimes, as self-inflicted nuisances. Doctors expressing an interest in their treatment risked being viewed as dilletantes compared to colleagues in more 'serious' specialities. Against this background, people were working hard lobbying medical colleges and government to permit the development of a separate speciality for sports medicine.

Sport and exercise medicine courses began to appear. The Royal London's offering began in 1983 and was the first in Britain and probably Europe. Other educational establishments also began to offer suitable qualifications, including Bath University.

In 1986 Scottish doctors established a Board for Sports Medicine and a syllabus for a diploma three years later. Enthusiasm for these developments was lukewarm at best from some of the big beasts of the British medical scene.

Eventually, in 1998, the Intercollegiate Academic Board of Sport and Exercise Medicine was founded, tasked with developing a syllabus for examinations and, ultimately, the establishment of the new discipline of sports medicine. Finally, in 2005, sport and exercise medicine was declared a specialty and a year later the Faculty of Sports and Exercise

Medicine (FSEM) became the UK's governing body for the discipline. Fittingly, because of the Scots' pioneering stance, it is based in Edinburgh.

To support this venture, a broad group of doctors already immersed professionally in sport were sought to become foundation fellows and members. I was honoured to be accepted as one of those fellows in September 2007. Ten years later the number of members and fellows had risen to 560. Training commenced the same year and finally British doctors could undergo training to become sports medicine consultants. By 2017, 115 doctors were registered as being qualified in sports medicine.

It has been a long road to recognition but at last we have a cadre of domestically trained doctors providing high levels of care to elite athletes and the rest of us. Their aim is the promotion of health and well-being with an emphasis on lifelong exercise. FSEM provides organisational skills for delivering training and education and, alongside bodies such as BASEM, it is a focal point for doctors to develop structures and governance principles to help clinicians in their work with sporting organisations.

However, the increased knowledge and expertise of doctors of sports injuries has not been associated with a parallel increase in their professional standing within sport. A 1966 Tottenham Hotspur football programme front cover gives club doctor Brian Curtin equal billing with their fabled manager Bill Nicholson. And on the opening page of a 1969 Northampton Town programme five people are listed as worthy of mention: the club secretary, manager, honorary medical officer, club surgeon and dentist.

In contrast, a 2019 Cobblers programme lists 34 important people including the ticket office manager and stadium safety officer. The doctor and dentist have disappeared without trace.

Chapter 27

THE CHRYSALIS
BECOMES THE BUTTERFLY

WHAT ABOUT physiotherapists and other colleagues involved in the care of our athletes?

The Society of Trained Masseuses was established in 1894 by four nurses and became the forerunner of the physiotherapy profession. By 1920 it had a Royal Charter and changed its name to the Chartered Society of Massage and Medical Gymnastics. Men were allowed to join the same year. It became the Chartered Society of Physiotherapy (CSP) in 1944.

The 1970s saw major changes in the physiotherapy profession. In 1976 the first physiotherapy degree course was launched in Belfast. The following year the Department of Health enshrined in law the professional autonomy of physiotherapy. Physiotherapists were allowed to see patients without a doctor's referral from 1978.

However, despite those developments, in the 1980s I still had to write on a 'physiotherapy prescription pad' details of rehabilitation to be undertaken. Now, this seems an act of professional arrogance – it suggested that a surgeon, especially a junior, had more in-depth knowledge of physiotherapy techniques than practitioners themselves. A decade later, physiotherapy became an all-graduate profession and physiotherapists were allowed to undertake injection treatments soon after. Almost 20 years on they were permitted to prescribe medicines after suitable training.

The ties between doctors and physiotherapists are vital to the well-being of injured athletes. The phrase 'a good physio can make a bad surgeon look good and vice versa' remains as true today as when I was first told it 40 years ago.

Remedial gymnasts and football managers

The Second World War saw significant developments in rehabilitation techniques; the phrase 'necessity is the mother of invention' could have been coined for the influence that military conflicts have had on patient care. Advances were made during wartime in areas such as plastic surgery, injured soldiers' transport from the battlefield, antibiotics and rehabilitation.

Most of the credit for the recovery of the injured servicemen and women can be ascribed to physical training instructors (PTIs), who are acknowledged to have been the inventors of aerobics. They promoted the importance of carrying out exercise in groups, for efficiency and camaraderie.

After the 1940 Battle of Britain the RAF established residential rehabilitation centres. Sites at Torquay and Blackpool were followed by others at Hoylake, Cosford and Loughborough to treat the growing number of injured. After the war, rehabilitation units were centred around specific industries, such as car production, docks and mining. Others were based around the emergency professions, such as the military and police services. Due to cost-saving and health reorganisations most have closed. Farnham Park Rehabilitation Centre was one of the last such civilian sites but closed many years ago.

Demobbed PTIs formed the backbone of these services. A course was established for further training at Pinderfields in Yorkshire. By the late 1950s, the PTIs' profession had changed their name to remedial gymnasts. Pinderfields continued as a source of civilian training but the military remained the dominant supplier of remedial gymnasts, many of whom later qualified as physiotherapists.

Later, as physiotherapy developed, remedial gymnasts' jobs became squeezed and a degree of inter-professional rivalry developed. By 1985 the Society of Remedial Gymnastics and Recreational Therapy merged with the CSP. It meant an end to remedial gymnastics, but not before it had populated sport with many excellent clinicians ... and football managers!

Bertie Mee, an ex-Royal Army Medical Corps remedial gymnast become Arsenal's physiotherapist. He was manager from 1966 to 1976. His team won 'the double' in 1970/71.

Harold Shepherdson was the part-time trainer of England from 1957 to 1974 including during the 1966 World Cup triumph. In 1947 the ex-wartime PTI re-joined the Middlesbrough FC staff where he had once been a player. Like Mee, he stepped into the manager's role, on four occasions, but only in a caretaker capacity. He worked at Middlesbrough until 1983. The word 'trainer' embraced the role of the remedial gymnast well. It emphasised the dual responsibilities of treating individual injuries while maintaining the fitness of the whole squad.

Bertie Mee's physiotherapy successor at Arsenal was Fred Street. He worked for 20 years with the England camp simultaneously, where he succeeded Shepherdson. Street was also a remedial gymnast before becoming a physiotherapist.

Bob Paisley succeeded Bill Shankly as Liverpool manager and achieved multiple national and European triumphs. He had joined the Anfield backroom staff as a 'self-taught physiotherapist' after stopping playing. He was reported to diagnose injuries by simply looking at the player.

Two remedial gymnast luminaries have worked in Northampton, Jack Jennings and Dennis Casey. Jennings was a trained masseur, wartime PTI and trainer to Northampton Town from 1945 to 1964. Like Mee and Shepherdson, he became manager of his club, albeit for a short while. Casey was physiotherapist at Northampton Town from 1985 to 2008. His longevity speaks eloquently of his skills and experience. By his retirement he was one of the most experienced physiotherapists in professional football. I was the club's honorary surgeon and it was an education to work with him and benefit from his encyclopaedic knowledge.

The physiotherapist-turned-manager did not die with remedial gymnasts' demise. In 1991, the PFA started a course at Salford University to retrain retired footballers as physiotherapists. Subsequently, several were promoted from club physiotherapist to manager.

Mick 'Baz' Rathbone became Halifax Town's 'physiotherapist' despite having only just started his undergraduate studies. He recalled events in his book, *The Smell of Football*. Within months, he was manager. Twenty-four games and six months later Halifax exited the Football League and Rathbone lost his job. It was my beloved Cobblers who were Rathbone's relegation rivals that May 1993 afternoon. He qualified subsequently as a physiotherapist and, via Preston, became head of Everton's medical department. Another graduate, Nigel Adkins, was promoted from Scunthorpe club physiotherapist to manager in 2006. He went on to manage Southampton, Reading, Sheffield United and Hull City.

As a youngster watching Northampton, it was always the trainer with his magic sponge restoring stricken players. It was never the 'physio'.

Team photographs from 1897 reveal that a physiotherapist appeared first in 1985 – the year Casey arrived. Previous incumbents were called 'trainer' or 'gymnast'. Liverpool did not appoint a qualified chartered physiotherapist until the 1990s – later than little Northampton. Post-1945, qualified physiotherapists' predecessors were often people with a remedial gymnast background or 'good old boys', often ex-players, whose primary responsibilities were to maintain team fitness and help with coaching. In 2000, Leicester University's sports researcher, Martin Roderick, stated that 'half the physios in football aren't qualified for a job in the NHS. Their appointment is a gift of the manager.'

Brian Clough led Derby County and Nottingham Forest to league titles and the latter to two European Cups. He began his post-playing career as Hartlepool United's manager and wanted his friend and sounding board Peter Taylor with him. To win Hartlepool's consent, Taylor agreed to add medical department responsibilities (without any experience) to his coaching duties; he manned the cold bucket during games. Later, the pair jettisoned the Ellimans Rub and forged wonderful over-achieving teams.

Up until the late 2000s I would encounter 'physiotherapists' from some of the 92 senior football clubs with no formal training – astonishing, given the number of talented chartered physiotherapists anxious for such opportunities. Did this reflect ignorance within football's hierarchy of the skills of a trained physiotherapist or a desire to keep support staff salaries low?

There are trends I find surprising. Increasingly, in some sports, pitchside physiotherapists wear tabards emblazoned with the title 'Medic' while others are identified as 'head of medicine'. Physiotherapists have worked hard for acceptance within sport. Why are they not prouder of their profession and why do they want to change their job descriptions? The CSP guards jealously the title and reputation of its members from untrained imposters. Rightly so. If I called myself a physiotherapist the CSP could prosecute. Using different terminology causes confusion with respect to roles and responsibilities.

Training stateside

The United States has always been different. The certified athletic trainer flourishes alongside physical therapists (as physiotherapists are known there). Athletic trainer training started in 1881 when my alma mater, Harvard University, employed James Robinson to condition the football team. The National Athletic Trainers Association (ATC) was formed in 1950.

The ATC's responsibilities are wide and include oversight of the health and well-being of their athletes. But they work under the direction of a physician. The 32 professional American football teams in the NFL employ many ATCs, with some salaries in excess of $100,000 per year.

The strength of Samson

The work of S&C coaches has become increasingly recognised and encouraged. The benefits of developing power and strength have been known for over a century. It helps with general well-being and success in sport, and in recent decades there has been a proliferation of sport science research and dissemination of successful techniques.

In the 1970s these coaches became increasingly sought in the USA, primarily in college football. Now they are used in all areas of sport. In 2004 the profession became organised properly here with the formation of the UK Strength and Conditioning Association, which now has over 2,600 members.

The aims of S&C coaching are to enable the athlete to maximise their performance potential, prevent injury and supervise and plan recovery programmes post-injury. The athlete's speed, power and technique are developed in a sport-specific fashion.

Steve Black built up an enviable reputation in rugby union with Newcastle Falcons, Wales and the British Lions working with Jonny Wilkinson among many others. His autobiography, *Blackie*, stressed the difference in conditioning for various sports. Team sports play week in and week out, while individual athletes have isolated targets – one, possibly two, annual peaks per year such as the Olympics. Each sport has different priorities. Keeping team players close to maximal fitness for prolonged periods increases soft tissue injury risks. It is better to be 'bubbling along just under' with limited peaks targeted. Conversely, the 'single-minded' athlete must progressively build towards their Olympic final or world title bout.

Centres of rehabilitation excellence

My experiences abroad suggest that other countries have put greater emphasis on rehabilitation than we have.

In the USA in the late 1980s a rehabilitation hospital was located next to our surgical unit. When patients were stable they were transferred to the hospital to benefit from the skills of the many physical therapists and medical rehabilitation specialists. Germany has greater availability of similar facilities, where, post-surgery, patients can be transferred for intensive work in units that resemble five-star hotels.

The ability of the British military and police to rehabilitate injured personnel is astonishing. They established rehabilitation units such as Headley Court in Surrey (military) and Flint House in Berkshire (police). In 2018 the military closed Headley Court after 60 years of service. It was replaced by a £300m state-of-the-art Defence and National Rehabilitation Centre at Stanford Hall near Loughborough.

In 1951 the Central Council of Physical Recreation (CPRE) rescued a crumbling Lilleshall Hall in Shropshire and turned it into a second national recreation centre after Bisham Abbey in Berkshire. Like Farnham Park it was a stately home set in parkland. Facilities by modern standards were spartan but were still an improvement on anything available elsewhere. Lilleshall was chosen by Alf Ramsey to prepare the England football team for the 1966 World Cup and from 1984 to 1999 it was the FA's school of excellence. Now it is an English Institute of Sport (EIS) high performance centre for archery and gymnastics.

As a youngster in the early 1970s I spent happy times at athletics training camps at Lilleshall. Memories of Bobby Moore and Bobby Charlton were still vivid. Today I see some of the elite gymnasts based there.

The FA opened St George's Park at Burton in 2012 at a cost of £120m. It is a central administrative setting and venue for squads to train and acts as the epicentre of sports science, medicine and rehabilitation.

Stanford Hall and St George's are populated with experienced multi-disciplinary teams working on the physical and psychological aspects of recovery. The military and football identified the human and economic costs of inadequately recovered injured personnel. It is a sad reflection on healthcare priorities that many more ordinary citizens had access to such facilities after the Second World War than we do three-quarters of a century later. I have wondered how many injured civilians with long-term disability would have been made more able with access to such facilities. This is health economics writ large but coming at cost to the more widespread national purse.

You have to be in it to win it!

UK Sport is a government organisation tasked with overseeing sport development. Established in 1997, it took over the roles of earlier organisations such as the Sports Council (established in 1972) and the CPRE (1935). Beneath it are organisations representing each nation – Sport England, sportscotland, Sport Wales and Sport Northern Ireland.

UK Sport's establishment followed the launch of the National Lottery in 1994. It distributes government funding and Lottery grants. This gives it enormous power over development and support for different sports.

This tough love has been a major element in the success of the UK in recent Olympics. At the 1996 Atlanta Olympics – the year before UK Sport was formed – we won one gold medal, at Lake Lanier where I cheered home Steve Redgrave and Matthew Pinsent in the coxless pairs. In 2012 we won 29 gold medals.

The National Sports Centre for Wales opened in Cardiff in 1971. It was renamed the Welsh Institute of Sport in 1994 and in 2010 became the Sport Wales National Centre. The Scottish Sports Council was established in 1972 and is known now as sportscotland. In 1998 the Scottish Institute of Sport was formed and in 2008 became the sportscotland Institute of Sport. Sport Northern Ireland was established in Ulster in 1973 as The Sports Council of Northern Ireland.

In 2002 the EIS was established through grants from UK Sport. It provides high-quality sports medicine and science and functions as 'the team behind the team'. Networks of specialists have developed in areas such as orthopaedic surgery and it has immeasurably improved athletes' care. The EIS has ten high-performance centres for different sports. Lottery funding has given a huge fillip to sport and has allowed experienced doctors and clinicians to be employed. Athletes now have a central reference point for support and continuity of care.

How things have changed. Northampton had one athlete at the 2000 Sydney Olympics. She returned injured with no continuing access to medical support and appeared in casualty asking for advice. The casualty consultant asked if I could help. Nowadays, elite athletes are advised by companies such as Health Partners Europe. This company was formed in 1996 in conjunction with the Premier League Medical Care Scheme. It manages the healthcare of more than 5,000 high-profile athletes and directs over 95 per cent of secondary (hospital-based) treatment in professional football and cricket. Similar arrangements exist in other sports.

The criteria for who qualifies for funding is strict and performance driven, which is the only way to be fair. It can create problems, though. Athletes sustaining long-term injuries cannot compete and lose funding;

they find it difficult to receive care when they need it most and it is heart-breaking fielding phone calls from such individuals. They are used to rapid access to MRIs, for example, but must now navigate the NHS, which comes as a shock. The removal of support from underperforming sports risks casting adrift entire squads from high-quality medical support; athletes are returned to the pre-millennium situation. Clinician turnover is another concern and the end of an Olympic cycle is a natural break. In the cauldron of high-level sport, clinicians want to change roles, sports and seek new adventures. For both athletes and specialists, it takes time to build relationships with new team doctors and physiotherapists.

Evolution and revolution

I have witnessed an enormous evolution of medical services in sport and we have moved a long way from when having a medic present on matchday was as much about crowd health and safety as player welfare. Progression in physiotherapy has improved expertise in injury management, and S&C coaches have taken their specialist area to a new level. They now form valuable partnerships with physiotherapists. Parallel to this has been education for GPs and improved levels of support from consultants, with access to national and international specialists now available. Finally, the arrival of sports medicine as a recognised speciality has allowed doctors to become well-trained in all aspects of athletes' care. Finances have played a major role in these changes – the huge contracts with satellite television and Lottery funding.

There are myriad disciplines within major sporting organisations' science and medicine departments – sports physicians, physiotherapists, physiologists, S&C coaches, nutritionists, psychologists, masseurs, biomechanicists and podiatrists. I apologise to anybody I have left out.

Are they all needed? In certain sports, such as rugby union, injury levels appear to be higher than 30 years ago, despite the exponential growth in the number of staff employed to prevent and treat injuries.

Modern athletes have higher levels of fitness, strength and skill, and sports science and medicine has had a major influence on these advances. Does improving performance levels ultimately become self-defeating from a health perspective as the body is pushed closer to its limits? The speed, frequency and power of impacts are increased which can lead to the breakdown of the most wonderful machines known to man – our own bodies and brains.

Chapter 28

YOU'RE SIMPLY THE BEST!

'You're simply the best
Better than all the rest
Better than anyone
Anyone I've ever met'

Tina Turner, 'The Best' (1989)

WHO IS the best sports surgeon? How do we know? Results are the simple answer but not that easy to come by. How do you compare hernia surgeons with their knee counterparts? From a psychological viewpoint the need for an athlete to believe they have entrusted their bodies and careers to the 'top surgeon' is understandable.

In 2016, James Haskell, the England rugby forward, underwent surgery. He said, 'When I saw the surgeon the other day for the first time since the operation, he was very pleased with how it looks – apparently it is way better than he thought it might be. I was concerned when I first saw him because he used words like "unique" and said things like "we don't get to see a lot of this". I had visions of him putting an instruction manual on my forehead during the operation as he tried to figure out what to do. But he's the best surgeon in the game and I am very pleased with the results.'

In 2018 Andy Murray explained why he underwent his first hip surgery in Australia: 'He's one of the best in the world.' A year later Murray was more reflective. His second surgery would take place in London. 'I chose her because she was honest. She told me the truth.'

Should surgical success be judged by time taken to return to play? Or perhaps return to pre-injury skill levels? Or speed and endurance recovery? Or long-term freedom from reinjury? However expertly put back together, some injuries will leave permanent reminders.

Injury-pattern monitoring should provide answers but is fraught with pitfalls and the potential for error. Often, I suspect that the aura of 'top dog' starts with the athlete's own clinicians. The medical team need to maintain the trust of the sportspeople under their care and their athletes expect them to have entrée to the best bone setters in the business. However, the selection criteria underpinning their recommendations often does not bear scrutiny. In the 1990s I was told that the definition of a sports medicine expert was a doctor who 'came from elsewhere and gave lectures'. Little has changed.

In contrast, the culture surrounding surgeons has changed enormously during my career and the development of the multidisciplinary team has dampened the 'surgeon ego', reducing their arrogance and overconfidence. Surgical conviction, based on experience and knowledge, allows timely and accurate decisions to be made. Unearned grandiosity can lead to poor decision-making and outcomes.

In any speciality the various facets that fit together to create a decent surgeon are as numerous as the pieces of a jigsaw. Very few surgeons are 'naturals'. Most hone their skills through years of training and repetition. We need to constantly appraise new techniques and reflect honestly on our outcomes. As in all walks of life, surgical failure is ever present. Like my colleagues, I counsel patients carefully about surgical outcomes and potential complications.

Mary Tudor, Queen of England from 1553 to 1558, said, 'When I am dead and chested you will find Calais written on my heart.' For every surgeon, the equivalent is the memories of patients you have not restored to health, mobility and comfort. I certainly bear those scars.

I strive to be that 'best surgeon in the world' but know I come up short. At times I imagine reaching the pinnacle, and out of my 600–700 annual procedures I might have a 99 per cent success rate. But this means that every year, six or seven patients consider me the 'devil incarnate' because they do not have the results I had hoped for. After decades of practice, this produces a large clan who are not your best cheerleaders – and that is if I am the absolute bee's knees.

Many of the best technical surgeons I have come across do not have the best 'bedside manner'. Their desire to complete a procedure perfectly is the main driver. However, their inability to schmooze up to the athlete and their entourage does not endear them to their visitors. There are also extremely talented surgeons who elect to concentrate solely on their NHS practices, which removes them from the orbit of professional sports organisations.

How not to choose your 'top surgeon'

The amount of advertising associated with the doctor and clinic should not be factors in choosing your surgeon. The geographical location of a surgeon also has little to do with their skill set – a Harley Street address, for example, is no guarantee of quality. Often a surgeon's operating base is determined by luck, family circumstances and the desire for a rural or urban lifestyle.

Nowadays, superb surgeons, capable of dealing adroitly with most sports injuries, can be found in all the UK's major hospitals. During my training it was Nottingham and later Oxford, rather than London, that led the way in trauma care.

In 1990, Prince Charles chose to have surgery in Robin Hood country following a polo accident. In addition, centres such as Oswestry on the Welsh borders have long been recognised as units of outstanding surgical and research expertise.

Mad men and medicine

In TV's *Mad Men*, which featured the 1960's advertising industry, our knowledge of products could only be accessed via print, radio and television. Knowledge about health provision was even more controlled and restricted. Now, information about available medical services via the web and social media sites is expected by all.

NHS and private medical establishments publish information about their personnel and expertise. Organisations such as Dr Foster work with many healthcare bodies and publish data on outcomes and doctors' qualifications and interests. The government wishes to publish similar data about surgeons. Patients want to be able to examine the merits of doctors they are contemplating consulting.

On top of that, national newspapers and magazines publish lists of 'top doctors' and run articles such as 'Meet My Surgeon'. Social media sites invite patients to review doctors. The absence of a silky online presence is regarded by some patients as a form of professional neglect. Many clinicians feel compelled to populate their professional website with colourful images, blogs and patient testimonials. Latterly, this has reluctantly included me.

Some surgeons add regular folksy Twitter messages about their day-to-day activities to convey the semblance of a modern mindset. Does this increase their allure? Nowhere are these impulses truer than in the world of sports-related medicine. In 2017, the GMC was investigating an average of one doctor per month in relation to Facebook, Twitter and WhatsApp activities.

We quickly forget how things have changed. It has long been held that a central doctrine of medicine is to refrain from self-promotion, and throughout most of the 20th century the GMC and other regulatory bodies regarded medicine as essentially different from other professions. Medical misadventure, due to inappropriate referral, can lead to irretrievable patient harm. Sir Donald Irvine, writing about the history of medical advertising in 1991, said that such catastrophic outcomes did not generally occur when engaging the services of lawyers, architects or financial advisors.

In 1905 the GMC warned doctors against 'the practices of canvassing and advertising for the purpose of procuring patients'. Any registered medical practitioner resorting to such practices risked being charged with 'infamous conduct in a professional respect' and erasure from the Medical Register.

This situation continued until 1990 when the GMC published new guidance about advertising medical services. Its rules were relaxed but only for GPs, who were warned about claims of superiority of services offered. This coincided with my appointment as a consultant.

Specialists, however, including orthopaedic surgeons, were deemed sufficiently different to bar them from public advertising. They were only permitted to provide information to other colleagues, not to patients, and could not claim superiority of qualifications, skills or experience. In 1997 consultants were allowed to advertise but the information had to be factual, verifiable and not make claims about quality.

When advertising was confined to newspapers and periodicals, monitoring of disreputable medical activities was easier to monitor. This changed at the turn of the millennium when the internet and the increasing profusion of clinical websites made this type of activity difficult to police. Often, false claims come to the attention of regulatory bodies only because of a direct patient complaint. Is the patient any better off? Is so much online medical information superior to a GP's recommendation?

Younger consultants ('the medical millennials') feel far more comfortable about self-promotion, but those raised in an era where specialists could be seen and heard but only in their clinics remain more reticent.

The medical merry-go-round

Physiotherapists who work for sports organisations and, more latterly, sports physicians have most influence on the direction of traffic to various sports surgeons' clinics. However, the tenure of medical and physiotherapy jobs often appears to follow a four-year cycle. Post-2012, several of our top sports physicians were poached, including a number who went to the superb Aspetar facility in Qatar. Particular orthopaedic surgeons can be sought by a club or a sport for years but excellent results do not render them immune from finding the referral tap turned off as medical teams change.

Surgeons should be best able to identify suitable colleagues – it's their professional life. However, when quizzed about their choice of referral a team's medical staff might refer to vague commendations (often from players) and internet surfing. On one occasion, 'the surgeon's website claims he has an interest in this injury' was the justification I heard for despatching an athlete hundreds of miles away. Forget the more local specialists with not only 'an interest' but a proven track record – they are not so exotic.

Leaving on a jet plane

'Cause I'm leavin' on a jet plane
Don't know when I'll be back again'
John Denver, 'Leaving on a Jet Plane' (1966)

It is understandable that overseas players in our soccer Premier League may choose to return 'home' when they are injured, to consult surgeons who have looked after them previously and who share a common language. The reverse also occurs. In 2016, Gareth Bale dislocated ankle tendons while playing for Real Madrid. There would have been a raft of capable Madrid surgeons available but Bale returned home for treatment.

My first overseas athlete arrived in the mid-1990s. He was a world top ten tennis player and travelled to Northampton from the French Open. At the time we operated out of a former nursing home and had no luxurious accoutrements. The player had keyhole surgery and next morning announced that he was flying to California for rehabilitation.

I blanched at the thought of the risks of flying so soon after surgery and took the necessary precautions. He spent just 48 hours in the Mecca of the East Midlands.

I never saw him again but he phoned to let me know how he was getting on. He returned to court quickly, beat Pete Sampras in his first tournament back and had another decade at the top. I have no idea why he came to Northampton; at the time, the best-known ankle arthroscopists were in California.

Top-tier English football has undergone a remarkable transformation since the Premier League was formed in 1992, and with it has come the cult of the foreign manager. Between 1992 and 2018, 385 managerial (including caretaker) appointments were made, including coaches from 20 different overseas countries. From 1992 to 2009, 85 per cent of those appointments were British. Between 2010 and 2018 that figure fell to 51 per cent.

It is not just Premier League chairmen who are in thrall to all things foreign – medical care at football clubs has become so as well. Players with overseas managers are now often directed to visit surgeons who have served their boss's previous clubs. Incoming coaches are not keen to understand the 'local surgical scene' or even to trust the experience and established contacts of the club's own medical team.

A new Premier League manager frequently imports a raft of technical support staff and this churn has been extended to medical teams. In business this is known as a 'corporate lift out': an organisation seeks to prosper quickly by engaging a group of proven successful professionals who have worked together previously. Even a talent as obvious as Pep Guardiola does not have inevitable success embedded in his DNA but by employing his henchmen he increases his chances of early success.

The arrival of overseas medical staff must be balanced by the removal of the experience and contacts of the incumbent clinicians. Over long periods they will have built up a network of specialists in various fields who newcomers will know nothing of.

In 2018 the ex-Watford physiotherapist Richard Collinge announced he was taking legal action against the club following his 2016 dismissal, 'I was sacked for being an Englishman,' he was reported as saying. Walter Mazzarri had been appointed Watford manager and had brought six Italian backroom staff with him. Mazzarri himself was sacked eight months later. West Ham snapped up Collinge as their head of medicine.

This practice increases the likelihood of lax ligaments and mangled menisci heading for the nearest airport; if a club appoints an Italian manager the chances are that your star striker will finish up on an operating table in Milan.

After Guardiola's arrival at Manchester City, the *Manchester Evening Telegraph* reported that he was 'taking a hands-on approach to City's medical department'. It was explained that he was helping reduce the injury toll. Was he not busy enough coaching?

In 2016, he appointed Dr Eduardo Mauri, the former Espanyol footballer, as the club's head of medical staff. Guardiola also appears to be able to call on the services of an orthopaedic surgeon in Barcelona who he described in the Manchester newspaper as 'the best doctor in the world'. Guardiola continues to use this appellation. Previously, the Spanish surgeon had treated numerous Barcelona and Bayern Munich players during Guardiola's tenures in Spain and Germany. There is no indication that the surgeon himself promoted or requested such an accolade. Interestingly, Rafael Nadal's troubled knees also find their way to Barcelona in times of trouble, but to another knee specialist. The city is clearly blessed with experts dealing with this specific joint.

What does Guardiola mean by his statement? Does he mean that the doctor's knowledge is better than any other physician on the planet? Manchester City should be concerned, because it suggests that their manager spends more time scouring the medical literature than reviewing football videos. It is of course arrant nonsense.

City players have suffered a catalogue of injuries. In 2016, Kevin de Bruyne was despatched to Spain with his troublesome hamstring only a month into the season. He was accompanied by the club's great, but injury prone, captain and centre-back Vincent Kompany, who had a groin injury. Fabian Delph's groin injury was not healed by the club's new medics and he, too, was despatched to Spain for surgery, returning to first-team action four-and-half months later.

In November 2016, Kompany returned to Spain with a knee ligament injury, which was reported to be his 35th injury in eight years at the Etihad Stadium. Guardiola insisted that his player was now 'in the best hands'. Unfortunately, despite Guardiola's reassurance, Kompany did not play for another ten weeks instead of the initially predicted three to four.

A month later, the German player İlkay Gündoğan ruptured a cruciate ligament in his knee. He was despatched to Catalonia. This highly talented player was Guardiola's first Manchester City signing but it was reported that the club had had doubts about the player's durability before he was signed, due to a catalogue of injuries including to his knees and back.

Gündoğan returned nine months later and has made important playing contributions to the club since. However, in an interview with the *Manchester Evening Telegraph*, under the heading 'Why he'll never be the same player again', the 27-year-old said, 'If I said I am the same player as I was a year ago, I would be lying … that was the second injury on my knee, so obviously my knee doesn't feel like the knee of a 20-year-old footballer … I need to do things to take care of everything, but especially the knee.'

Following the exodus of injured Manchester City players to see medics in Barcelona, the *Daily Mirror* revealed in November 2016 that Arsenal were also sending their players to Spain for treatment. Santi Carzola's Wikipedia page chronicles the unfortunate tale of his Achilles injury, on which he had 11 operations and which, in November 2017, Arsène Wenger described as the worst injury he had come across. The little Spanish midfielder had lost a large section of his Achilles and had come close to amputation. He said that his doctor in Spain had 'never had a case where two different bacteria eat away at eight to ten centimetres of an Achilles tendon'. It was another 686 days before the player returned to club football – now in Spain. He eventually represented his country again.

Meanwhile, back at the Etihad, Manchester City's trail of injury blues continued. In February 2017, Gabriel Jesus broke a metatarsal in his right foot. The club ignored the half-dozen orthopaedic surgeons in the area skilled in this surgery and flew him to Spain for surgery by the man Guardiola rated as the 'best in the world'. The player came back ten weeks post-surgery – two weeks longer than the original estimate and par for the course. In April 2019 Chelsea joined in, despatching Callum Hudson-Odoi to Catalonia for treatment on his ruptured Achilles.

Guardiola is not alone in making bold claims about medics. Jose Mourinho claims to have the best dentist in the world; I doubt if his dentist makes the same claim. Probably Mourinho doesn't genuinely think this but it is his way of telling the world, and himself, that he can identify and utilise the best molar filler on the planet. And if his special skills extend this far then his judgement on football matters must be unchallengeable too.

People are experts in narrow fields and Guardiola, Mourinho and Wenger are great football managers. Full stop. Even the best, most astute tactical and man-management coaches cannot always prevent players' injuries or accelerate their return to play. Surgeons such as Guardiola's friend have well-deserved reputations for their clinical skills. But even when great coaches are assisted by the 'best doctor in the world' miraculous healing is not guaranteed nor the prevention of complications. Medical successes and misfortunes are no respecters of national boundaries. Hyperbole in elite sport is commonplace but when it is applied to medicine it threatens integrity and invites suspicion.

Another major problem in English football is the likely tenure of the manager. In 2015 it was estimated to be on average 15 months. This creates turmoil in clubs. Usually the manager's expensively assembled staff leave with him, including the medics – the new boss wants his own team – and players have to keep up with the turbulence. Lost is the experience of the clinicians who knew intimately the long medical history of specific players, because there is no continuity.

Many countries, including the UK, have surgeons of international standing based upon research, education and surgical outcomes. These surgeons do not work in the most expected places. AC Milan sent David Beckham and his torn Achilles to see Sakari Orava in the town of Turku in Finland. In Sweden, outstanding work has come from Hakan Alfredson, who is based in the small town of Umea, 400 miles north of Stockholm.

There are potential hazards in undergoing surgery by overseas doctors, however, whether in sending patients abroad or in the recent trend for surgeons to fly to the UK (and out again in short order). One is circulatory problems, such as deep vein thrombosis, from travelling too soon after surgery. Patients have a right to expect immediate help from their surgeon if they have post-operative problems and British surgeons have had to pick up the pieces after much-vaunted overseas surgical stars have flown the nest. A surgeon's duty of care does not cease when the final suture is in place.

I have experienced athletes' reluctance to return to see their chosen specialist because of the distances involved. Even if they have worrying wounds or persistent pain athletes can turn up on the door of the local surgeon. This is the same poor sap that they (or their manager) did not trust in the first place to undertake the work.

In the mid-1990s I heard a radio programme involving several major sports names of the day. One, an Olympic champion, discussed his frequent trips to Germany for treatment. He was asked how he judged the quality of a clinic and its staff and included ease of parking, coffee quality and freedom from autograph hunters in his reply. The sportspeople felt that 'top surgeons' should be identified and located at centres like Loughborough, where many national teams were based, and be immediately accessible for operating on injured athletes.

This suggestion ignored the sheer number of surgeons this would involve because of increasing specialisation. It would also lead to deskilling because of the small number of operations required. The surgeons would be twiddling their thumbs most of the time.

So, do away goals count double?

Elite sportspeople tend to sustain the same scope of injuries as a Sunday morning park footballer and a critical review of injury outcomes and return time to sport does not always reveal results significantly different between the privileged few doctors globally and the local 'jobbing surgeon'.

Information on sports players has been revolutionised by computer analysis. The work by Billy Beane and the Oakland 'As' baseball team, celebrated in the book and film *Moneyball*, is a prime example of this. From his work we know that combining information from many sources, including statistical analysis, will help with player acquisition, team selection and tactics. However, objective data determining the world's best surgeon is less clear than the rationale for giving Sam Allardyce or Alan Pardew the next available managerial vacancy in the Premier League.

To be able to determine differences in outcomes between surgeons it is necessary to have huge numbers of patients to study. Such numbers are available, for instance, in cancer surgery and in aspects of orthopaedics with common procedures such as hip and knee replacements generating large databases from which some surgeons will emerge more skilled than others. However, differences may become apparent only after five to ten years of study. Even then, it is unlikely that Chelsea will sign their next centre-back from a pensioner group with hip replacements.

Even those surgeons looking after the elite will undertake most of their surgery on weekend warriors. Using one surgeon's results only from prime athletes would, in most cases, reduce the sample size to low levels, rendering them unsuitable for analysis. Perhaps only knee ligament repairs and keyhole (arthroscopic) surgery would escape such difficulties.

It is obvious that the demands made of a Barcelona midfield dynamo after surgery will be different to those of your Wednesday-night, five-a-side insurance salesman. Most surgeons will probably have good outcomes for the latter but minor differences in surgical prowess are more likely to be obvious in the outcomes for the sporting elite. However, for most conditions, information is not available.

Achilles injuries are a prime example of these differences and ruptures of this tendon can have fearful consequences. Soccer players such as David Beckham, John Barnes, Mark Lawrenson, Neil Webb, Yakubu Aiyegbeni and Christian Benteke are illustrations of elite athletes suffering this damage.

I was faced with a group of Achilles ruptures in elite teenage gymnasts. World literature gave no indication of how teenagers or high-performing high bar exponents would recover and research suggested a general return to the same standard of any sport varying from 54 per cent to 73 per cent. Outcomes for elite athletes following Achilles rupture had hardly reached clinical consciousness. The *Daily Mail* attempted a non-scientific review of felled soccer players following David Beckham's Achilles rupture in 2010. It made depressing reading. Phrases like 'never the same player again' and 'retired prematurely' dominated. In America, 36 per cent of footballers (NFL) and 39 per cent of basketball (NBA) victims did not return professionally after such injuries. Many more prematurely retired or had reduced performance. However, these were not the outcomes of one or two surgeons – they were the pooled results of many. Nobody knows who was the best stitcher.

In my gymnastic group I was aided by colleagues and did not publish the results for years. I needed to follow the athletes' careers first. Fortunately, all resumed their careers and several won numerous national and international medals. However, soccer, rugby and cricket do not have years to consider outcomes – they live in the now.

There are important differences for elite athletes which are denied to most: they have rapid access to knowledgeable doctors and an array of imaging tools; they can have surgery at a time to suit them and the injury; they have entrée to the best post-operative science and rehabilitation personnel and equipment; and they are fit and extremely well-motivated patients.

Given those advantages most surgeons would like to think they could achieve comparable results: 90 per cent of acute elite sports injuries can be managed by 90 per cent of well-trained local surgical units and the increasing trend to denigrate local expertise is unwarranted. The key is recognising the injuries that fall outside your comfort zone.

So, there is no UEFA Champions League for shoulder, knee or spinal surgery. The Holy Grail of finding the best surgeon in the world is akin to finding the end of the rainbow. To saddle a medic with this title is putting undue pressure on that individual and degrading the thousands of excellent surgeons out there.

Football managers might announce that they have identified the greatest doctor/surgeon/dentist in the world but it is all hot air arising from the fevered furnace of elite sport. It burnishes those managers' reputations for infallibility and omniscience but does nothing beyond that.

Chapter 29

'SISTER! BOIL ME
UP A SOLICITOR'

Words attributed to the late George Bonnie
(1920–2007), orthopaedic surgeon and raconteur,
St Mary's Hospital, London, spoken while
addressing his theatre sister when faced with a
challenging surgical case

Flirting with the law

No one wants a clash with the legal eagles, least of all sports doctors, but legal actions against doctors have never been more common despite medical expertise and technology having never been more sophisticated.

It is claimed that we imported this litigious culture from America. When I worked in Massachusetts in the 1980s my insurance (paid for by the hospital) exceeded my salary. In the last 30 years, the UK has caught up but not everywhere is so ready to take to the law courts. A Peruvian surgeon told me that doctors in her country have no insurance. 'Why should anybody sue me? I always do my best for my patients.' Unfortunately, I anticipate that Lima will soon resemble London from a legal perspective.

For over a century doctors in the UK have insured themselves with medical defence organisations (MDOs). These cover medics against legal actions by patients. To understand the impact on the sporting world one must start in the context of the legal challenges facing the wider British health economy.

'The one great principle of the English law is, to make business for itself.'

Charles Dickens (1812–1870), *Bleak House* **(1853)**

The number of claims against the NHS for injury and negligence is soaring. The NHS spends around 15 per cent of its annual budget settling actions. That sum would build a lot of hospitals and improve staffing numbers enormously.

In March 2016 the NHS Litigation Authority reported that it had set aside £56.4bn for known and predicted future claims. The next year, legal fees increased by 19 per cent. The NHS Litigation Authority renamed itself NHS Resolution that year. It should not be confused with its near namesake HMS *Resolution*. The irony of giving the organisation the same name as a First World War Royal Navy battleship was not lost on me. The ship was one of the Navy's Revenge class boats.

The private health sector fares no better. In 2016 an MDO referred to a 'toxic claims culture' with 'rocketing compensation costs'. Claims-inflation was rising 10 per cent annually with costs doubling every seven years.

The compensation culture in this country developed quickly from the mid-1980s, fuelled not least by the advent of conditional fee agreements or 'no win no fee' deals. Effectively, open season was declared on medics and other healthcare professionals; costs of MDO subscriptions had risen dramatically within five years. To help doctors working within NHS hospitals, Crown Indemnity was introduced in 1990, under which the responsibility for handling and financing claims of negligence against hospital medical staff fell to their employer, the NHS. Doctors remained responsible for paying insurance for work outside of their NHS-based hospital – including work with sporting organisations such as pitchside cover. This made it difficult and expensive for young doctors to gain experience in the sporting sphere.

In 1991 my annual insurance was less than £2,000. Twenty years later it had risen to over £43,000. Colleagues with specialty interests in other areas, such as spines, had annual premiums exceeding £100,000. These eye-watering sums have caused some doctors to stop working in elite sport.

Pricing themselves out of a decent opinion?
Writing large personal cheques every year for such huge sums is certainly chastening. Does it give you peace of mind? No. The ceiling

for a single medical negligence claim is set at a maximum of £10m by most MDOs.

Sporting superstars earn colossal amounts of money. A claim for loss of earnings resulting from alleged medical negligence would exceed the £10m ceiling within months for these athletes. Furthermore, these players have considerable worth to their clubs.

In 2008, an 18-year-old Manchester United youth-team player received £4.3m in compensation following a broken leg from a 2003 playing incident. He had made a further 50 appearances abroad before retiring in 2007. The payout was based on future lost potential earnings.

By 2009, I felt that the challenges faced by sports doctors had reached critical levels and wrote an article in our professional organisation's newsletter entitled 'Elite Sport, Indemnity and the Orthopaedic Surgeon'.

Inevitably the story has moved on significantly since then.

Where is a duty of care owed?

'I do perceive here a divided duty'

William Shakespeare, *Othello* (1602–1604)

Before the mid-2000s, club doctors (even of major soccer clubs) were usually part-time local GPs. Remuneration from the clubs may have been minimal or nothing. They saw players in their own practices or at the club and liaised with local specialists and club physiotherapists. The latter may also have been part-time. A GP's presence at home games was welcome, not least because it fulfilled health and safety requirements. International teams of major sports followed similar models.

This situation continues in the lower echelons of sport. However, the organisation and expertise of medical support for more wealthier outfits has become increasingly sophisticated. In 2005, following the introduction of sport and exercise medicine as a separate speciality, senior clubs began to employ sports doctors on either part-time or full-time contracts. By 2008, some of the MDOs had become very concerned about the position of medics employed by these organisations, aka 'the club doctor'.

Do such doctors have a dual responsibility to the player and the club? Could negligent medical treatment risk legal action from both the player and the employing organisation, to recoup the financial loss of their asset? More recently a footballer criticised his club doctor in the media. He felt he was cajoled into playing with an injury by the promise of seeing 'the best people in the world' at the end of the season and that the 'doctor's agenda was different to mine'. The implication was that the medic was siding with the club's interests rather than those of the patient.

In the 2008/09 season, some MDOs started refusing to insure doctors employed by football clubs in the higher echelons – the existence of sports medicine doctors was being threatened by the unintended consequences of the huge wealth and worth of the players under their care. One MDO reiterated that its upper ceiling for a successful claim remained limited to £10m. The purpose of compensation was related to the needs of the patient – not the financial concerns of the club. It warned that 'sports clubs should not rely on recovering their investment, in the event of negligent treatment', from the insurer of the doctor.

Legal problems are not confined to soccer. Rugby union faced its first case of a player suing his club for clinical negligence in March 2013, following two concussions sustained by a player in the same match. The player was forced to retire having failed to recover and the action was taken against the club as the employer. The actions of the club's clinical staff were also investigated. Such scenarios can involve the sporting organisation bringing their clinicians into any legal action as a third party and doctors and physiotherapists have needed to ensure full cover for such eventualities. However, most MDOs will not insure against claims made by employers, agents, sponsors, sporting organisations or organisers or owners of a sporting event. The MDO SEMPRIS was formed in 2010 to plug the gap in cover left by the other MDOs. It provides indemnity, advice, and support for doctors whose work brings them into professional contact with athletes. Critically, it provides a higher ceiling of cover for sports doctors.

The sports team environment does not lend itself to potential dissection by a forensic barrister. Hospitals, clinics and GP surgeries have provided medical care as their *raison d'être*. Their systems should be well oiled. Information recording and providing safe interventions are subject to constantly evolving audit, review and inspection by outside agencies such as the CQC.

A sport's organisation's core activity is winning games or developing champions. Medicine must fit around this central ambition. Premier League football clubs and their ilk spend millions on state-of-the-art medical facilities, but for the majority the funding of clinical departments comes a long way down the pecking order.

The nature of team sport is that half the games are played away which means that ailing athletes will be treated in all kinds of facilities, including away dressing rooms, hotel rooms and luxury coaches on the motorway. This also means that the travelling physiotherapist cannot always have to hand all their clinical records and favourite bits of equipment.

Chelsea away from home in a Champions League fixture or athletes at Olympic holding camps will have experienced sports physicians in attendance. Northants cricket visiting Weston-super-Mare will not. In a clinical sense, the physiotherapist is 'Billy no mates'.

Sports injuries happen unpredictably and require rapid management. Coaches need to know whether players can continue and whether to alter their tactics. Within this maelstrom of decision-making, accurate medical note-taking often takes a back seat. Frequently the team physiotherapist is multitasking, especially in those few minutes before the team takes to the field – dealing with a request for a painkiller from the fast bowler while simultaneously strapping the wicketkeeper's ankle. The retrospective note of each activity may be forgotten. However, when matters turn sour it is this documented evidence that forms the basis of a clinician's legal defence.

Lack of records can cause problems for both the doctor and athlete. It makes a doctor look sloppy, raises suspicions over the intended use of the treatment, and leaves a cloud over the recipient. Poor record-keeping has come home to roost in recent high-profile cases such as Mo Farah's L-carnitine injections and British Cycling and Team Sky's use of TUEs for Bradley Wiggins' asthma.

Farah's 2014 injection came under scrutiny from Parliament's Digital, Culture, Media and Sport Committee. 'We believe the General Medical Council should investigate any incident where doctors working in sport have failed to properly record the medicines they are supplying to athletes,' the Committee said. The doctor's defence was that he was responsible for the care for 140 athletes and was understaffed. He received little support from his boss. 'Inexcusable' was the verdict.

The United Kingdom Anti-Doping investigation into the Wiggins Jiffy Bag affair heavily criticised British Cycling and Team Sky. Among many misgivings was the fact that the British Cycling medical room was 'chaotic and disorganised'. There was no record of medicines given to athletes or those sent to events – home and abroad. Papers were found piled up in cupboards.

Working in sport, clinicians can have difficulties protecting their independence. At the core of their work is the well-being of the athlete-patient. It takes a combination of knowledge, experience and confidence in a doctor's abilities to confront tricky issues appropriately. Challenging problems arise, such as the withdrawal of a player from a game through injury, pressures from coaches for an athlete to return to play, and deciding when an athlete-patient's right to medical confidentiality is endangered. Confidentiality is difficult to maintain in an organisation that frequently leaks like a sieve. Everybody from the kit man to the chief executive wants to know if the star striker will make Saturday's game.

Like any business, sport is governed by health and safety regulations. Doctors within sport fulfil many of the roles of an Occupational Health (OH) doctor and employers have the right to know if an employee is fit to undertake the work expected of them. However, they have no right of access to medical records. Doctors need explicit consent from players to reveal medical information to non-clinical colleagues, including coaches. Usually this is not a problem but a doctor should not automatically assume an athlete's consent.

Sports doctors must manage injuries and illnesses. They must advise when a player is ready to return and, critically, on the probability of injury recurrence. Players must know future health risks even if recovery seems complete. For example, arthritis detected in a joint may have no present symptoms but the player must be advised on whether continuing sport might accelerate matters. Usually an explanation suffices for the athlete to make an informed decision but sometimes the risks may be significant. The doctor may feel that the risk to health – present and future – for the athlete is high and refuse to sanction continued involvement in the sport on medical grounds. Such decisions are rare and usually taken only after discussions with colleagues.

The case of Hamed versus Mills, Tottenham Hotspur and Cowie in 2015 bought this issue to public attention. Radwan Hamed was a teenager who had undergone cardiac screening like all young professional footballers. The purpose of the screening was to discover heart problems that might lead to future serious concerns. Everybody in football remembered Fabrice Muamba's near fatal collapse at White Hart Lane in 2012.

Hamed's tests raised suspicions which needed following up but, unfortunately, a year later, the youngster developed an irregular heartbeat during a youth game and sustained brain damage. Hamed and his parents were not aware of the concerns raised by the tests and so did not have the knowledge to allow them to decide whether he should accept the risk and continue with sport or stop. Spurs joined their own in-house doctors in defending the case.

In 2016 Hamed received £7m in compensation. In the judgement 30 per cent of the blame was apportioned to the cardiologist for inadequately communicating concerns. Spurs and their doctors were held 70 per cent responsible for not acting on the cardiologist's concerns. The club doctors agreed to indemnify the club for damages.

In September 2019 the signing-on spectre surfaced. It 'will send a shiver down the spine of every doctor and physio working in sport', *The Sun* announced. Sunderland were suing their former doctor for £13,182,647.93p after signing a player with troublesome knees. The club doctor was in London for a first-team fixture at the time of the examination and delegated it to other experts. Knee problems were identified but the doctor told the club that they were not significant. The case is ongoing and the club contends that the doctor was in breach of contract and negligent as he 'did not oversee the medical appropriately, or act with best practice'. The ramifications either way could be widespread. The doctor was not a 'knee specialist' in the sense that an orthopaedic surgeon might be. In future, should doctors only give advice in areas in which they are acknowledged experts? If so, signing-on medicals will be protracted affairs. Will sports doctors join the 'defensive medicine society'? Any sniff of an old injury could cause them to advise the club to back off, in which case will they then face legal action if the player joins a rival club and has a successful career? Doctors will struggle to win this game.

'Cured yesterday of my disease,
I died last night of my physician'

English Poet Matthew Prior (1664–1721), 'The Remedy
Worse than the Disease'

While doctors employed by clubs are most in the firing line when things go wrong, specialists providing back-up at games, undertaking pre-signing medicals or sitting in their clinics are not immune. Back in 2006 such dangers were clear. A footballer successfully sued his surgeon after failing to recover sufficiently from an injury and subsequent operation. Simultaneously, the player's club brought a case against the same doctor. The club wanted millions of pounds to replace the player and to cover the loss of his transfer value and wages. Even though the club had recommended the surgeon and arranged the consultation, it was established that there was no contract between the club and surgeon. The club lost the case. The surgeon was ruled to owe no duty to the club and his duty of care to the player not the employer was reinforced.

Clear advice has been given by MDOs to specialists seeing elite sports people. Doctors are advised to accept referrals principally from other medical practitioners, although if other clinicians such as physiotherapists are well known to the sports specialist they also may refer. Requests from other members of sporting organisations are not acceptable.

The FSEM has advised that any professional fees should be addressed directly to the patient, even if the bill is subsequently forwarded by the athlete to their employers. This can come as a surprise to highly paid footballers, used to finances being taken care of by their clubs or agents.

Fringe benefits

'A gift consists not in what is done or given,
but in the intention of the giver or doer.'

Seneca, Roman Stoic philosopher (4 BC–AD 65),
Moral Essays: Volume III

Many specialists maintain an honorary position with clubs and sporting organisations. This has advantages for both doctor and club. Critically, independence should be maintained in both clinical decision-making and employment status for the former.

However, there can be fringe benefits and specialists may be in receipt of complimentary match tickets, season tickets, car park passes and hospitality. GMC guidance states: 'You must not allow any interests you have to affect the way you prescribe for, (or) treat … patients … You must not ask for or accept any inducement, gift or hospitality which may affect or be seen to affect the way you prescribe for, treat or refer patients …' These guidelines relate mainly to gifts received from patients, but there are two important points to consider in the world of sport.

The specialist may not be seen as entirely impartial in decision-making for an athlete if they are receiving gifts from a sporting organisation. There may be a conflict between what the athlete feels is the best course of action for themselves and what is best for the club. Secondly, such benefits may be construed by others as compensation for services to the club. If they are accepted, a reciprocal arrangement could be seen to have been made between the club and the doctor.

It is a hard road to follow when people in business and commerce can enjoy the largesse of sporting organisations without risking censure, and it can be difficult to decide when your professional input at a sporting event justifies the acceptance of a seat or car park place to allow you to fulfil your duties. Not wishing to fall foul of probity guidance, I paid for my own season tickets for 11 years at Northampton Saints while performing unpaid pitchside duties and post-game injury assessments.

Take cover!

How might these changing times affect other busy doctors? They might offer to provide medical cover at a local club or ask for advice on participation in a sporting event.

In 2010, the FSEM issued a code of conduct for doctors working at sports events. They emphasise that any doctor agreeing to provide cover has a professional duty of care. With this carries a legal responsibility, even if they are doing it for love and not money. If they agree in advance to attend such events, either voluntarily or for payment, they are considered to be private practitioners. As such, there exists a contractual obligation and requirement for professional insurance. This should be discussed by the doctor and the relevant organisation prior to the event.

This is a long way from the customary model for organising medical cover for sporting events in this country, such as the local under-11s rugby or cricket tournament. The traditional scenario involved something like a phone call to the local doctor a week before; often the medic was a friend of a parent on the organising committee. If any remuneration existed it was commonly a pint and pie in the bar after the conclusion of hostilities. Very few of these sporting events have the financial means to arrange specific indemnity cover, even if the need for such cover occurred to the organisers and press-ganged doctor.

The awareness of medicolegal banana skins has increased enormously in recent years. Political correctness, risk assessments of public events and Disclosure and Barring Service certification have alerted everybody's antennae. However, many events continue to fly by the seat of their pants. An inadvisable intervention by a doctor to a stricken player outside their level of expertise can land them in hot water. It may not be judged as a 'Good Samaritan act' in the eyes of the law.

Professional comfort zones

In modern times, we desire experiences to fulfil physical and psychological challenges beyond our normal day-to-day lives. However, our ambitions to step beyond our own comfort zones can create dilemmas for medical advisors who may be forced to step out of theirs.

Concerns over advice to sportsmen and women is certainly not confined to elite circles and problems have arisen from the popularity of mass participation events. These include marathons, tough mudders and extreme physical challenges such as Ironman races. Organisers want to minimise the sudden demise of participants and, often, require applicants to seek medical clearance from unsuspecting general practitioners. It's a clear case of passing a potentially very hot potato.

The first marathon in 490 BC led to the death of its sole participant, Pheidippides. However, perspective is needed. In 2007 it was estimated that the risk of death during a marathon was eight per million people – ten times safer than giving birth. Triathlons had double the risk at 15 per million contestants.

In 2017, an MDO reported many enquiries from doctors who felt underqualified to assess the medical readiness of a patient to undertake various challenges.

Its website advised that 'GPs may not always have the required expertise to deem the patient fit to take part without risk and will understandably be worried about the implications of signing such a form. GMC guidance requires a doctor to do their best to ensure reports they write are not misleading and says they should not undertake assessments beyond their area of clinical competence.'

The fit-to-compete requests were not confined to marathons. They included such diverse events as 'fat camps' hosted in the desert, mock hostage situations and even events where the participant had to undergo psychological torture.

Closing remarks for the defence

Legal costs will rise and 'no win no fee' solicitors proliferate. Settlements for claims will increase exponentially; sports doctors will face the extra 'jeopardy' of being implicated in 'third-party' actions.

However, enthusiastic and knowledgeable clinicians will still want to care for athletes of all ages and skill levels, within and without the NHS. The enjoyment can wear off, though. One highly experienced surgeon has in recent times stopped treating professional footballers.

All doctors will receive complaints from patients. Many result from a breakdown in communication, misinterpretation of information and unrealistic expectations. Such accusations can be hurtful, especially when you have tried to give of your best. They create anxiety; doctors' reactions to such events are no different to the rest of society.

Medics should resist exhortations from non-clinical managers and politicians to reduce face-to-face time with patients. They need to accurately record consultations and interventions. Case law has established that claiming an NHS clinic was overbooked is not a mitigating factor in misdiagnosis. Using the defence that you were trying to look after multiple athletes simultaneously may not win much sympathy in the courtroom.

Complaints leading to legal action are not confined to the few. Although accurate data is hard to acquire I anticipate that most doctors presently working in this country will become involved in a legal action during their careers. This risks developing a culture of defensive medicine and increases national health costs from investigations ordered 'just in case'.

The British legal system is adversarial and doctors and patients with their many advisors are forced to withdraw to their respective bunkers and throw grenades at each other. Cases involving health concerns take an intolerable time to resolve, because traditionally the law works at a pace that would be totally unacceptable in any other profession. Delays can cause resentment and frustration for the claimant.

Frequently, this serves neither the patient nor the doctor but only lines the pockets of rapacious lawyers. I was involved in a case that lasted nearly seven years and endured three gruesome days in court before the truth was established. I can attest to the toll such actions take on all parties while still holding on to the certainty that I tried to do the right thing for my patient.

Chapter 30

PUBLISH AND BE DAMNED!

Confidentiality in sport

'... in thee have I trusted: let me
never be confounded'

Morning Prayer Te Deum

MAINTAINING PATIENT confidentiality is a central principle of medicine. Patients expect that only clinicians directly involved in their healthcare should be privy to sensitive information without their consent.

In December 2018, Salford Royal Hospital announced an enquiry into whether uninvolved staff had accessed the records of Sir Alex Ferguson. One newspaper headline read, 'Doctors spied on ailing Sir Alex Ferguson'. Staff stood accused of breaching patient confidentiality and data protection laws. In extreme cases doctors can be struck off for this activity.

Sir Alex did not comment but would have had genuine cause to feel violated. If the details were relayed to third parties it would represent a serious infringement. Where does this place athletes when their football manager broadcasts their injuries to the media without explicit permission?

In 2019 Manchester United had a medical emergency during a pre-season tour to Australia. A club statement revealed, 'A member of our backroom staff was taken ill overnight and has been sent to hospital ... We request that medical confidentiality be respected.' Sadly, such niceties are not often observed for sportspeople.

The GMC lays down the circumstances required before medical information can be disclosed. This includes when required by law, if a patient gives consent or if in the public interest. To that might be added preventing the patient coming to harm. Similar strict guidelines are published by governing bodies of allied health professions including physiotherapy and nursing.

The athlete-patients mentioned in this book are only those of people who granted specific permission or where details were already available within the public arena such as media articles, autobiographies, broadcast interviews or the internet, including social media.

I have had misgivings about patient confidentiality in sport for some time and the subject came into sharp focus during a conference in Cardiff in 2009. During a discussion, an experienced physiotherapist, heavily involved in elite sport, expressed the view that medical ethics within sport should be regarded as different to other areas of healthcare. No.

Terry's all gold surgery

Imagine the *Daily Tabloid* leading with the headline, 'Mrs Toni Terry has undergone a successful operation for her haemorrhoids today, claims colorectal surgeon Bill Ribbans'. Mrs and Mr John Terry would be mortified. Most likely, a complaint to the GMC would follow – assuming that the patient had not given consent for a public broadcast.

So why do we think that a similar headline about her husband published by the BBC under the headline 'Terry has surgery on back injury' in 2006 is acceptable? The report said: 'Chelsea and England captain John Terry has undergone successful surgery to cure his troublesome back injury. But Blues officials have yet to reveal how long they expect the 26-year-old centre-half to be out of action. "The operation to remove a sequestrated lumbar intervertebral disc was successful," said a Chelsea statement.'

The timing of Chelsea's press statement made me think. The BBC report was posted at 17.21 on the day of surgery. The player was still in the early post-operative hours, probably with fluctuating levels of consciousness. Was he capable of providing consent for this information to be shared with the outside world? Terry could not have authorised the release of the statement pre-operatively because he could not have predicted the outcome of the procedure.

Fatuous press communiqués

How many of us have read an immediate post-surgical bulletin on a sports star claiming that the operation has been a failure?

'Wilshere undergoes successful ankle surgery,' trumpeted West Ham in 2018. The midfielder had seen his career stall at Arsenal following a series of injuries. He had joined the Hammers before his latest setback was announced. With relief it was announced that 'the surgeon was happy with the procedure'. The club believed he could be back within four weeks. Unfortunately, it was ten weeks before he was back on the subs' bench.

John Orchard, the Australian sports injury researcher, re-tweeted a comment credited to Dr David J. Chao MD. "Surgery is success" now, is like "Excellent pick" right after the (American football) draft. Time will tell. Hope it's true?' Such immediate optimism is inevitably speculative.

Andy Murray underwent keyhole hip surgery in January 2018 in Australia. After surgery, he said that the 'surgeon was very happy with how it went' and that 'my plan is to be back playing around the grass court season, potentially before then'.

Twelve months later the player admitted that he was likely to remain in pain for the rest of his career. BBC Radio interviewed his Melbourne surgeon who confirmed that at the time of surgery Murray's joint 'wasn't really at a stage where we could attempt to make his hip normal, it was just to try and make it as good as we could'. It is better for the media not to press athletes or doctors on return-to-play schedules. This only heightens speculation when hastily plotted comeback dates are not met.

Leaking sieves, plugging holes and avoiding being stitched up like a kipper

The safe holding of athletes' confidential medical information has never been more difficult to control. Social networking sites allow the spread of individuals' personal details, and dedicated online sites monitor closely sportspeople's injuries.

In 2016 a group called The Fancy Bears hacked the WADA computers and leaked medical files. Athletes' details were published, many of which were related to TUEs, which are applied for by athletes' medical teams when prohibited drugs are required for genuine health problems. Some may regard these leaks as necessary investigative work. They generate debate and expose difficult grey areas, such as the bending of TUE rules to enhance sporting performance. I share concerns about the misuse of TUEs but many of the athletes had committed no offence and had a reasonable expectation that such information would stay within the medical room or on their doctor's hard drive.

A lot of media space was devoted to the TUEs used to treat Bradley Wiggins' asthma before major cycling events. The BBC reported that the doctor involved, Dr Richard Freeman, 'did not respond to a request for comment'. The implication was that the doctor was in some way being evasive but, rightly, he was following professional-body advice in not replying to media questioning of his actions without the patient's permission.

Concerns have been expressed by numerous organisations, including the British Olympic Association, FA and British Medical Association. Investigations have reported clinicians being pressurised into releasing medical information to team management against athletes' wishes and there have been calls for the development of an ethical code.

A physician's first responsibility is to the athlete-patient. The GMC states that, 'If you are asked to provide information to third parties, such as a patient's employer, you should ... obtain or have seen written consent to disclosure from the patient.' The FSEM recognised that this requirement could cause medical problems. 'This may bring the member or fellow in breach of his/her employment contractual obligations and employer expectations.' One MDO has stated that, 'Even confirming to the media that someone is a patient, without their explicit permission, is a breach of confidentiality,' and the Chartered Society of Physiotherapists confirms, 'Physiotherapy information is only released to sources, other than those immediately involved in the patient's care, when there is a signed patient consent form to allow this process.'

In 2010 I realised how easy it can be to become entangled in an unwelcome story. Our local further education college asked if I would become the medical director of their wonderful new sports rehabilitation centre. A year later I was asked to turn the first sod on site. I was accompanied by various college dignitaries and local worthies. The local newspaper was there to record the happy occasion.

The next day the newspaper published a photograph of my cheesy grin and the spade sinking into the mud. The strapline proclaimed, 'Local residents up in arms at new centre development'. It appeared that the local villagers were unhappy about the traffic implications. I had just become the public face of their wrath.

Fishing expedition

In March 2010 my daughter and I trawled through every national newspaper published that month – 333 editions in total. Obsessive-compulsive, I know.

We identified 5,640 medical bulletins, with each paper averaging 19 medical reports each day. Saturdays were the worst, when 84 per cent of revelations dealt with soccer players' woes. Acute injuries and historical wounds were described, together with details such as the fact that a sportsman had had steroid injected into his testicles. Inevitably there were errors, with 'fibias and tibulas' abounding (it should be tibias and fibulas). On the same day, a cricketer's absence was attributed to ankle surgery and a chronic knee injury by different newspapers.

Two soccer injuries dominated the back pages one month – David Beckham's Achilles, torn while he was playing for AC Milan, and Aaron Ramsey's fractured tibia sustained while playing for Arsenal. There were 145 and 185 medical bulletins respectively on the two injuries. We observed a trend. The newspapers reported the initial press releases from clubs and followed up with information from treating clinicians. 'Medical experts' were wheeled out. Club officials, ex-players, families, friends and even referees provided further comment. Archives were trawled for similar injuries. Players with the same injury described their own experiences.

The era of the personality cult ensures that certain individuals' problems are documented in precise detail; no medical problem seems too trivial when it involves the great and the good. Even in the absence of a major problem Wayne Rooney warranted 125 medical bulletins in 31 days. These included various injuries and illnesses, including minor viral problems.

The contemporaneous 2010/11 Football League/Premier League Contract (Form 13A) supposedly covered the release of medical information: 'The club shall not without the consent in writing of the Player use or reveal the contents of any medical report or other medical information regarding the Player obtained by the Club save for the purpose of assessing the Player's health and fitness obtaining medical and insurance cover and complying with the Club's obligations under the Rules.'

Whether players knowingly waive this right is a moot point. Even if they do, it does not necessarily follow that clinicians are exempt from their own professional responsibilities regarding patient confidentiality. Little has changed since then. The collective gnashing of teeth that greeted Andy Murray's premature announcement that the game was up because of his hip problems followed a similar media montage endured by Beckham in 2010.

Indeed, the tennis player had to run the gauntlet twice following surgical interventions in 2018 and 2019. He was pictured, clearly distressed, at a press conference and there were interviews with fellow players. His treating surgeon was interviewed in print and on the radio and non-involved surgeons described his options and treatment. His mother revealed that her son's punishing regime had worried her throughout his career. Finally, there were interviews with former and contemporary sportspeople who had undergone similar problems and found solutions. At least Murray tried to control the story by his postings on social media, including his post-operative hip X-ray.

Fonts of knowledge?

My daughter and I found that the legitimacy and sources of authorisation of medical press releases were not always clear. Clinicians were directly quoted in less than 1 per cent of the stories. Non-clinical staff were much more responsible for the majority of identified medical bulletins which were credited to any individual. The latter are not constrained by professional norms or disciplinary deterrence. Their source of information is usually the treating medical staff, who may experience conflicts of interest with both patient and employing organisation. In this respect, it is significant that in many organisations the manager/coach has a controlling influence that extends to decisions over the continuing employment of clinical staff.

Our original review took place before the explosion of social media outlets such as Twitter. At that time, athletes in individual sports were more likely to be responsible for personally discussing their own health with track and field athletes responsible for over half of their sport's bulletins. In contrast, individual footballers (5 per cent) and rugby union players (8 per cent) were less likely to address the media themselves. Their sports were likely to have press offices and a culture of having day-to-day activities controlled by their sporting organisations.

The advent of social media in the last decade has changed this. Even when athletes decide to speak directly to the press or their fans, their utterances can be surprising and misleading, which can be unhelpful to the treatment and reputation of those looking after them as revealed in Chapter 9.

Within elite sport, the pressures to leak confidential patient data by clinical staff are considerable, and coaches have manipulated medical situations for tactical gain before events (by distorting injury information) and during game-time (to gain tactical advantage). Clinician participation in providing misleading information runs counter to GMC guidelines to 'only disclose factual information you can substantiate'.

The power of the media must be considered along with its insatiable need to fill the back pages and sports journalists are eager to receive and report sensitive medical information. Stories can be grossly misrepresented by reporters and football managers alike while never achieving the appropriate level of evidence-based commentary. Misleading stories risk fuelling perceptions of the low status of sports medicine professionals.

Some commentators have advocated guidelines to help and support sports' physicians. Others advise a return to an older model of preserving clinical independence from sporting organisations. The multiple gold medal Paraolympian winner Tanni Grey-Thompson's report of 2017 called for precisely this. However, it is difficult to imagine Premier League football clubs agreeing to neutral physiotherapists and doctors at games or for appointments to be made for ill or injured players at the local medical clinic.

I hoped that the publication of our newspaper analysis would contribute to the debate on the ethics of professional boundaries regarding athlete-patient data release and lead to a call for more specific guidelines for reporting on athletes' medical problems. It became required reading on one of the master's courses in sports medicine. Whether it had any effect on sporting organisations is very doubtful.

Clinical staff are bound by the seven principles enshrined within the 1997 Caldicott Report. These include 'access to patient identifiable information should be on a strict need-to-know basis' and 'everyone with access to patient identifiable information should be aware of their responsibilities'. Breaching these codes risks dismissal but many sporting organisations and their staff still choose to drive the proverbial horse and cart through such recommendations.

Stop press?

Sports coverage is traditionally at the back of newspapers and end of television news bulletins, perhaps for good reason. If newspapers were read in the direction intended we would have to wade through columns of doom and gloom; sports stories come as a welcome relief and means of escapism. The problem is that many of us turn to the back first, making sport our world. Its characters, victories, defeats and controversies take on an importance not always warranted in the greater scheme of things.

Injuries to national icons have always attracted detailed attention. The three stitches in Jimmy Greaves' left leg that took him out of the 1966 World Cup were reported in the national press of the time. Tommy Simpson's death on Mon Ventoux during the Tour de France in 1967 made the next day's front pages. The Munich air disaster of February 1958 and updates on the injured and deceased Manchester United players and fellow passengers dominated newspapers and television bulletins.

The media has always had an unhealthy interest in the sick and injured. Michael Green, the best-selling author of *The Art of Coarse Rugby*, recalled his duties as a young journalist at the *Chronicle and Echo* in post-Second World War Northampton. He was one of my late father's colleagues at the time. Each day a scribe would go to Northampton General Hospital and be furnished with the names, addresses and injuries of emergency admissions, enabling the young journo to visit patients' relatives at home to gather information for the local rag. The concept of confidentiality had not reached the East Midlands by the early 1950s.

There are arguments on both sides for both maintaining or decreasing the present level of media intrusion into medical matters. Questions of what is 'in the public interest' and 'what the public is interested in' abound. Those in favour of maintaining the status quo might reply that 'no one has come to any harm', 'its's been going on for ages' and 'sports people court publicity and must accept intrusions into their lives, including the publication of medical details'. Some have argued for a more liberal view to enable the monitoring of injuries and, ultimately, reduce injuries. One 2002 research paper stated, 'Professional athletes are celebrities working in a segment of the entertainment industry, and when they suffer injuries, this is part of the entertainment.'

The obverse would include views that 'media intrusion is increasing', 'sports' contractual clauses are being broken', 'clinical professional guidelines are being breached' and 'clinical management is being misrepresented'. At CAS in 2019 Caster Semenya accused the IAAF of breaching confidentiality rules by releasing the names of medical experts involved in her case.

Accurate information consented by the athlete should reasonably be released. This can be via means of personal interview, social media sites or the employer. Similarly, injuries witnessed on the sports field by journalists and spectators are a matter of public record. However, the unsanctioned disclosure of detailed information at a press conference by a coach offends the norms of medical confidentiality and consent.

Perhaps the mood is changing

In 2018 it was reported in *The Times* that the Munster and Ireland rugby scrum-half Conor Murray 'had not played for Munster this season because of an injury, the nature of which has not been disclosed to the media'. The lack of public information led to wild speculation, described by the player as 'mad injury rumours'.

A year earlier, Dan Roan, sports editor for BBC News, had written an article in the Northampton Town programme under the heading 'Patient confidentiality applies, unless you are a footballer'. He asked, 'Is it fair on footballers to have their ailments broadcast all over the news?' and 'We do know, but do we have a right to know?'

Clinicians working in sport are faced with ethical dilemmas not normally experienced by other medical colleagues. Training in preparation for meeting these situations should be enshrined in sport and exercise medicine education for junior doctors. Athletes' consent to the release of their own medical information is central to this issue. Often, athletes are young and unaware of their rights regarding the control of medical information.

Employers and supporting professional associations should advise athletes appropriately. Medical staff should play a key role in supporting, protecting and educating their patients. Everybody needs reminding of what has been signed in contracts – agents, management, players and medical staff. Would the development of a code of conduct by sporting authorities be helpful?

The press, sporting organisations and clinical and non-clinical staff should be more aware; there are threats to athletes' rights and clinicians' professional status.

Chapter 31

WHAT GOES ON TOUR
COMES BACK FROM TOUR

'O this learning, what a thing it is!'
William Shakespeare, *The Taming of the Shrew* **(1592)**

SURGEONS CANNOT sit on their hands. To do so is to fossilise in an uncomfortable position.

Our profession moves on at a pace. Innovations occur annually and they will not be found by looking under a rock in the East Midlands. Surgeons can never be complacent at any time in their careers and must demonstrate their commitment to continuing professional development.

Each surgical unit has dedicated time for education and audit. Every surgeon must present their 'activity figures' to their peers. They must be robust. There is no time for mutual backslapping. Instead, problems and complications are forensically dissected as would be expected from a collective of cutters. Feedback and the identification of trends from pooled experiences are important for ensuring safer and more successful outcomes for our patients, even if the glare of publicity on your own shortcomings is uncomfortable.

In the 1980s I attempted to lighten up such a session at the Massachusetts General Hospital in Boston by using a cartoon of President Ronald Reagan in my presentation. It was received with deafening silence by the ranks of glittering Harvard professors sitting on the front row. Afterwards I was taken aside and told that, 'We would never parody your Queen.' *Spitting Image* had not yet arrived in the United States.

Doctors can spend entire evenings and every weekend reading the many medical journals available, although the most intense and stimulating activities are found in attending conferences and visiting colleagues. There are numerous meetings and courses for surgeons and, while mandatory for doctors, they are not always fully budgeted for by the NHS. The quality of such congresses in Britain is excellent and interspersed with these meetings are visits to other surgeons, usually doctors respected in the field and developing new techniques. Watching colleagues' approaches to operations that you are embarking on or find challenging can be enlightening.

Breakfast in America
Album by Supertramp (1979)

The more specialist your interests become the further you may have to travel, which inevitably involves seeking out best practice abroad. I appreciated this first at Harvard, in 1987.

My first inkling of my 'transfer' to the States was a letter from my seniors. 'Your career has been discussed. You would benefit from a year in America. Please pass the necessary examinations and present yourself in Boston on July 1st.' OK! Travel expenses and organised accommodation had not been invented, and I had six months to satisfy the Massachusetts medical board that I could speak English and correctly answer 850 multiple choice questions. The latter contained more questions on geriatric sexual preferences than orthopaedic surgery. Surprisingly, I passed.

The house was packed up and my wife resigned her position as a senior ward sister, and with our two-year old daughter we headed off into the unknown. My impressions of America had been gained from episodes of *Bonanza* and *Kojak*. We landed with six suitcases to last a year and tried to find somewhere to live. An apartment was found on Beacon Hill close to the pub featured in the TV comedy *Cheers*.

For a first visit to America, we were lucky. Boston is a great city, full of history and tradition and most importantly sports mad. Despite the upheaval, relative poverty and the sobering experience of being registered as an alien, the year there was a career changer.

America had moved on from the British apprenticeship model of surgical training – 'see one, do one, teach one'. Surgeons now specialised in specific areas, such as hands or feet, and displayed great technical skills combined with advanced, structured teaching superior to that in most hospitals in Britain.

Trainees were expected to practise surgery on cadavers before being let loose on breathing specimens. This was a revelation to me then but it is mainstream now. Ward rounds took place before 0600. Teaching took place over breakfast at 0630, Monday to Friday. Compulsory Saturday morning education began with a written test.

Reading scientific journals changed from being a solitary domestic experience to one that involved sitting with the editor of the most prestigious orthopaedic journal in the world. Everybody sat an annual national examination and each trainee was ranked countrywide. There was no hiding place. Work was intense and the hours were long. Most specialists wanted their patients looked after by their own juniors, which could mean 168 hours' on-call work per week. You slept when you could and crept home when all was quiet.

The hospital on-call sleeping arrangements were novel – a communal, functional room behind the emergency room, where multiple bunk beds hugged the walls and a solitary telephone occupied a coffee table in the centre. It was bedlam – bleeps going off, doctors traipsing wearily in and out in scrubs they had worn for 24 hours. One time I returned from assessing a patient and found that another medic had snuck into my bed.

I worked for several sports surgeons including those responsible for the New England sports teams – New England Patriots (American football), Boston Bruins (ice hockey), Boston Red Sox (baseball) and Boston Celtics (basketball). Ice hockey and basketball featured at the old Boston Gardens, only a stone's throw from the hospital and our apartment. Baseball took place at the iconic Fenway Park and football was out of town in Foxborough.

Felled tree trunks masquerading as defensive linemen arrived in the emergency room via the back of ambulances on autumn Sunday evenings. It could take four of us to man the stretcher. One of my bosses, Bert Zarins, travelled home and away with the Patriots and was also surgeon to the Bruins. On one ice hockey road trip, Bert became so incensed by the physical and verbal goading from opposition fans that he seized a hockey stick and attempted to club the miscreants – all caught live on television.

I adored the skills and athleticism of the Celtics, who were led by the wonderful Larry Bird and who battled with their perennial rivals Los Angeles Lakers led by Magic Johnson. I also saw the astonishing performances of Michael Jordan from the Chicago Bulls. However, it was the Red Sox and Fenway Park that provided my quintessential American experience. Sitting in the bleachers – the uncovered stand – on a balmy

July evening watching Roger Clemens pitching his changeup ball against all comers was close to sporting heaven.

On my few spare Saturday afternoons I turned out for the local rugby team. The standard was decent; two players played in the inaugural Rugby World Cup in Australia in 1987. We changed in cars, played on local parks and went home for a shower.

I learnt a lot about adult sport stateside. American football was king in high schools and colleges but very few players would be drafted into or become multimillionaires in the NFL. There was no organised post-college football infrastructure of junior clubs; probably it was too dangerous. If an impromptu park throw-about did not rock your boat you needed an outlet for your sporting juices. Rugby anyone? Our team comprised exiled Commonwealth players and frustrated local Bostonians. The latter struggled with the nuances of line-outs and throwing the ball backwards but nailed you in the tackle.

American surgeons maintained their power within hospitals long after it had been expunged from our NHS. It massaged their egos but also ensured the best outcomes for patients, for whom the surgeons were strong advocates. When one illustrious surgeon celebrated his 60th birthday he commissioned Sir David Frost to narrate a commemorative video – with opening shots outside the White House. We sat through it before starting surgery. Several times. He also commissioned a new self-portrait. A three-line whip was issued to attend its unveiling at the Harvard Club. How would NHS managers react to similar antics?

'Even while they teach, men learn'

Seneca the Younger (c.4 BC–AD 65), Roman philosopher and poet, *Epistulae Morales*

During my career I have been fortunate enough to teach and lecture on five continents. You always return with more than you have given and the exchange of ideas and challenges to your own beliefs leave you energised.

'When you have caught the rhythm of Africa, you find out that it is the same in all her music'

Karen Blixen, *Out of Africa* (1937)

In 1996 I was asked to host a Saturday morning meeting in Northampton to be addressed by the celebrated South African knee surgeon Daan du Plessis. Our guest had represented the Springboks at rugby in the 'wilderness years' – when South Africa was barred from international competition because of apartheid – and was never on the losing side for Northern Transvaal in six Currie Cup finals. His surgery had saved the careers of numerous subsequent Springboks. His trip to the UK had been miserable – he had given many lectures but had had little hospitality and was developing cabin fever from staring at hotel bedroom walls.

After a stimulating presentation I took Du Plessis to Franklin's Gardens. Professional rugby in the UK was only months old and he sat in the directors' box while I undertook sideline duties. Saints beat Bath 9-6 in a game to be savoured by an ex-prop-forward and in the dressing room afterwards, Tim Rodber, the England international, presented Du Plessis with his match shirt. After dining with several local sporting luminaries, his week had been rescued. It was the start on an enduring friendship.

Four months later I found myself addressing the South African Knee Society in Sun City and visited Loftus Versfeld in Pretoria, a citadel of South African rugby. I returned three months later for the 1997 Lions series. Springbok pride was so wounded by that series defeat that I had to promise to return for the next Lions tour – 12 years hence.

Between these tours I made numerous visits to South Africa. Only a small minority of surgeons are naturals but Du Plessis was one. With the strength and endurance of a front-row player he undertook 20 knee operations daily. In the evenings he retreated to his home workshop to create beautiful pieces of furniture from various African woods. He was a true master craftsman. His work, and my American experiences, made me realise the futility of being a jack of all trades. No orthopaedic surgeon can keep up with every technical development in every part of the body.

As promised, I returned for the 2009 Lions tour and was invited to a gathering of ex-Springbok internationals in Pretoria before the second Test. I was surrounded by heroes of my youth including two members of the South African 1960/61 British Isles and French tour. During the amateur era careers were put on hold for rugby tours. Players travelled by boat, played 34 matches in four months and defeated all four home countries before succumbing to the Barbarians. I listened to the players recall their first experience of snow while playing in Scotland, heard of their punishing schedule and primitive medical support.

The National Institute of Sport in Cape Town was led by the formidable Professor Tim Noakes, whose numerous and varied contributions to sports science and medicine had educated and challenged me. The institute had become the research leader investigating the role that genetics (inherited factors) play in increasing risk for developing sports-related tendon and ligament injuries. The subject had fascinated me since my early days when Steve Jones had tutored us in genetics at university. He became one of the great communicators on science, in books, scientific papers and in the media.

The institute is in Newlands, between the Test grounds for cricket and rugby. The National Rugby Museum was housed in the same building. With the majestic Table Mountain close by, I felt there could not be a more inspiring location for work in sport and exercise. In 2007 I emailed the institute's principal researchers ahead of a South African visit. We met and they generously allowed the University of Northampton to join their inner sanctum of collaborators. This has led to a rich body of ongoing work that has helped improve our understanding of how vital tissues involved in sport function sub-optimally in some people. Three years earlier the Human Genome Project was declared complete, although much more work was needed. It provided a road atlas of the 20,000-plus genes that control our lives. Rightly, most work has gone into improving our understanding of life-threatening disorders such as cancer. However, within this mind-boggling mass of information lie many of the answers as to why certain athletes are more prone to injuries that others.

Jewels from India

In 1995 I visited India for the first time and immediately fell in love with it. It is full of sounds, sights and smells that never sleep.

Our combined London and American delegation were to undertake clinics and lectures on haemophilia, an inherited disorder causing bleeding into body parts. It affects boys and is inherited from their mother. The most celebrated cases affected numerous European royal families in the 19th and 20th centuries, including some of Queen Victoria's descendants. Prevention, by replacing missing clotting factors, is the best treatment for haemophilia but is very expensive. If successful, however, it can allow a young boy to enjoy sport and exercise and to reach adulthood without arthritic joints or withered and contracted limbs.

In the 1980s a lot of factor replacement had been imported from the US but many human donors were drug addicts, many of whom had been infected with HIV and hepatitis by sharing needles. Their blood infected the blood of recipients. The toll on our patients was immense and the stress on my colleagues enormous. Many of our patients lost their lives.

The following decade I became orthopaedic surgeon to the haemophilia unit at the Royal Free in London, one of the major national haemophilia centres. It was a difficult time. The treatment for HIV was in its infancy and there was uncertainty as to whether major surgery might negatively affect a patient's chances of survival. We published research, which became a significant part of my subsequent PhD thesis. Surgery to joints and muscles could only take place safely with infused blood factor replacements to prevent patients bleeding to death. One knee replacement I undertook cost over £100,000 in blood products alone. As the surgery began, I told myself, 'Don't mess that one up, Ribbans.'

I accidentally cut my finger on a chisel during one operation on an HIV-positive patient and wondered if I had infected myself. The operation was only half complete and I could not leave the job to a junior. I had regular blood tests for two years before being given the all clear.

One of our roles on the Indian trip was to advise our local colleagues on the best use of their limited stock of blood factor replacement. One night we found ourselves evicted from our Delhi hotel rooms which had been reallocated to President Mandela's delegation. The great man was the chief guest of honour at the capital's Republic Day celebrations. How could we quibble? Having found new accommodation, we managed to get ourselves invited to the parade on the Rajpath. It was one of the most amazing sights to witness. Representatives of each of India's 36 states and union territories were present, adorned in regional traditional costumes. Elephants and camels were paraded too.

The experience in India was eye-opening. Many of the children did not even have a haemophilia diagnosis and there were not enough funds to undertake a simple blood test – something routine in the UK. The deformities and disabilities caused by haemophilia were more severe than anything witnessed in our leafy Hampstead Heath hospital. Mostly the kids had no access to any treatment. In some units, funds were so short that needles had to be reused on successive patients.

There was a small sub-group of boys with haemophilia, from wealthy families. The parents had dug into their pockets and imported factor replacement from America. HIV and hepatitis followed.

We were asked not to mention HIV at public lectures and clinics. Several boys were reaching eligible age and arranged marriages were commonplace. The families were unwilling to acknowledge to future daughters-in-law that the prospective groom had either haemophilia or HIV. Into the breach strode our wonderful counsellor Riva Miller, who from a height of 5ft would take no nonsense. An interesting clash ensued as we tried to influence culture and tradition.

Clinics were chaos and many rooms had no examination couches. Old desks sufficed instead but there was no patient privacy as 40 to 50 inquisitive souls crowded round. Some had travelled by train for over 24 hours and slept overnight on pavements. It was humbling.

How best to use scarce resources – in this case, the blood factor replacements? Some surgeons wanted to perform heroic operations on a few patients with dreadful deformities, which would have quickly exhausted the supplies. Alternatively, the products could be used in smaller doses on more healthy children to preserve their limbs. The case for the greater good prevailed. However, it was rationing and making choices we never faced at home. It was heart-breaking.

In 2008 I returned to India and addressed the orthopaedic conference of one of India's states, Maharashtra, whose capital is Mumbai. The state is 27 per cent larger than the UK and has a population of 122 million people. I was the annual meeting's first-ever overseas speaker. After beening embarrassingly garlanded on arrival I travelled to the meeting venue, Mahalebeshwar, an old colonial hill station used by the British during the Raj to escape the heat. Inadvertently I managed to generate some heat of my own.

I took two Northampton Saints rugby jerseys with me as presents for the organisers. They were curious about rugby and, with them adorned in the club's black, green and yellow hoops in front of 500 delegates and their spouses, I tried to demonstrate scrummaging, finishing up with my nose scraping the ground. I could only attribute this to illegal binding learnt by my hosts from their own sport of wrestling.

My discomfiture did not stop there. The conference dinner entertainment was provided by a well-known female singer and local custom had it that the invited speaker join her on stage in an exhibition of regional dancing. Despite my clear discomfiture at exotic dad dancing, my attempts to 'throw some shapes' rarely seen in Bollywood musicals appeared to win some admirers. Several male surgeons encircled me and joined in as their wives looked on bemused. Perhaps it was to save my embarrassment. It was certainly a new take on ladies dancing around their handbags in the nightclubs of my youth.

Technical exhibitions run alongside the educational content at most surgical meetings. In Europe and America we look at new hips and knees on trade stands. In Mahalebeshwar a great many exhibitors produced herbs and other medicinal plants. I lost count of the number of invitations I received to visit farms.

The scientific content of the meeting was fascinating. I chaired several sessions and listened in awe – the range of problems surgeons had to deal with was beyond the scope of nearly all British counterparts. They included tuberculosis, tropical infestations and severe congenital and nerve-related disorders, all treated with the most basic surgical equipment and implants. I felt my work at home was pampered and wondered what I could possibly add to their knowledge. The answer was 'Western society-acquired disorders' – first-world disorders resulting from leisure activities such as running.

I talked about Achilles disorders, which are at epidemic levels in North America and Europe where elite long-distance runners have a more than evens lifetime risk of developing swollen, stiff tendons. One in 13 runners in big-city marathons experience painful Achilles before their event. My Indian colleagues had minimal exposure to such issues.

Most of Indian society did not have an unquenchable desire to pound the roads at weekends and towns were not festooned with health clubs and gyms. Distance running and health and fitness were simply not on their radars. However, I predicted that such problems would emerge as sporting tastes changed when the advantages of India's booming economy filtered through. On more recent travels to the Indian subcontinent the increased number of gyms was noticeable. They appeared well used and, reassuringly, attracted women and men. However, beware that first warning sign of early morning stiffness in your Achilles!

Many of the conditions on my operating lists in Britain had little priority for my Indian counterparts. Wobbly ankles and painful tendons were low in the pecking order compared to the serious conditions their patients suffered. I wondered if my Western colleagues and I had made an industry out of issues that had no resonance in countries such as India?

*'Leadership and learning are
indispensable to each other'*

**John F. Kennedy, US President, part of a speech due to
be delivered in Dallas, 22 December 1963**

The surgical departments of major American hospitals continue to produce quality research and the teaching and clinical experience for trainees remains magnificent. The volume of excellent work they undertake makes them people to listen to and respect.

American sports medicine and surgical conferences are bigger and better than most and can attract tens of thousands of doctors. Several years ago I was invited to give several presentations at a national sports injuries meeting in Texas and was the only Brit on the podium over the three days. I wanted to leave a good impression and rashly decided to demonstrate certain injuries by showing videos of cricketing calamities. The audience looked bewildered.

An open question and answer session followed and I sat with three past-presidents of American surgical societies – the great and the good whose research I had marvelled at for years. Imposter syndrome succinctly describes my anxieties, although I reckoned correctly on not having to answer questions on the health dangers of a reverse sweep or ramp shot and managed to wing my way through the other curveballs coming my way.

You meet interesting people at such congresses. At the Texas meeting I was fascinated by meeting Dr Elliott Schwartz, an experienced team doctor for the Golden State Warriors and the Oakland Athletic baseball franchises. The latter appointment coincided with Billy Beane's use of sabermetrics to analyse and maximise the potential of his squad when working on a limited budget. His work intrigued me and his story was turned into the film *Moneyball* in 2011.

Leading American sports surgeons are always in great demand at international congresses. In my own field, doctors such as Jim Nunley, Bob Anderson, W. Hodges Davies and Tom Clanton have been very generous with their time and knowledge. With their vast experience, particularly in the NFL and elite college sports, there is not an injury they have not seen and dealt with, yet their explanations are given in a low-key, unassuming manner that never leaves the audience feeling inferior. True class.

I have arranged many conferences myself but for one, staged in Warwick, two American surgeons were grounded at home by bad weather. Instead, they got up at home at 3am and delivered their lectures by Skype. We made it up to them in later years by putting them in the stocks at Warwick Castle and subjecting them to warm beer and morris dancing on a green in the Cotswolds.

On another occasion I asked an American guest to address the assembled surgeons at dinner. He did so, comparing NHS healthcare with that in the States. He was witty and erudite. At 3am in the morning he phoned my hotel room to announce that he was dying. I got him to the local casualty where senior consultants diagnosed a kidney stone. As the ID tag was placed around his wrist I told him that he was experiencing the NHS first hand. Opiates were required to numb the pain, rendering my guest 'away with the fairies'. This meant, however, that my star lecturer could not give the meeting's keynote lecture hours later. His American buddies stepped in and delivered an excellent alternative for us.

'The First Cut is the Deepest'

Cat Stevens song (1967)

The use of cadaver surgical workshops was well established in America before my stay there in the 1980s. There are few such labs or specimens available in the UK and most of the latter must be flown in from the US. In 2010 I was organising one such meeting but it coincided with the eruption of the Icelandic volcano Eyjafjallajökull and subsequent build-up of a volcanic ash cloud. My specimens were grounded stateside and the conference postponed until the ash had cleared. You never know what's in the hold of transatlantic jets.

Mainland Europe has better facilities and I have spent much time in Munich using their labs. For 20 years, in Switzerland, Professor Beat Hintermann ran wonderful cadaver teaching sessions. He is one of the most respected orthopaedic surgeons in the world and has brought Swiss precision and logical thought to his operating and teaching.

In 2012 he invited me to join the international faculty for his course and it was clear I'd be working hard during my four-day visit. Hintermann announced a pre-congress 'experts meeting' in St Moritz to help bond those drawn from Europe and North and South America. I reckoned I knew what a 'bonding exercise' in St Moritz entailed and the ski gear was packed. Our hotel gave beautiful vistas over the Upper Engadine valley but as we checked in our host announced that the meeting would start in 30 minutes – in a requisitioned conference room rather than at the base of the nearest piste. Panic! I was not prepared. For three days we discussed the most complex cases and I spent each spare hour preparing my own cases for presentation. The closest I came to alpine recreation was to be taken to the cleaners at curling by my Peruvian and Chilean colleagues. Somehow I survived and became a permanent contributor at the annual meeting. It proved to be the most educational week of my year.

'Isn't it good Norwegian wood?'
The Beatles, 'Norwegian Wood (This Bird Has Flown)'
from the album *Rubber Soul* (1965)

Norway has a rightful claim to be the most successful global sporting nation.

This is probably due to three factors: its small population (5.3 million in 2018); the Scandinavian characteristic of doing what is asked of it (if explained reasonably); and the foresight to establish a national Olympic training centre in Oslo in 1985. It also helps having a population with the fourth-tallest people in the world, one of the lowest obesity rates at 6 per cent (compared to 28 per cent in the UK) and being the sixth-richest per capita country.

The Olympic training centre offers all aspiring Norwegian athletes support and has produced a uniformity of purpose and approach overseen by clinicians and scientists of the highest calibre. In 2014, after addressing a Norwegian surgical society, I contacted Professor Lars Engebretsen, who had the best job in the world combining work as professor of orthopaedic surgery with that of chief of sports medicine for the Norwegian Federation of Sports and Olympic and Paralympic committees. For good measure, he was also head of medical sciences for the IOC. His clinical and pioneering research work was acknowledged throughout the world.

He showed me around the centre and discussed his work and that of the unit. His office overlooked the athletics track and had ready access to indoor training facilities. The research department had personnel from all over the world and the immediacy of athlete, scientist and medical staff gave an almost tangible energy to the whole enterprise. It has been recognised by the IOC as one of its global flagship centres.

It was not only the quality but the breadth of research that impressed me most. Most orthopaedic surgeons concentrate on surgical procedures but after years of work at the coalface you end up wishing not to see so many injuries.

Engebretsen and his colleagues have shown how changes in training regimes can reduce injury and, with other Norwegian researchers, found that an interventional programme of exercises can reduce ACL knee injuries in female handball players. This sport has cult following in Norway and at the 2012 Olympics I watched thousands of fanatical Norwegians celebrate as their women's team won gold.

The beauty and sadness of the research emerged after the training programme ended. It required athletes and coaches to buy into the schedule but, once the research was over, the exercises were discontinued and soon the injuries mounted. Once reinstated, injury occurrence dropped again and remained low for years. It was a perfect example of the worth of sport-specific, targeted conditioning and strengthening.

Will Norway soon be overrun by overseas coaches? Will they insist on athletes being medically assessed in Madrid, Milan or Montevideo, with Oslo merely an embarkation point? Will the good work and success be lost? I think the Norwegians have more sense.

Surfing and sounding out

Like much else, the internet has transformed the world of surgery and sports medicine. Previously, hours were spent in hospital libraries searching for suitable articles. A database, Index Medicus, was published since 1879 to aid such quests but it could take weeks for the requested scientific paper to arrive in the post.

Now, at the press of a button, electronic searches can provide the answers. In 2004, Index Medicus was supplanted by online resources such as PubMed. The best clinical practice can now be disseminated worldwide. Surgeons can go online and watch operative animations and live surgery.

However, there remains a place for attending conferences and visiting colleagues, allowing for animated discussion and the establishment of networks of colleagues that enrich your life personally and professionally. Out of these bonds come better outcomes for patients.

Chapter 32

COVID-19 AND SPORT

ON 5 March 2020, the first official death from COVID-19 was recorded in the UK. The nation had been watching for weeks as the virus crept closer. Media footage depicted the toll that the virus was taking in China, Italy, Spain and various cruise ships dotted around the globe. The first cases in Britain had been confirmed in York on 29 January but the disease was probably in circulation for some time before that. By the end of February, the crisis seemed to be developing an unstoppable momentum.

Serie A Italian football was suspended on 8 March and, within four days, six of that league's players and one of the teams' doctors had tested positive for coronavirus.

So what was the early impact of COVID-19 on sport, how did sport and the medical teams respond, and how might sport have impacted the development of the disease?

9–16 March 2020 – A week in politics and sport like no other; 100 days and counting ...

When Leicester City thumped Aston Villa 4-0 on Monday, 9 March 2020, the Premier League season still had 92 games left to complete and the FA Cup and European club competitions had three and four stages to finish respectively. A day later, the three divisions of the English Football League played a handful of games, leaving 341 outstanding matches before champions, promoted and relegated sides could be determined. On 11 March, Scotland witnessed its last pre-COVID professional football match.

No one could have anticipated that it would be 100 days before the English Premier League would restart, when Aston Villa re-ignited the season taking on Sheffield United on Wednesday, 17 June to the backdrop of a deserted Villa Park. The clubs battled out a goalless draw.

Anfield and Cheltenham

On Wednesday, 11 March, Liverpool entertained Atlético Madrid in the second leg of the Champions League round of 16. Over 40,000 home supporters were joined by 3,000 fans who had travelled from the Spanish capital, despite Madrid being the epicentre of the escalating crisis in that country and its schools having closed the day before.

The Anfield game took place on the day the World Health Organization (WHO) declared COVID-19 a pandemic: 'We are deeply concerned both by the alarming levels of spread and severity, and by the alarming levels of inaction,' a WHO statement said. Professor John Ashton, ex-north-west regional director of public health and Liverpool season ticket holder, declined to attend the game, claiming that the government's strategy at the time 'was clinical and policy negligence'.

Spain went into national lockdown three days later.

The *Liverpool Echo* reported on 3 June that Merseyside had experienced a spike in deaths one month after the football match. Although this coincided with peak national mortality figures, one company (that analysed NHS data) suggested that the local hospitals had experienced 41 extra deaths between 25 and 35 days after the game.

The annual Cheltenham Festival is the pinnacle of jump racing in the British Isles and, every March, around 150,000 horse racing fans descend on the Cotswolds course from Britain and Ireland. In 2020, the four-day equestrian extravaganza was scheduled to run from 10 to 13 March. Despite warning notices and hand sanitiser facilities, the stands were packed and the bars full to overflowing.

By mid-April, Gloucestershire Hospitals Trust had recorded more than double the number of deaths compared to nearby hospitals in Bristol, Bath and Swindon.

The government defended its decision to allow the Festival to go ahead. The Culture Secretary, Oliver Dowden, said that the risk at mass gatherings was no greater that it would have been in pubs or restaurants. One local resident later described the race meeting as a 'petri dish' and 'breeding ground for COVID-19'. It is possible that the exact contribution of the event to the pandemic spread will never be known, due to the absence of effective testing, tracking and tracing at the time. Therefore, the source of the infection that led to the deaths of such people as a local publican and the chairman of Lancashire County Cricket Club, David Hodgkiss, who attended the meeting, remains unclear.

However, at least one expert was scornful of the decision-making. King's College, London professor of epidemiology, Tim Spector, was quoted as saying that the Liverpool and Cheltenham events had 'caused increased suffering and death that wouldn't otherwise have occurred'.

Friday 13th

On Friday, 13 March, the Premier League and English Football League announced a suspension of football in the senior four divisions.

The previous evening the Premier League had announced that the forthcoming weekend games would go ahead. However, the announcement that Arsenal manager Mikel Arteta had tested positive for the virus, closely followed by a similar announcement about Chelsea player Callum Hudson-Odoi focused minds. A suspension was announced with an initial 'hoped for' return date of 4 April. Scottish football made the same decision simultaneously.

Arsenal announced that around 100 club players and staff would need to complete a 14-day self-isolation period. Chelsea closed their first-team training ground for deep cleaning.

Other sports were considering their positions.

In Australia, the Formula 1 Melbourne Grand Prix was cancelled 48 hours before the event, after a McLaren mechanic tested positive for the virus.

In Galle, Sri Lanka, at 3.40pm local time, the England cricket team were in the middle of a four-day game against the Sri Lankan Board XI. Before tea, the players left the field and returned to their hotels to pack for the flight home.

The rugby union Six Nations had already announced that Italian games in Dublin on 7 March and in Rome against England on 14 March would be cancelled. However, internationals staged in London and Edinburgh on 7 and 8 March went ahead. The prime minister was at Twickenham to see England play Wales.

Many Cheltenham racing followers had intended to prolong their sporting party by joining fellow fans at the Millennium Stadium in Cardiff on 14 March to watch Wales vs Scotland. As with its Premier League football counterparts, the Welsh Rugby Union (WRU) performed a rapid volte-face. On the Friday morning (before the Premier League football suspension announcement), the WRU declared that the game would go ahead. Less than five hours later, it announced the game's cancellation, with the two sides in the middle of their final training sessions.

Rugby league closed its doors after the Castleford Tigers vs St Helens game on Sunday, 15 March.

The scene was set. Within five days, sport had gone from packed stands at Cheltenham and Liverpool to closure.

16–23 March 2020 – March to lockdown

Over the weekend of 14–15 March, the British government and its scientific advisers undertook a dramatic policy U-turn for tackling the pandemic. New modelling calculations from Imperial College suggested that over half a million deaths in Britain could occur if the government persisted with its approach.

The original policy, outlined by England's chief scientific officer Sir Patrick Vallance, was based on the assumption that 'the vast majority' of the population would suffer only a mild illness and 'generate' herd immunity, while the most vulnerable needed protecting.

The week between sport's closure and the government's lockdown announcement left many sports in limbo. Many sought guidance on what was permitted to maintain players' fitness, while some sports medicine colleagues told me that a few coaches wanted to 'push the envelope' in terms of team training. On Tuesday, 17 March, UEFA took the decision to postpone Euro 2020.

The nation was shutting down.

On Friday, 20 March, educational establishments closed. The entertainment, hospitality and indoor leisure industries, such as gyms, were shut. The optimistic hope that some entertained of elite sport restarting within weeks began to fade and was extinguished three days later.

In response to the Imperial advice, the UK 'locked down' on 23 March in line with most other European countries – but between one and two weeks after Italy, Spain and France. The day after, the IOC and the Japanese government jointly announced that the Tokyo Olympics, scheduled for July, would be postponed by a year.

Sport lies stunned

As NHS and care home staff battled bravely with the consequences of the virus and the British population grappled with isolation, illness, the loss of loved ones and fears of economic meltdown, the huge beast that is professional sport initially lay stunned and silenced.

Powerful figures within the sporting world, used to getting their own way, had to come to terms with the 'new order'. The government and its medical advisers simply did not have the time to consider sport when it was wrestling with constructing Nightingale hospitals, obtaining enough PPE for NHS, private hospital and care home staff, and developing strategies to contain the pandemic.

The furlough announcement by chancellor Rishi Sunak on 20 March was an economic lifesaver for millions of workers and companies nationwide. Likewise, much of professional sport.

Many sports clubs took the furlough route. However, it was a new playing field with different rules. All had to be careful not to breach employment law and to avoid requests to already furloughed staff and players that could be construed as generating revenue for the sporting organisation. However, maintaining social links and keeping tabs on welfare concerns was part of our medical duty of care.

A few Premier League clubs toyed with the idea of accepting the government's beneficence but withdrew in the face of a social media backlash revolving around the wealth of many of the club's owners and staff. Further down the sporting food chain, many sporting organisations had no choice but to furlough staff or face ruin; sports administrators and leading athletes agreed to take significant pay cuts. In professional cricket, only Surrey and Lancashire out of the 18 first-class clubs continued to pay the salaries of their players. Many well-known sports organisations limped along with only a handful of essential staff working.

The media looked for scapegoats when the salaries of sports stars attracted the ire of many whose livelihoods were threatened. Inevitably, some sacrificial lambs came forward 'meekly'. On 29 March, Aston Villa's Jack Grealish was involved in a car accident while breaking lockdown rules soon after using social media to implore people to stay at home. Two days later, Manchester City's Kyle Walker was reported to have hosted a 'party' for friends. The next week, Tottenham Hotspur manager Jose Mourinho was filmed undertaking a training session with a player in a public park.

However, most sportspeople reacted magnificently. Manchester United's Marcus Rashford raised £20m for food charities and, later, persuaded the government to change its policy on meals for poor children during school summer holidays. Liverpool's Jordan Henderson and Andy

Robertson and countless more players worked tirelessly for other causes, and tens of thousands of isolated supporters received phone calls of support from their heroes. Many clubs showed their connections with their communities. Watford's chief executive, Scott Duxbury, and his staff converted executive boxes into bedrooms and counselling rooms for hospital staff and fed NHS employees. There were many similar examples across the country.

As the crisis deepened, the nonsensical business plans of many sports clubs came home to roost. Most obvious was the spiralling wage bills for footballers that, in some instances, exceeded the annual turnover of the clubs. Those clubs had speculated (and spent) future anticipated revenues in the belief that the gravy trains would keep arriving. The threatened non-arrival of Sky television revenues for non-completion of the season threatened the survival of some famous and historic clubs. The Premier League, facing an economic apocalypse, wanted to negotiate with the government separately from the rest of sport. To its credit, the government resisted and put the Premier League firmly back in its box.

For sports such as cricket, the crisis broke as professional clubs were in their final stages of preparation for the 2020 summer season. There had been a lot to look forward to. The increased media coverage following the triumphant 2019 England World Cup win and exciting Ashes series was designed to promote the sport to young and old alike. The innovative 100-ball competition for men's and women's cricket was due to be launched in July 2020. It was hoped it would swell the coffers of the ECB and the 18 first-class counties. All hope lay in tatters.

Performance machines to welfare outfits

Previous chapters have described how sporting organisations normally function as well-oiled performance machines. They had been brought to their knees in one fell swoop and had to metamorphose overnight into welfare establishments – a role for which they had minimal experience or understanding.

In Chapter 15, the theme of feudalism within sport was developed; this unseen virus was forcing clubs to emerge from the Dark Ages. From late March, uppermost on sports clubs' agendas had to be the physical and mental well-being of their employees – furloughed or not.

To facilitate this, the various doctors engaged within sport began to organise and liaise quickly and widely. Links had to be established with doctors in specialities such as public health and microbiology, who traditionally had little to do with sport. My first-hand experience and colleagues' recollections indicate that these specialists gave up their time and knowledge fulsomely, even when working ridiculous hours, to manage the national crisis. Help came from senior medical experts (frequently found flanking politicians in Downing Street press conferences) through to medics working near to individual clubs.

The numbers of doctors involved within sports medicine nationally remains relatively small for reasons described earlier, and many are known to each other. This helped, as colleagues from different sports were able to easily exchange experiences, problems, plans and policies. Major medical journals such as the *British Journal of Sports Medicine* fast-tracked well-researched articles that helped foment our knowledge.

The ECB swung into action impressively early, led by its medical lead, Professor Nick Peirce, and from 17 March, all first-class county doctors and physios were involved in weekly conference calls. The information given was comprehensive and far-ranging. These calls also allowed experiences to come in from around the country. Priorities and problems altered as the pandemic developed and the government announced its updated strategies. Supplementing these sessions were phone calls with friends and colleagues at other cricket clubs. Each county clinical team supplied weekly medical updates to the ECB to allow a national picture to be developed and help formulate planning for a return to training and, ultimately, competition.

The Northants CCC board was kind enough to invite me to its Zoom meetings to provide updates on the welfare and health situation. Our chairman, Gavin Warren, remarked that five years previously he had an insolvency expert advising the board but now he needed a doctor to do the same. Different times, different priorities. Supporters were not forgotten, and an online Fans Forum was organised to answer questions and disseminate information.

Sport in the recovery ward

It was always clear that the timing of the return of sport in the UK would depend primarily on national control of the virus and protection of the NHS from being overwhelmed and, secondly, the specific characteristics of every sport and its financial circumstances. The latter included the level of facilities and each sport's normal seasonal dates. Where there was a significant degree of interdependency with team-mates or contact with colleagues or opponents in games such as football and rugby, the potential problems were greater.

As the national situation began to improve during April, the government was able to turn its attention to planning the return of elite sport. It drew together a working party, which included senior doctors from all major sporting organisations and representatives of Public Health England (PHE), UK Sport, the Department of Culture, Media and Sport and the Department of Health and Social Care. The working party for sport was spearheaded by cricket's Nick Peirce.

Elite sport was being shown a priority not seen in other sectors of the economy and society. Both sporting organisations and the government were determined that sport should be seen to act responsibly and reasonably.

Doubting Thomases

Some people at home and abroad remained concerned about sport returning too soon.

In late March, the *British Journal of Sports Medicine* published an impassioned article from Italian doctors imploring football not to restart until the crisis was under control. They explained that Italian law conferred team doctors with ultimate control over players' health problems and a letter had been sent from all Serie A doctors warning football administrators about planning too early a return.

As late as 29 April, *The Times* was reporting that the chairman of the FIFA medical committee, Dr Michel D'Hooghe, was advising that it would be unwise to consider playing competitive football until 1 September.

Premier League footballers also expressed concerns, with the Bournemouth captain Simon Francis saying on 30 April, 'I'm not sure why the return of a contact sport is being considered,' and a day later, Manchester City's Sergio Agüero, Chelsea's Antonio Rüdiger and Brighton's Glenn Murray stating similar anxieties. Andy Murray said that tennis 'is not the most important thing at the moment'.

Sport put on amber

With the input of many diverse experts the government was finally able to publish its initial guidelines on 13 May. They contained the principles of a 'road map' that would govern all sports in their quest to come back to training and ultimately competition.

Five steps were laid out: 1: individualised training; 2: return to small-group training; 3: return to behind-closed-doors competition; 4: return to cross-border (international) competition behind closed doors; 5: normal sport in front of spectators without restrictions.

It was up to each sport to study the document and consider whether it was able to comply and what risks might be encountered. Various sports took to analysing 'pinch points' within their sport to calculate likely 'close encounter' times such as rugby scrums and mauls.

Some sports were easier to recommence than others. These included sports that could be undertaken individually such as running and cycling. Other sports could be sanctioned so long as social distancing could be maintained. This allowed recreational golf courses to reopen in England on 13 May, albeit with clubhouses closed and rakes removed from bunkers. Lawn tennis at local clubs and angling restarted the same day.

The equestrian industry never stopped working, due to the welfare requirements of the horses. It was the obvious elite sport to be first to return to television screens on 1 June, with jockeys wearing the obligatory face coverings. Later the same day, professional snooker returned, having created its own biosecure bubble in Milton Keynes.

What were the main concerns for fit young athletes returning to sport?

National statistics suggested that the dangers to fit young athletes from COVID-19 were minimal. However, dangers clearly existed within elite sport.

Young athletes were not the only people involved in 'getting the show back on the road again'. For example, staff involved were likely to be older and more at risk – one Premier League manager was 72 years old. Players and staff may have had vulnerable family members at home who needed shielding. In addition, elite sport has a high percentage of BAME athletes whose racial groupings (for reasons not fully understood) made them particularly vulnerable to the complications of the virus.

As we have seen in previous chapters, elite athletes are more likely to suffer from asthma than the normal population. Furthermore, elite athletes in high-intensity training may be at increased risk of altered inflammation and immunity, potentially affecting their response to viral exposure – particularly if their training load is increased quickly. This includes the potential for cardiac inflammation. The medical world was having to learn quickly about this new disease. The long-term effects (even following mild exposure) from the virus were unclear – for example, young people with minimal symptoms were suffering lung damage.

There was every reason to be concerned for the sports world and its participants, and sport had to develop carefully planned protocols for the assessment and gradual return to exercise of anybody suffering symptoms of the disease.

Looking after body and soul

Compared to the anguish of the relatives of people who had lost their lives, and the psychological trauma and exhaustion of the NHS and care-working community, the well-being concerns of young, fit professional sportspeople might seem insignificant. However, peak mental toughness in the elite sporting arena does not always equate to resilience in confronting problems caused by a miniscule foe measuring 0.1 micron in diameter. Problems could and would arise.

The loss of the potential pinnacle of their careers following the cancellation of the 2020 Tokyo Olympics must have been profound for many, and the rescheduled date of 2021 did not come with any guarantees of selection, optimal form, funding and freedom from injury.

Many professional sportspeople faced being out of contract during lockdown or during its aftermath. Professional football contracts traditionally end on 30 June and professional cricket contracts usually expire in early autumn. Players faced the prospect of not being 'able to prove their worth' before receiving their P45s.

That was not all. Out-of-contract professional footballers could potentially be involved in games after the official end of their contracts, and the worry of sustaining injury could affect their ability to find a new club.

In cricket, the 18 first-class counties had 134 players out of contract at the end of the 2020 summer – probably close to one-quarter of the profession. Furthermore, some players had only red-ball contracts and others only white-ball contracts. The delay until 7 July of an announcement regarding the format for the truncated season gave some cricketers doubts as to whether they still had a future in the sport. Players previously selected for the inaugural 100-ball competition had anticipated excitement, increased media exposure and a substantial boost to their incomes. Its cancellation removed all their hopes.

For all professional sportspeople, the downturn in the economic health of their sports created concerns about their ability to support their families – a fear they shared with many millions of people throughout the country. Most found their incomes diminished during the lockdown, through either voluntary salary cuts or furlough arrangements. They also knew that some reductions would be permanent. This led to players and their professional representatives (the PFA, PCA and Rugby Players' Association) having to work hard with the sporting organisations. Some players, such as Manu Tuilagi at Leicester Tigers, could not agree new terms and left their clubs.

Many players had concerns about family members with medical conditions with whom they were shielding, and athletes from the BAME community, reasonably, had heightened concerns for themselves and their families from increased risks due to their ethnicity. In football, Watford's Troy Deeney and Chelsea's N'Golo Kanté had legitimate anxieties and delayed their return to training until the first testing results were revealed and early experiences of training-ground organisation could be gauged.

In many sports, players and staff members come from abroad. Some are accompanied by families while others leave loved ones on the other side of the world. All needed regular contact from club officials to make sure they were coping with their confinement. Some lost loved ones, such as Pep Guardiola, whose mother died in Barcelona.

Academy players were a special consideration because of their age and potential vulnerability from a sporting standpoint. This particularly affected those about to graduate from academy to senior ranks. Many were trying to pursue simultaneous academic and sporting goals. Not only were sporting ambitions thwarted: with schools closed and exams cancelled, there was a risk of double disappointment.

Elite sport has a fast-moving conveyor belt of talent, being constantly assessed, promoted and rejected. Gifted youngsters are fast approaching from the years behind. It is a ruthless business. It was clear from the early stages of the pandemic that there would be a financial fallout from the crisis with unknown effects on youngsters who may not have the final opportunity to demonstrate their skills and earn a senior contract. These youngsters and their parents needed support from the club's clinical team. When a return to cricket training was announced for July, it was important that both players and their parents were fully briefed on the safety arrangements that would be in place to allow them to make an informed decision on whether to 'opt in'.

In my experience, at club level, the priority was support and knowledge dissemination for staff and players. Chairmen and chief executives were frank and open with their staff about the financial consequences to their sport as a whole and their own club during the crisis. Everybody was left in no doubt that they would be fully supported if they opted not to return to training or competition.

At Northants cricket, regular Zoom meetings of our welfare group were organised and involved the club chaplain, sports psychologists, a representative of the PCA and clinical staff. Matters discussed included players from overseas, isolated individuals and players whose contracts were due to expire. Staff made sure that players were contacted.

I sent out 15 weekly newsletters to keep players and staff abreast of developments. It was important to interpret and distil the information coming from various sources – government, PHE, sporting bodies, educational journals, etc., and make it relevant for the players and their sport. They are intelligent people and needed to be kept informed. Additionally, advice needed to be given to them – making sure the asthmatics had plenty of inhalers, explaining the local medical situation and what a return to training might look like.

With so little sport to write about and discuss, media outlets became interested in player welfare and the plans for restarting professional sport. I found myself spending two Sunday afternoons on talkSPORT radio discussing the issues of the day with Mark Saggers and his guests. BBC television's *Look East* required pieces to camera on various professional sports clubs' plans and their progress.

Northants cricket organised remote social events such as quiz nights, which were useful in maintaining morale and monitoring those fully engaged – and those who were not. It was here that having a mature and long-term backroom staff paid dividends. These staff had got to know the players (and their families) well over the years and understanding different personalities helped to interpret their messages.

What does it take to put a team on the park?

Sport had to work hard to produce its own sport-specific protocols and football published its guidance to clubs within 24 hours of the government's announcement that training could resume. Other sports followed with voluminous documents for each of the government's five stages.

Each individual club had to lay these 'blueprints' on their own facilities and personnel and develop detailed risk assessments and mitigation strategies.

I spent days developing policies for Northants cricket and going over the plans with our chief executive Ray Payne. It takes time to work out the safest way to flush a toilet and the order in which the lid and basin should be cleaned afterwards!

Testing times and difficult decisions

The question of COVID-19 testing was always going to be a major factor in the return of elite sport.

On 19 March, Prime Minister Boris Johnson had promised the nation that an antibody test would be available as soon as possible in industrial quantities. 'A game changer' was how our leader described it. Sadly, his words were hot air. Tests to determine if a person had been exposed to the virus and developed immunity proved elusive and it would take months for reliable tests to be approved. Even then, our understanding of the length of immunity and varying individual responses to viral exposure made it an unsound test on which to base sport's return.

The antigen tests performed by swabbing noses and throats was used to detect the presence of the virus in our respiratory passages. However, the chronic undercapacity of the nation's laboratories and other sourcing problems meant that the country was struggling to swab key workers and exposed patients in sufficient quantities.

There was a moral debate over prioritising sports people for testing – even if undertaken privately. A few days after the country reported its first daily 100,000-plus tests on 30 April, Chelsea manager Frank Lampard was quoted, saying, 'It's important for football to take its place … I don't think it would sit well with me or anyone if we didn't make sure people were being tested on that front line.'

Performing such tests was not without problems. The tests only had about 70 per cent accuracy and some people continued to test positive after recovering from the infection. A negative test one day did not mean a person was not in the early stages of incubating the disease. The only way to be sure was repeated testing … and then we come to the cost. At around £100 per test the bills mount up quickly.

The Premier League committed to twice-weekly testing. The first round was undertaken on 17 May with six positive tests from three clubs. The League's swab test bill was around £200,000 per week.

While these financial sums might have been loose change for the Premier League, such amounts made English Football League (EFL) clubs blanche. And while top-tier clubs got players back into training, the EFL debated the pros and cons of continuing with the season. How could 341 league games and play-offs be safely negotiated and costed? The EFL calculated that they needed 66,000 tests (at a cost of £6.6m) to conclude the season for all its clubs. This was in addition to the costs of unfurloughing players and staff and staging behind-closed-doors games. Only 17 per cent of Manchester United's annual revenue of £627m was derived from ticket sales and matchday revenues, but for League One and League Two clubs this figure rose to 40 per cent.

On 15 May, League One and League Two clubs bowed to the inevitable and agreed to abandon the season – except for the ten play-off games involving only eight out of the 47 clubs. All football leagues below the National League had already been expunged on 26 March. On 22 April, the National League had confirmed the end to its regular season, leaving only play-offs to complete.

The Championship agreed to bring players back into training on 25 May having already conducted two rounds of virus testing, and started competitive football on 20 June – only days after the Premier League restarted.

The need for testing was shown by the results. By the end of June (six weeks after testing began), 77 positive tests had been returned from 52 English football clubs. Fortunately, none of the identified players or staff appeared to have become severely ill, caused a major outbreak in their clubs or caused a delay to the season restarting. However, it was an indication of the continuing presence of the disease in the community – even in asymptomatic individuals.

When football returned to our screens, the waiting audience was informed that certain behavioural changes had been requested of the players and staff. These included avoiding gathering around referees to dispute decisions, avoiding spitting, and celebrating goals in a socially distanced manner. It was immediately noticeable that these requests were being ignored. Similarly, images appeared of opposition managers 'elbow greeting' but then hugging each other, and some staff wore face masks while others eschewed the coverings in seemingly bare-faced defiance.

Abroad, different countries came to different conclusions. France, The Netherlands and Belgium made an early decision to abandon their seasons. However, better control of the pandemic allowed the German Bundesliga to return players to training in mid-April, with the first games played on 16 May. The Italian Serie A restarted at the same time as the English Premier League, on 20 June, with the Spanish La Liga resuming a week earlier on 11 June.

Meanwhile, English women's football was stopped. On 25 May it was announced that the Women's Super League 2019/20 season would be abandoned with immediate effect. It was a dispiriting end to a season that had started so promisingly in the afterglow of the 2019 World Cup and increased media attention and match attendances.

Rugby union was always going to be a difficult sport to make safe, given the close-contact nature of the game. On 2 June it was announced that Premiership rugby players could come back into individualised training. Five weeks later, on 6 July, the players were allowed to start close-contact training. By then the 12 clubs had tested 804 people and returned ten positive cases. The League recommenced on 14 August with a punishing fixture list including several midweek fixtures to be shoehorned in.

At the recreational end, rugby union bowed to the inevitable: no testing meant no tackling, and junior club rugby would have to commence with a sanitised ten-a-side touch-rugby format.

Within professional cricket, the priority (for obvious financial reasons) was restarting international games. The schedule had the West Indies first up, although two of their star players declined to travel because of health concerns regarding the virus. The team arrived on 9 June and were the first overseas sporting side to arrive in the UK since lockdown began. England's squad had started training with the fast bowlers on 21 May. They trained under tight precautions at seven grounds around the country.

The ECB developed two biosecure bubbles – at Old Trafford for the visitors and at the Ageas Bowl in Southampton for the home squad. Both had the advantages of a hotel on site. Their tight security would have done justice to Fort Knox. COVID-19 testing machines (costing over £80,000 in total) were stationed at both venues. The tight planning was justified and the ECB was able to report no positive tests out of several thousand undertaken before cricket recommenced. The Test series started on 8 July. The ill-advised detour of Jofra Archer to Brighton while en route to Manchester from Southampton after the first Test led to him being dropped for the second Test. The speed and seriousness of the sanction underscored the ECB's determination to complete the series without any health scares.

The sensible precaution of pre-travel testing of overseas athletes was emphasised by the initial screening of the Pakistan men's cricket team, England's next opponents. On 23 June – only five days before departure for England – ten players (out of a squad of 29) and a masseur tested positive. Those infected had to remain at home until they had tested clear and completed the necessary quarantine periods. The Test series commenced on 5 August at Old Trafford without further alarms.

In the House of Commons on 23 June, the prime minister described a cricket ball as 'a natural vector of disease' prompting Dukes, which manufactures cricket balls, to call the remarks 'inexplicable'. The company believed that if hands were regularly sanitised, balls cleaned and no saliva was put on them, the risk of disease transmission was minimal.

Within professional county cricket, most first-class clubs started training around 1 July. The weeks before were hectic behind the scenes. Players and staff had to be screened for health risks for themselves and their families, I delivered an online presentation to explain the training arrangements, and all had to watch ECB educational programmes. I spent one weekend undertaking one-to-one calls with all staff and players to discuss individual concerns. Everybody then had to return opt-in statements if they wanted to train. Players had checklists to complete every day before leaving the house and each was provided with a set of personal cricket balls – to comply with the ECB's mantra of 'one skin, one ball'. For the players arriving at the ground it was a novel experience to be greeted by a physiotherapist in PPE pointing a thermometer at their foreheads through the opened car window. Typically, after glorious spring weather, it seemed to rain nearly every training day for the first week. I spent part of the first morning of training checking that the various loo hand dryers had been decommissioned (for fear of spraying the virus widely) and that gel bottles were operational. Sometimes our jobs can be very glamorous.

Despite all these precautions the players still came back to training with no idea of a fixture list or even which of the three competition formats would be played. Test cricket started a week later but players had to retrieve balls hit over the boundary ropes themselves. Amateur club cricket returned on 11 July. Professional first-class cricket found itself in the middle and would not restart until 1 August. The decisions were all financial: the clubs could not afford to unfurlough staff before July.

Despite swab-testing all international cricketers, the ECB decided on a strategy of non-testing for the rest of the first-class game because its assessment suggested that the game itself carried minimal risk. The distinction between international and domestic cricket measures caused some consternation among the latter group of players in discussions I had with them.

False starts

On schedule, the Bob Willis Trophy four-day cricket competition started on Saturday, 1 August, but not without a last-minute hiccough. Trophy games at Edgbaston (Warwickshire and Northants) and at the Oval (Surrey and Middlesex), Goodwood horse racing and the World Snooker Championship had been designated as pilot spectator events by the government and 2,000 fans were expected in Birmingham to watch the cricket. However, less than 24 hours beforehand ministers cancelled the experiment due to rising concerns of positive COVID-19 tests nationally and the games were played in front of empty stands. The financial costs to the respective hosts was not inconsiderable and cast fresh doubts on an eventual return date for viable spectator numbers to watch professional sport.

On the same weekend, driver Sergio Perez was ruled out of the first of two Silverstone Formula 1 Grand Prix races. He had contracted the virus during a trip home to Mexico.

Tennis resumed tentatively but the Madrid Open was cancelled eight days before its scheduled start on 12 August. The US Open (delayed until the end of August) was shorn of the many competitors unwilling to travel to New York – particularly the European contingent.

On 11 August it was announced that Aberdeen and Glasgow Celtic would have their next two football games postponed for infringing lockdown regulations. Players had visited pubs that had become the centre of a viral upsurge and another player had visited Spain, not quarantined on return, and turned up to play. Scotland's First Minister Nicola Sturgeon said, 'Consider today the yellow card. The next time it will be the red card because you will leave us with absolutely no choice.' On 15 August, a COVID-19 outbreak at the Hull rugby league club led to the postponement of the club's games. On 6 September, the Gloucestershire–Northamptonshire cricket match in Bristol was abandoned when a non-playing member of the latter's squad tested positive for the virus.

These were all signs of how far the sporting world had to go to return to normal.

The view from 'long on'

From a medical point of view, there were always two problems to face when considering the return of elite sport in the summer of 2020. Most important was the safety of players and staff – preventing them contracting COVID-19 and carrying it back to vulnerable family and friends.

Secondly, there was the potential for increased injury risk, during the weeks after return and, as important, in the longer term when concerns related to increased workload and potential fixture congestion over the next couple of years could arise.

Elite English football elected to bring its players back to complete the 2019/20 season and protect the integrity of its competitions – and to ensure it received millions of pounds in satellite television revenues. However, as football restarted, accountants Deloitte estimated that the Premier League would still lose £1bn due to the pandemic.

The rescheduled Premier League season needed to complete 92 league games and finish on 26 July. Six FA Cup ties had to be slotted in before the FA Cup Final on 1 August. Most of August would be devoted to the completion of the European club competitions – the Champions League and Europa League. Both had still to finish their rounds of 16 at the time of the pan-European lockdown, and the final rounds were rescheduled to be played in Portugal and Germany to minimise travel and health risks. Successful clubs faced the possibility of playing up to 16 games in under ten weeks.

Early results from the resumed Bundesliga in Germany showed (as expected) a rise in game-time injuries. Triple the number of expected injury problems arose – albeit based upon a small sample of games. In England, similar injuries to hamstrings, groins, knees and ankles were predicted. Dutch conditioning coach Raymond Verheijen, who had worked at Barcelona, Chelsea and Manchester City, believed that football was playing 'Russian roulette with the health of players'. In the FA Cup Final, Chelsea players Azpilicueta and Pulisic sustained serious hamstring tears and substitute forward Pedro dislocated his shoulder. All could have occurred during a 'normal' season but the hamstring injuries, in particular, raised concerns over the degree of muscle fatigue suffered by the players despite their enhanced sports science conditioning.

As important a question as the resumption of football was when (and in what format) would the 2020/21 season start.

The previous season had begun on 9 August 2019 and, throughout that summer, various start dates for the 2020/21 Premier League season had been mooted. Media outlets speculated on the start for the next season – dates as early as 22 August were suggested when English clubs might still be involved in the previous season's European games. At last, sense prevailed and a start date of 12 September was agreed, with the intention of ring-fencing a guaranteed 30-day rest for players involved in European competition. The season was scheduled to finish on 23 May 2021. Additionally, 2020/21 European club competitions required new timetabling.

The UEFA Euro 2020 summer football competition had been rescheduled for 2021, just 19 days after the new end of the English Premier League. And the FIFA 2022 World Cup in Qatar was proposed to run from 21 November to 18 December 2022 to avoid the highest temperatures, prompting the Premier League to schedule the start of the 2022/23 season a week earlier and the finish a week later to allow for the World Cup taking place halfway through.

Players' schedules would also have to accommodate the UEFA Nations League, starting with group stages between September and November 2020, finals in the autumn of 2021 and relegation play-offs in the spring of 2022, and World Cup qualifiers between March 2021 and March 2022.

Whatever decisions were made there was no doubt that elite footballers would be playing a lot of football over a two- to three-year period with limited periods of rest. There was no reason to expect that the injury toll post-COVID-19 would be any less than recorded after other major international tournaments historically. With this evidence, it was particularly disappointing that the English Premier League announced that it was scrapping the players' winter break for the 2020/21 season – just when they needed it more than ever.

Football was not alone. Elite English rugby union players faced 51 weeks of unrelenting play after the season resumed on 14 August. That season would culminate in the most attritional Test series of all – a Lions tour in South Africa finishing on 7 August 2021.

The evidence for injury risks following enforced sporting shutdowns is hard to come by. The investigation most often quoted during return-to-training planning is the effects on American football of the 14-week lockout of players from the NFL during an industrial dispute in 2011. The players had only 17 days in training camp before two weeks of pre-season competition. There was a fourfold increase in the number of Achilles ruptures in this time. The authors were also concerned that the lockout prevented players receiving the rehabilitation they required to recover from pre-existing injuries or surgery, thus increasing their risk of reinjury.

In my own practice during lockdown I saw professional footballers who were unable to access treatment from furloughed physiotherapists who would otherwise have helped with their post-operative recoveries.

The time footballers needed to be match fit for the resumption of games was a matter of debate. Many Premier League football clubs returned to stage 1 training from 19 May. This gave them between four and five weeks' preparation. Prior to the restart, the Watford manager Nigel Pearson said four weeks was too short a period and requested six weeks. I debated the issue with ex-internationals Danny Mills and Ray Houghton on talkSPORT. Temporary changes had already been put in place, such as a drinks break in the middle of each half and increased numbers of substitutes, to help reduce injuries.

In cricket, fast bowlers risk injuries such as muscle tears and spinal stress fractures and a normal pre-season of 10 to 12 weeks is considered ideal. In 2020, Test cricketers returned after fewer than seven weeks of training and other first-class cricketers with just over four weeks' preparation. The dangers were clear. To counteract the risk in domestic first-class cricket, the limit on total overs bowled per day and overs bowled per player were reduced.

It will be some years before we know whether these measures were successful in reducing injury risk but it was clearly important that, as a medical group, we did everything we could to protect the players in our charge.

Conclusions

The COVID-19 pandemic has been a shock to the health and economic welfare of the country. From government down, it has challenged and made us reflect on our priorities within our personal and professional lives.

It has reminded us all that 'no man is an island' and that we sink or swim collectively as a society. Major sports organisations came to appreciate how their survival at these difficult times was dependent upon the skills and support of people from many disparate walks of life, whose activities would not normally affect them. In sport, this pandemic will produce lasting changes; the financial impact should require sports to become better planners of their budgets. It will cause many sports to reconsider their financial models, which may be reflected in salary wage caps, more part-time professional sport and, unfortunately, cuts in areas such as academy funding.

Normally, 90 per cent of my professional life is spent working in clinics and operating on patients. All of that was put into abeyance for months. Like others, I needed to adapt and 'retool'. I had to bring up to date my knowledge on epidemiology (the study of the determinants of illness and health) and virology – both taught to me as an undergraduate in the 1970s. In doing so I had to ask colleagues in many different specialities to provide the knowledge to best help me advise my sporting organisation and its players and staff. Normally the work of a team doctor will take place quietly, out of sight on the wings; this crisis thrust sports doctors centre stage. As the Northants CCC chairman said to me, 'You are currently the most important person in this club.' No pressure, then.

After difficult experiences we often vow to learn and take out the positives, although many resolutions disappear as life returns to normal. On a wider front, hopefully the COVID-19 pandemic will kick-start a debate on society's priorities in terms of health spending and care of the elderly and disabled.

While the pandemic and lockdown risked isolating individuals within sport, it did bring many closer together in their desire to protect and support others and secure the future of their sporting organisations. Clubs realised that there were other important parts of their machine than just what 'happens on the park'. The increased understanding of the psychological side of coping with a crisis has allowed the discussion of such issues to become more acceptable. Hopefully, this will translate into better tolerance of mental problems in sport.

Overall, the increased focus on staff and player welfare should be maintained. This will improve the overall health of sports participants, ultimately improve athletic performance, and lead to improved transitions from sporting careers to post-retirement lives.

COVID-19 is here for the foreseeable future and all of us will have to adapt. Like others, I was moved by the actions and words of Captain Tom Moore (now Sir Thomas Moore) during his fundraising walk at his home in Bedfordshire in April 2020. He spoke with the experience of a centurion who had endured many national and international crises when he said, 'the sun will shine on you again and the clouds will go away.' The dark clouds will surely lift but the revealed landscape below will have changed irrevocably. How sport will have changed can only be speculated on, but its enduring appeal to both participants and followers will remain undiminished.

Chapter 33

GREAT (AND NOT SO GREAT) STRIDES FORWARD

HOW HAVE the changes in the medical landscape affected orthopaedic surgery, sports medicine and athlete care over the last 40 years?

There have been seismic changes in the development of sports medicine as a respected medical speciality. Orthopaedic surgery has gone through similar upheavals.

Flogging the dead horse

When I was a newly qualified doctor in 1980, British orthopaedic surgeons considered themselves largely 'jacks of all trades' – they prided themselves on being able to handle anything that came through the door.

Prior to being let loose on bones they had to prove themselves in other anatomical areas by removing appendices, gall bladders, testicle swellings and foreign bodies secreted up noses. Once allowed into orthopaedic training, a single operating list might include knees, hands, slipped discs and bunions. Being on-call for casualty trauma was all-encompassing and could mean switching from a safe opinion on a child's broken arm to a head injury and then a complicated spinal injury, all during a busy Friday night. The 100-hour-plus weekly schedules have already been described and meant that experience was gained rapidly. As a senior trainee and young consultant, I operated on around 700 patients per year.

Jobs for the boys?

There was only one female among the 862 orthopaedic surgeons in England and Wales when I became a consultant in 1991. It was a male-dominated domain. Medical folklore claimed that orthopaedics was the last sanctuary of the beer-drinking, rugby-playing male medic. Some may have thought I fitted the stereotype. Like all medicine, the male/female balance has changed dramatically, making the profession more civilised and reflective.

In 1992, Western Europe had 5.3 orthopaedic surgeons for every 100,000 people; the UK had 1.62. We are still playing catch-up and have not reached yet the staffing positions American and European countries enjoyed 30 years ago. UK doctors have resembled firefighters compared to the ultra-specialised medics from abroad.

Jacks of all trades and masters of very little?

The punishing timetables for junior consultants made it difficult for us to become 'masters of something'. Change was in the air, though, and my own experiences of working and travelling abroad made me appreciate the advantages of surgeons concentrating on limited anatomical areas, such as the knee or hip, or specific topics, such as children or tumours. This concept was rapidly gaining acceptance in the 1990s and specialisation has since enabled huge improvements in knowledge. Medicine is all about pattern recognition – previous problems and solutions seen in clinics or surgeries are stored in your memory bank for later recall.

Education does not stop when a doctor becomes a consultant. Becoming a specialist is only the beginning – it is like a pilot gaining their wings. You are qualified to fly solo but that does not mean you should be entrusted with a fully laden jumbo jet first time out. Gladwell's theory of 10,000 hours of practice to attain more than mere competence in a skill was explored earlier and is a reasonable description of the time spent at the coalface during a surgical apprenticeship. This time allows for knowledge acquisition, the mastering of techniques and for rehearsing situations that might arise during your later daily schedules.

Unlike the television programme depictions in *Holby City*, *ER* or *Casualty*, most of a surgeon's week does not involve operating theatres. I spend double the time in clinics that I do in surgery. Choosing the right operation for the right patient is as important as your surgical skill set. You can complete the most technically wonderful surgery but if it is not appropriate for your patient you will fail. I undertake less surgery now than 20 years ago. It may be the natural development of conservatism that comes with age but also I better understand those conditions that get better without surgery, by using conservative options such as physiotherapy, injections and bracing. It may take longer but it avoids an operation.

A medical or surgical specialist is an expert who knows more and more about less and less. Has the development of super-specialist surgeons in the last 30 years advanced the care of our athletes and the general population? The answer is undoubtedly yes. Our sportspeople are better served by access to clinicians with considerable and specific surgical mileage under their belts. The old maxim holds as true in surgery as it does in sport:

'The harder I practice, the luckier I get'

**Attributed to Gary Player, nine-time golf
major championship winner**

Surgical expertise

I have nothing but admiration for the skills of my mentors and the surgeons I have met in underdeveloped countries. All have had to work with inferior diagnostic tools and surgical equipment, and without access to the rehabilitation facilities that our patients enjoy today. They performed wonders while trying to undertake surgery from one end of the body to the other. The scope of surgery has changed dramatically since 1980. This is perhaps best illustrated in two areas with which I have long been involved – knee surgery and the treatment of trauma, such as fractures and dislocations.

In many specialities (not only orthopaedics) surgeons do more and more through smaller and smaller incisions. The first keyhole surgery of the knee (an arthroscopy) was attempted in 1912. Despite important technological advances in the 1950s, such as optical fibres, arthroscopies were still not universally practised in all UK hospitals by 1980. Nowadays, sports people enter hospitals daily for minor day-case knee surgery. The media report such interventions lightly with the expectation of the athlete's rapid return. In the not too dim and distant past, such outcomes could not have been taken for granted. Patients would stay in hospital for two weeks after knee surgery and sported a large battle scar on their knee. Whole cartilages were removed, even if only a small section was damaged. Rehabilitation was slow and future knee arthritis common.

NHS hospitals were not sufficiently convinced about keyhole surgery to fully fund it. In the mid-1980s we undertook charity fun runs to raise money for keyhole equipment. Knee day surgery was in its infancy but in 1987 my boss Robin Allum and I published one of the first British research papers confirming that knee surgery was safe in day units. Major London teaching hospitals still did not budget for keyhole equipment in the early 1990s when I was asked to buy my own equipment for my NHS lists, including a £600 instrument to remove cartilage tears. It still does the job nearly 30 years later. Who claimed NHS restraints are a modern invention?

Keyhole surgery revolutionised the treatment, rehabilitation and return to sport of those with knee injuries. The skills were quickly transferred to other joints such as the shoulder, elbow, wrist, hip and ankle. Understandably the demand for these procedures increased from all quarters. In June 2015 the *Daily Mail* reported that 'more than 150,000 British people undergo arthroscopic keyhole surgery to their knees every year – many of them in the 50s, 60s and 70s'. Over 1.5 million over-45s in Britain have knee arthritis. It is twice as common as before the Second World War. Many of these arthritic over-45s undertake some form of sport to stay fit. They see sports stars undergoing such treatments and hope that a similar 'small op' will be the panacea for their ills. However, evidence is accumulating that such operations may have only small, inconsequential benefits for our middle-aged, worn-out weekend warriors. It can be difficult to explain this to the patient sitting in front of you.

ACL injuries are dreaded by athletes and have been referred to earlier in the book. The ACL is a vital internal strap between the thigh and shin bones, providing stability. In the 1950s and 1960s, ACL injuries were often missed and were frequently career-ending for professional sportspeople. Brian Clough, the prolific Middlesbrough, Sunderland and England centre-forward, ruptured his ACL in 1962 aged 27. After two years of rehabilitation, a three-game comeback ended in retirement. His later successful career in football management is well documented.

Thirty years on, progress remained slow. A 1993 survey of ACL surgery on players at 75 English Football League clubs found that 150 ACL ruptures and operations had taken place in ten years – on average each professional English football club experienced one ACL injury every five years. Only 42 per cent of players returned to the same level and a further 22 per cent to a lower level. One-third never recovered sufficiently to return to their sport. Those results were woeful and put orthopaedic surgery in a poor light. The injury rates are much higher now.

Have we improved? Coaches and players confidently predict a return to play within six to nine months after these injuries. However, multiple studies suggest that only two-thirds of patients return to their previous level of sport after ACL surgery. Over half a century after Cloughie snapped his cruciate there is still room for improvement.

In the 1980s I would spend the first hour of every morning doing ward rounds with colleagues. Male wards were full of youngsters who had come to grief on their motorbikes or on sports fields. Their legs were suspended on traction. Pins were skewered through their thighs, shins and heels. It could have been a scene from *Carry on Doctor*. Patients remained in our care for months and daily we adjusted the weights, pulleys and position of their supporting frames. Slowly the bones knitted. Blessed release from this torture for the patients was followed by months trying to coax seized joints and withered muscles back into action.

Modern fracture fixation is more proactive. Stabilising fractures and allowing early movement benefits the patient's joints, muscles, bones and general well-being. Bed is a dangerous place – perils lurk under the bedclothes such as deep vein thrombosis, stiff joints and melting muscles. Early activity leads to quicker and fuller recoveries and the increased probability of patients returning to their beloved sport.

The sports physician

There has been a sea change in the attitude of many health professionals and medical purse holders towards exercise. In the 1980s and before, many clinicians regarded sports injuries as avoidable and self-inflicted; they were not always given the priority they deserved. Today, from our politicians downwards, there is a realisation that encouraging exercise is essential for an efficient workforce and to the nation's health.

Doctors wishing to follow a career in sport and exercise medicine and surgery are not now treated with the suspicion that their forebears endured, when colleagues felt that such doctors should be involved in more worthy activities. The final and belated recognition of sports medicine as a medical speciality in 2005 was an important landmark in changing these attitudes. However, it will take time to train the numbers of specialists required in this area.

A sports physician's training is all-encompassing. Many medical problems can befall people participating in sport and specialist doctors need to be knowledgeable in such diverse areas as altitude medicine, asthma and allergies as much as pitchside emergency care. Doctors become involved in the planning and execution of pre-event holding camps for athletes around the globe. Most challenging is the welfare of paraolympians, with their diverse medical requirements. Sports doctors advise athletes on the appropriateness of medicines. They must enact screening programmes for heart and melanoma screening and lead in matters of drug abuse or psychological stress. Their experience in leading the planning for return to safe sport during the 2020 COVID-19 pandemic has been impressive. In my experience, the leading exponents of sports medicine are some of the most remarkable doctors encountered.

The clinical team

The number of clinicians and scientists involved in athlete care has mushroomed in recent times. As well as doctors, there are physiotherapists, S&C staff, masseurs and sports scientists. Input may be requested from nutritionists, biomechanicists and other medical specialists at various times. Trying to assimilate so many different professions into one efficient unit can create problems.

The extensive training of pitchside staff in rapid and efficient responses to medical emergencies such as cardiac arrests, concussion and serious spinal injuries has been a positive contributor to player safety. Most of these people make significant contributions to the team effort. However, the accumulation of backroom staff in wealthy organisations does smack occasionally of being the same as stockpiling centre-backs – 'We will because we can.' The nadir may have been reached in 2009 with Manchester City's attempt to hire the Serbian afterbirth therapist. Sometimes, sports organisations less awash with cash make more astute hiring decisions.

Sports science

In 1970 it was rare to study sports science subjects at a UK university but within five years I had an unusual opportunity to take a BSc in biomechanics and exercise physiology. In 2019, 81 colleges offered undergraduate sports science courses. The country is turning out thousands of graduates annually with a good grounding in the basics of sport-related anatomy, physiology, biochemistry, nutrition, psychology and many more associated areas. Not everybody will follow careers in the sports field, but enough will do so to provide support and education to people involved in exercise at all levels of expertise and execution.

Our understanding of the basic biology of sports injuries has increased enormously even down to the cellular level. My research group has spent years studying genetic influences on injury. Our knowledge of how environmental factors, such as nutrition and training load, can influence the way our genes respond to training and injury is evolving.

To draw meaningful conclusions from this work needs collaboration and large numbers of subjects – no inferences can be made from the isolated treatment of one or two players at Manchester United. Injury surveillance reveals patterns of injuries and outcomes in sport. The RFU and ECB have been among the leaders in accumulating this data.

Programmes for the safe and speedy recovery of athletes have been developed by expert physiotherapy and S&C staff. Injured athletes progress through stages and the completion of each phase has become more criteria (rather than time) driven. There has developed a continuum from the operating table to the physiotherapy treatment table and on to the gym and practice field. The athlete progresses from general rehabilitation towards sport and position- or discipline-specific activities. Rehabilitation does not finish with a return to sport – maintenance programmes are devised to minimise breakdown. All of this is designed to put back into sport a fully functioning athlete ready for the fray.

Prevention is always preferable to treatment. Screening programmes and appropriate prehab work reduce specific injuries such as ankle sprains and knee ligament tears. Workloads are monitored in all sports. Whether you are a cricket fast bowler, soccer centre-back or rugby tight-head, you are likely to be monitored electronically, often by telemetry. Measurements of velocity, acceleration, distance and all variety of stresses and strains are assessed.

Post-activity sessions are carefully managed. Rehydration, nutrition, warm-downs, massages, and ice baths or cryotherapy chambers at minus 140°C await the tired athlete. Our research has been focused on the benefits of the last. Overall, these measures should ensure a safer sporting environment.

The medical information superhighway

When Tim Berners-Lee invented the World Wide Web in 1989 he would have had no idea of the impact it would have on everybody's lives. Medicine is no different.

Beyond the lecture theatre and hospital every bit of medical knowledge I gleaned as a student and junior doctor came from textbooks and laborious visits to the hospital library. I've mentioned the benefits of immediate access to medical data, and in writing this book I needed to check numerous medical and sporting facts to make sure my recollections held true. Sometimes they did not! Without search engines I would have been at the task for years to come.

The internet has allowed an international community of doctors with similar medical interests to develop. Problems can be shared and experiences and solutions pooled. The development of digital imaging – X-rays, MRIs, etc. – has transformed our ability to collaborate. At a touch of the keypad, encrypted medical information and images of an athlete can be winged around the world for a colleague's opinion and patients, colleagues and clinic staff can stay in touch with me when I am abroad. One of my radiology (imaging) colleagues is a keen skier. His favourite slopes are in Alaska and every evening, after schussing down the piste, he switches on his laptop and reviews the day's MRIs and X-rays and sends back to me his reports.

The internet has allowed athletes to become much better educated about the nature of their injury and management options – everybody from the occasional gym user to the Olympic competitor. If their information is accurate and relevant it helps plan treatment.

Image is everything?

Forty years ago our ability to 'look inside' our patients without surgery was limited, although X-rays had been around since 1896 and remain a staple form of investigation of bones and joints. As a junior doctor, the new imaging kid on the block was the CT scanner, invented in 1972. It gave us helpful information about heads, spines, bones and joints. Muscles, tendons, ligaments and cartilages were not so easily seen and patients were still subjected to exploratory operations.

The first human MRI scan took place in 1977 but it was not until the 1990s that these scanners were routinely available, although their availability was still woefully short of demand. It took another 20 years to catch up. MRIs revealed new problems with bones, joints and soft tissues we had no idea of.

They took some of the guesswork out of sports injuries and have allowed patients to be better counselled before any proposed surgery about the likely benefits and limitations. They are sensitive and pick up abnormalities that athletes had no idea they possessed and which, in all probability, cause them no problems. It is here that the experience of the doctor in interpreting these findings is vital – sorting the wood from the trees.

Imaging should never replace clinical assessment for sportspeople. That way lies lazy and expensive medicine. If clinicians start adopting a scattergun approach to MRI scanning we will break the budget of our health economy and lose our patient's respect for our own clinical skills. An MRI is not mandatory or desirable for every sports injury and may not provide any answers. I have seen many elite athletes with multiple MRI images whose cost would stress the GDP of a small country. An initial, inexpensive X-ray would have provided the diagnosis months before.

The use of knee MRIs is a good example of these conundrums. A 2014 study reported that knee MRIs were only 90 per cent accurate in detecting cartilage problems. A year later another study revealed that 43 per cent of knee scans were useless, a figure that rose to 82 per cent if our amateur athlete had knee wear. In 2015, surgical associations warned against over-reliance on MRI scanning compared to examining a patient and taking an X-ray. Simply put, MRI is not the objective, independent arbiter of all that is wrong with an athlete, as many assume. Sorry.

Ultrasound was developed around the time of the Second World War and was sufficiently established for clinical use by the 1960s. The machines are not as large and sexy as a multimillion-pound MRI or CT scanner but are often more helpful. They play an important part in the diagnosis of many sports injuries despite their often small size.

The range of methods of looking inside our patients has increased hugely in the last decades and doctors must understand what is most appropriate for each of the problems they will encounter. They must avoid becoming a slave to imaging, for by doing so, the clinician will never develop the experience and confidence from using their most sensitive assessment tools – their ears, eyes and hands.

Where does all this leave healthcare in sport?

Where do various clinical professions fall in a modern sporting club's organisation and its ambitions?

Within many sports the head coach's philosophy, personality and ambition colour the whole enterprise. Many of these people have massively increased profiles nowadays and although the attention can bolster their self-esteem, many are riven internally with their own insecurities and desire for sporting immortality. Anything or anybody that threatens their position can be ruthlessly swept aside.

Over 99 per cent of doctors are based in GP practices, clinics or hospitals. These establishments have embedded strict governance arrangements and are subject to scrutiny from a national independent regulator, the CQC. Everybody working within it should be aware of the lines of reporting and their roles and responsibilities in the hierarchy. The performance of individuals is guided by long-established professional principles and subject to annual rigorous appraisal. The process of removing a staff member from post for poor performance or breaches of discipline must follow a pre-determined path and accord with employment law. The methods for recruiting and retaining clinical staff to sport frequently lack the tight structures of mature, conventional health establishments.

All activities within health organisations should have at their core the welfare of the patients they are serving. As discussed earlier, problems occur when the main employer of clinical staff is a sporting organisation. The development of major medical and science departments within these enterprises is relatively recent. Before that, physios and doctors worked in a manner akin to a cottage industry – usually on a part-time basis with few resources and minimal financing. Many teams and sports further down the food chain still operate in this manner.

Achievement, fame and fortune for the sporting organisation and its individuals has become all-consuming and performance optimisation must be its principle objective. There is clear potential for conflict between two of the principle pursuits of any organisation, whether it be Manchester United or the local widget factory – performance of the business and the welfare of employees.

The role and relationship of clinicians who are not employed fully by the club or sport needs better understanding. They are bought in on a consultancy basis to provide expertise for specific problems and to guide and liaise with core clinical members on injury and illness management. Their independence should be respected and encouraged, for the objectivity it brings to often difficult problems that ultimately affect athlete performance and health.

Confusion exists in the minds of the media and athletes as to the function of certain clinical professions within sports organisations. In a *Sunday Times* interview with Sam Peters, the Welsh and British Lions rugby player, George North expressed his thoughts: 'The touchline physio with a magic sponge has been replaced by hordes of S&C experts and a small army of nutritionists, dieticians and medical people all analysing data in a bid to improve players' performance.'

This viewpoint concerns me. The welfare role appears to have been sacrificed on the altar of sporting success. What are the roles of the principle inhabitants of the sports medicine and science departments?

Certain groups sit comfortably within the performance side of the sport. S&C coaches help athletes acquire the necessary strength, endurance, agility and skills. Although a relatively new profession, S&C has become vital for athletes rehabilitating from injury. However, their expertise is required for the whole squad, to maintain essential levels of performance.

Physiotherapy appears to straddle the divide between performance and welfare. The physio in modern sport is more than the conveyor of the magic sponge, and new knowledge, techniques and equipment have usurped this bath-time accoutrement. Eddie Jones alluded to the modern scientific replacements for the old 'reviver' when purring about the skills of the England rugby union medical team. 'Remember in the old days [when] they used to have magic sponges? You would be down and out and the guy with a yellow sponge put it on you and you'd recover. Well they're back. The (modern) magic sponges are back.'

Pre-season, physios will be heavily involved in screening programmes for the returning squad. Who has lost strength, flexibility and fitness or returned with niggling injuries? With the S&C team, vulnerable athletes can be identified. The physiotherapist provides the daily treatment for players' injuries and is well-placed to assess the overall well-being of the athlete. Anxieties over and above the immediate injury frequently surface on the treatment table, which can resemble the psychiatrist's couch. Physiotherapists metamorphose from performance to welfare-orientated healthcare professional and back again. The physio is usually the first point of contact for the coaching staff. Is that player ready for Saturday? The physio needs to balance the needs of the organisation with the rights of the athlete.

I believe that the doctor's role falls within the welfare aspect of the athlete and their sport. Medics must support the physiotherapists, the S&C team and sports scientists. However, when the doctor ceases to regard the athlete first and foremost as their patient there is a risk of altering priorities and the sense of perspective. Doctors must be empowered to take a lead in ensuring that maintaining a duty of care is uppermost for all in authority in every sporting organisation.

Sports doctors must retain their own critical faculties. Is the enormous expenditure showered on medical and science departments in the ultimate interests of the athlete? Has our expertise reduced injury and long-term disability? Are we patching up players and sending them back to receive the next big hit? Are we improving their resilience to avoid future damage or has our ability to make stronger, faster and fitter athletes made them more likely to sustain long-term disability? Some of these big questions are avoided or not considered in the frenetic atmosphere of elite sport.

There must be overlap and dialogue between the performance and welfare elements of any sporting outfit. We know poor communication diminishes performance by jeopardising the health and availability of the key elements – the athletes.

'Will it make the boat go faster' was the mantra of the gold medal-winning men's rowing eight in the run-up to the 2000 Sydney Olympics. It was applied to any adjustment or addition to their training and performance programme. For the doctor, this approach means not only helping individual or team fulfilment within sport but safeguarding the welfare of its participants.

ACKNOWLEDGEMENTS

THERE HAVE been several medical books released in recent years. Each has provided insights into different areas of our profession and some have been written by friends and colleagues. However, there has been little written about the medical and surgical input into an area of life that provides enjoyment and fascination for so many millions – sport. I hope that this book adds to that knowledge.

The decision for a doctor to write a book is a difficult one, restricted as we are by professional boundaries, which mean that some of the more outlandish experiences cannot be retold and other experiences have to be heavily camouflaged. I am grateful to those athletes who have given permission for their names to be mentioned.

Throughout my career, I have received instruction and support from so many talented mentors and colleagues at home and abroad. A consultant surgeon's skill set is hewn from many different facets of experiences and knowledge that are gathered along the way. These gems do not come solely from other doctors; they also come from the many other healthcare professionals who contribute to the care of our patients. It is the latter group who provide a doctor with most enrichment and education and it is an honour to meet people from so many diverse walks of life and achievements. Daily I am reminded that people's medical problems cannot be considered in isolation. Frequently, the solutions will not be achieved without taking a holistic approach to the patient and working with the colleagues who surround me.

I would like to thank Sir Ian McGeechan and Greg Rutherford for providing the forewords from both the coach and athlete's point of view. They have both inspired me.

No book sees the light of day unless a publisher is prepared to take a leap of faith. I am indebted to Jane Camillin at Pitch Publishing for providing that impetus. Once taken on board I felt that I had been accepted into their band of brothers. Cath Harris provided the expert editorial support and was extremely patient as she cajoled a naturally long-winded writer into producing a manuscript of acceptable length. Their team is enhanced by the input of Duncan Olner and Graham Hales.

I have received much encouragement from many sources in developing the book. I would especially like to thank Andy Roberts, Bill MacKay, Phil Pask, Mark Saggers, Neil Redman, Richard Bath, Joanna Koster, Jackie and Gordon Mackay, and Kirsty and Tony Wade for pointing me in the right direction at critical times. The book makes clear that I spend as much time reading the back pages of the newspapers as I do the scientific literature. I would like to thank everybody from the media who has entertained and educated me in equal measure.

My career has been enabled over the last quarter of the century by Gill Hurnell and Caroline Stewart. They have had to keep my surgical practice on an even keel while I have added to their burden by embarking upon numerous meetings and conferences at home and abroad, undertaking countless research projects and then adding insult to injury by deciding to write this book.

I hope the book makes clear my indebtedness to and love for my family. My parents, Maurice and Sheila, gave me a lifelong passion for sport and were unstinting in their support throughout my educational and professional endeavours. The encouragement of my two sisters, Kim and Elisabeth, of this specific project typifies the camaraderie we have shared throughout our lives.

Finally, I must thank my wife, Siân, and my three daughters, Rebecca, Hannah and Abigail. All surgeons need a strong, supportive, understanding and loving family. Mine has been all of those things throughout these last 40 years.

BIBLIOGRAPHY

Chapter 1

Ben, K., 'In complex world of rising wages, clubs face very tough calls', *The Times*, 13 January 2018.

Jacob, G., 'Ronaldo quits Real for Juventus in four-year deal worth £310m', *The Times*, 11 July 2018.

Kharat, K., 'England National Team Cricketers Salary 2017', Sports India, 12 October 2016.

Kuper, S. and Szymanski S., *Soccernomics* (London: Harper Collins, 2018).

Liddle, R., 'You'd be smiling too if you got £75,000 just for starting', *Sunday Times*, 13 May 2018.

Peters, S., 'Manu Tuilagi sparks wages war as "*£300,000 is new £200,000*" for Premiership elite but the rest suffer', *Mail on Sunday*, 5 December 2015.

Slot, O., 'Time to ring-fence players' salaries', *The Times*, 12 December 2017.

Souness, G., 'Lampard's Youth Club', *Sunday Times*, 6 October 2019.

www.bbc.co.uk/sport, 'IPL: Ben Stokes bought by Rajasthan Royals; Joe Root unsold', 27 January 2018.

Chapter 2

Conn, D., 'Northampton Town: scandal of missing millions from Council's stadium loan', *The Guardian*, 6 November 2015.

Foster, R., '1966: what you might not know about the most famous year in English football', *The Guardian*, 11 February 2016.

Marsh, H., *Do No Harm* (London: Weidenfeld & Nicolson, 2014).

Times Higher Education, 'Participation rates: now we are 50', 25 July 2013.

Vaughan, H., 'Inquiry into NHS infected blood opens', *The Times*, 24 September 2018.

www.bbc.co.uk/news, 'Northants Cricket Club given £250,000 loan by borough council', 22 October 2015.

Chapter 3

Ammon, E., 'Ethics report says Australian sides have "culture of disrespect for opponents"', *The Times*, 29 October 2018.

Ammon, E., 'It was David Warner's idea to tamper with ball, says Cameron Bancroft', *The Times*, 27 December 2018.

Ammon, E., 'It was Warner's idea, says Bancroft', *The Times*, 27 December 2018.

Atherton, M., 'Game's balance lost between wild 1980s and joyless present', *The Times*, 31 October 2018.

Atherton, M., 'It's sport, not business. This report is vital for administrators everywhere', *The Times*, 30 October 2018.

Fraser, S., 'Murray playing through the pain', *The Times*, 31 December 2018.

Lowe, A., 'Munster doctor Jamie Kearns charged with misconduct for Jamie George comment', *The Times*, 24 December 2019.

Mott, S., 'Liverpool's iron man, Tommy Smith', *Daily Telegraph*, 22 March 2008.

Smith, T., *Anfield Iron* (London: Bantam Books, 2008).

Smith, T., *I Did It the Hard Way* (London: Arthur Baker, 1980).

www.bbc.co.uk/sport, 'Cricket Australia "partly to blame" in ball tampering scandal. Report by The Ethics Centre', 29 October 2018.

Chapter 4

Benson, M., 'In depth with Nick Blackwell: former boxer discusses life-altering injuries and long road to recovery in rare interview', www.talkSPORT.com, 13 September 2018.

Borg, G.A., 'Psychophysical bases of perceived exertion', *Med Sci Sports Exercise*, 1982; 14(5): 377–381.

Bull, A., 'Turner was one of the athletes who helped Liu Xiang off the Olympic track. It could easily have been him!' *The Guardian*, 29 January 2012.

Ferdie Pacheco Obituary, *The Times*, 28 November 2017.

Fraser, S., 'I don't know how long I'll last, says emotional Andy Murray after beating James Duckworth at Brisbane International', *The Times*, 1 January 2019.

Gouttebarge, V., et al., 'Prevalence of osteoarthritis in former elite athletes: a systematic overview of the recent literature', *Rheumatology International*, 2015; 35(3): 405–418.

Hammond, L.E., et al., 'The impact of playing in matches whilst injured on injury surveillance findings in professional football', *Scand J Med Sci Sports*, 2014; 24(3): e195–200.

Jones, M.E., et al., 'Osteoarthritis and other long-term health conditions in former elite cricketers', *Journal of Science and Sports Medicine in Sport*, 2018; 21: 558–563.

Jones, S., 'Tuilagi. The strength comes from within', *Sunday Times*, 16 December 2018.

Kevin Beattie Obituary, *The Times*, 18 September 2018.

Laurance, J., Clark, N., 'The pain game: sports stars risking their careers', *The Independent*, 5 June 2012.

Lowe, A., 'A witchdoctor found three lady spirits who wanted to punish me', *The Times*, 9 November 2017.

Lowe, A., 'Almost half of world's top players felt pressured to play while injured', *The Times*, 4 December 2018.

Lowe, A., 'I feared another injury in every session, says Tuilagi', *The Times*, 26 November 2018.

Lowe, A., 'Painkillers became "habit" for Brian O'Driscoll – and modern players are no different', *The Times*, 6 December 2018.

MacFarland, R., *Roy Mac: Clough's Champion* (London: Trinity Mirror Sports Media, 2014).

Noakes, T.D., Peltonen, J.E., Rusko, H.K., 'Evidence that a central governor regulates exercise performance during acute hypoxia and hyperoxia', *Journal of Experimental Biology*, 2001; 204: 3225–3234.

O Raghallaigh, C., 'Medication is not being handed out willy-nilly', *The Times*, 7 December 2018.

Robertson, G., 'Footballer's painkiller problem: why many can't get by without them', *The Times*, 13 October 2017.

Rugby World, 'International Survey Highlights Player Concerns', January 2019.

Smith, T., *I did it the hard way* (London: Arthur Baker, 1980).

The Guardian, 'England's Manu Tuilagi struggling to be fit for Six Nations', 14 January 2014.

Tran G., et al., 'Does sports participation (including level of performance and previous injury) increase risk of osteoarthritis? A systematic review and meta-analysis', *British Journal of Sports Medicine*, 2016; 50: 1459–1466.

Turner, A.P., et al., 'Long term health impact of playing professional football in the United Kingdom', *British Journal of Sports Medicine*, 2000; 34: 332–327.

Tveit, M., et al., 'Former male elite athletes have a higher prevalence of osteoarthritis and arthroplasty in the hip and knee than expected', *American Journal of Sports Medicine*, 2012;40(3): 527–533.

Westerby, J., 'Harry Ellis: I was lost after I retired. There is no quick fix for depression', *The Times*, 2 March 2019.

Wiegland, T.J., et al., 'Nonsteroidal anti-inflammatory drug (NSAID) toxicity', *MedScape*, 20 December 2017.

Windsor Insurance Brokers Limited, 'Investigations into career ending incidents to professional footballers in England and Wales from 1987–1988 to 1994–1995', 1997.

Winter, H., 'Footballers on anti-inflammatories play with their health', *Daily Telegraph*, 31 March 2009.

www.bbc.co.uk/sport, 'Warrington Wolves: Paul Wood has testicle removed', 7 October 2012.

www.leicestertigers.com, 'Tigers v Racing 92: match report', 21 January 2018.

Ziegler, M., 'Why top athletes really do suffer more from asthma', *The Times*, 24 September 2016.

Chapter 5

Hellen, N., 'Willpower wilting? Get a fitness buddy', *Sunday Times*, 21 January 2018.

Ingraham, C., 'People keep sticking their hands in snowblowers without turning them off first, data show', *Washington Post*, 27 January 2015.

Chapter 6

Ammon, E., 'Transgender rules can't stop me – I'm eligible for England', *The Times*, 27 November 2019.

Bermon, S., Garnier, P.-Y., 'Serum androgen levels and their relation to performance in track and field: mass spectrometry results from 2127 observations in male and female elite athletes', *British Journal of Sports Medicine*, 2017; 51: 1309–1314.

Broadbent, R., 'Athletics torn over treatment of one of its biggest stars', *The Times*, 2 May 2019.

Broadbent, R., 'IAAF must let Semenya run', *The Times*, 22 October 2018.

Broadbent, R., 'I was Caster Semenya of the 1980s', *The Times*, 6 May 2019.

Broadbent, R., 'Semenya: I've been targeted', *The Times*, 2 May 2019.

Clark, R.V., et al., 'Large divergence in testosterone concentrations between men and women: Frame of reference for athletes in sex-specific competition in sports, a narrative review', *Clinical Endocrinology*, 2019; 90: 15–22.

Diane Leather Obituary, *The Times*, 18 September 2018.

Dugan, S. A., 'Sports-related injuries in female athletes: what gives?' *Am J Phys Med Rehab*, 2005; 84(2): 122–130.

Eirale, C., Ekstrand, J., 'Epidemiology of injury in football', *Aspetar Sports Medicine Journal*, 2: 144–149 (April 2013).

Epstein, D., *The Sports Gene* (London: Random House, 2014).

Healy, M.L., et al., 'Endocrine profiles in 693 elite athletes in the post-competition setting', *Clinical Endocrinology*, 2014; 81: 294–305.

Hudson, M., 'Action on women's' injuries', *The Times*, 14 September 2019.

ICC document, 'Gender recognition policy', 20 February 2017.

Ito, E., et al., 'Sex-specific differences in injury types among basketball players, *Open Access of Sports Medicine*, 2015; 6: 1–6.

Killanin, Lord and Rodda, J., (eds) *The Olympic Games 1984* (Detroit, MI: Willow Books, 1983).

Kooman, K., *Een Koningin Met Mannenbenen*, (Amsterdam: L.J. Veen, 2003).

Miller, D., *The Official History of the Olympic Games and the IOC: Athens to Beijing, 1894–2008* (Edinburgh: Mainstream Publishing, 2008).

Mountjoy, M., et al., 'The IOC consensus statement: beyond the Female Athlete Triad – Relative Energy Deficiency in Sport (RED-S)', *British Journal of Sports Medicine*, 2014; 48; 491–497.

Myers, R., 'Quins Starlet blazes a trail', *Sunday Times*, 4 March 2018.

Pielke, R.Jr., Tucker, R., Boyle, E., 'Scientific integrity and the IAAF testosterone regulations', *International Sports Law*, February 19 (e-pub, 2019).

Ristolainen, L., et al., 'Gender differences in sport injury risk and types of injuries: a retrospective twelve-month study on cross-country skiers, swimmers, long-distance runners and soccer players', *Journal of Sports Science and Medicine*, 2009; 8: 443–451.

Sebor, J., 'The History of Women's Running', www.activekids.com

St Helens the reporter, 'Trailblazing women's football side honoured', 8 June 2017.

Syed, M., 'Men's deep-rooted bias holding back women's football', *The Times*, 5 December 2018.

Sönksen, P.H., et al., 'Why do endocrine profiles in elite athletes differ between sports?', *Clinical Diabetes and Endocrinology*, 2018; 4: 3.

Syed, M., 'No stopping boom in women's football', *The Times*, 2 August 2017.

Tannenbaum, C., 'Sex, gender and sports', *BMJ*, 474, 23, March 2019.

The Citizen, 'IAAF holds off on controversial "Semenya rule" change', 16 October 2018.

The Scotsman, 'Non-binary categories to be introduced in national Scottish Athletics', 23 January 2019.

Thibault, V., et al., 'Women and men in sport performance: The gender gap has not evolved since 1983', *Journal of Sports Science and Medicine*, 2010; 9: 214–223.

Turner, J., 'Male bodies don't belong in women's sport', *The Times*, 23 February 2019.

Wilson, B., 'Mexico 1971: when women's football hit the big time', www.bbc.co.uk/sport, 7 December 1971.

www.theconversation.com, 'So what if some female Olympians have high testosterone?' 15 August 2016.

www.topendsport.com', 'Women at the Olympic Games'.

Ziegler, M., 'ECB transgender policy under review', *The Times*, 15 August 2019.

Ziegler, M., 'Radcliffe: countries will exploit intersex athletes', *The Times*, 19 April 2019.

Ziegler, M., 'Transgender policies could alter after hormone research', *The Times*, 24 August 2019.

Chapter 7

Adams, A.L., et al., 'Associations between childhood obesity and upper and lower extremity injuries', *Injury Prevention*, 2012; 19(3): 191–197.

Adetunji, J., 'Michael Gove overruled experts to sell school playing fields', *The Guardian*, 17 August 2012.

Ardern, C.L., et al., 'Fifty-five per cent return to competitive sport following anterior cruciate ligament surgery: an updated systematic review and meta-analysis including aspects of physical functioning and contextual factors', *British Journal of Sports Medicine*, 48(21): 1543–1552 (2014).

Baer, D., 'Malcolm Gladwell Explains What Everyone Gets Wrong About His Famous "10,000 Hour Rule"', *Business Insider*, 2 June 2014.

Beck, N.A., et al., 'ACL tears in school-aged children and adolescents over 20 years', *Pediatrics*, 139(3): e20161877 (March 2017).

Brenius, B., Ponzer, S., et al., 'Increased risk of osteoarthritis after anterior cruciate ligament reconstruction: a 14-year follow-up study of a randomized controlled study', *AmJSM*, 42(5): 1049–1057 (2014).

Brogdon, B.G., Crow N.E., 'Little Leaguer's elbow', *Am J Radiol*, 83: 671–675 (1960).

Brophy, R.H., et al., 'Return to play and future ACL injury risk after ACL reconstruction in soccer athletes from the Multicenter Orthopaedic Outcomes Network (MOON) group', *Am JSM*, 40(11): 2517–2522e (2012).

Bysouth, A., 'Winter Olympic stats: Norway's record haul, Germany's Golden Games and more', www.bbc.co.uk/sport, 25 February 2018.

Calvin, M., *No Hunger in Paradise: The Players, The Journey, The Dream* (London: Penguin Random House, 2017).

Campbell, D., 'Michael Gove's Political Own Goal on School Sports', *The Guardian*, 6 August 2012.

Cao, J.J., 'Effects of obesity on bone metabolism', *Journal of Orthopaedic Surgery and Research*, 2011; 6: 30.

Cerny, C., 'Obesity is one of the biggest public health challenges facing the UK today', *The Guardian*, Supplement by Media Planet, 15 June 2018.

Dunman, N., 'We spotted Yarnold and Deas on the same day', *The Times*, 19 February 2018.

Ekstrand, J., 'A 94% return to elite level football after ACL surgery: a proof of possibilities with optimal caretaking or a sign of knee abuse?', *Knee Surg Sports Traumatol Arthrosc*, 19: 1–2 (2011).

Engebretsen, L., 'Are we destroying talent? 25% reinjury rate among children who have ACL reconstructions', *BMJ* blog, 16 June 2017.

Finkelstein, E.A., et al., 'The relationship between obesity and injuries among US adults', *Am J Health Promotion*, 2007; 21(5): 460–468.

Freeman, S., 'Obesity still eating away at the health of the nation', *Yorkshire Post*, 14 December 2010.

Grover, S.A., et al., 'Years of life lost and healthy life-years lost from diabetes and cardiovascular disease in overweight and obese people: a modelling study', *The Lancet Diabetes & Endocrinology*, published online 5 December 2014.

Ilich, J.Z., et al., 'Interrelationship among muscle, fat, and bone: Connecting the dots on cellular, hormonal, and whole body levels', *Ageing Research Reviews*, 2014; 15: 51.

Lambert, V., 'How women's bodies have been transformed in the past 60 years ... with huge implications for our health', *Daily Mail Online*, 15 September 2009.

Lay, K., 'Childhood obesity in primary schools is a growing problem', *The Times*, 11 October 2018.

Lean, G., 'Is it over for school playing fields?' *Daily Telegraph*, 12 September 2014.

Macnamara, B.N., Hambrick, D.Z., Oswald, F.L., 'Deliberate practice and performance in music, games, sports, education, and professions A meta-analysis', *Psychological Science* 25(8): 1608–1618 (2014).

MacNamara, B.N., Moreau, D., Hambrick, D.Z., 'The Relationship between deliberate practice and performance in sports: A meta-analysis', **Brooke N. Macnamara1Princeton University**

Myer, G.D., et al., 'Sports Specialization, Part I: Does early sports specialization increase negative outcomes and reduce the opportunity for success in young athletes? And Part II: Alternative solutions to early sport specialization in youth athletes', *Sports Health*, 7(6): 437–442 and 8(1): 65–73 (2015).

Myers, R., 'Alberto Salazar almost drove me to suicide, says former Nike runner', *The Times*, 7 November 2019.

National Paediatric Diabetes Audit 2016–2017, August 2018.

NHS Digital, 'Statistics on Obesity, Physical Activity and Diet – England, 2016', 2820:36 May 05, 2017 – 09:30 April 28, 2016 April 2016.

'Obesity and Injury: A review of the Literature', Australian Government publication, 2011.

Rana, A.R., et al., 'Childhood obesity: a risk factor for injuries observed at a level-1 trauma center', *Journal of Pediatric Surgery* 2009; 44(8): 1601–1605.

Reason, J., *Human Error* (Cambridge: Cambridge University Press, 1990).

Ribbans, W.J., Henman, P.D., Bliss, W.H., 'Achilles tendon ruptures in teenagers involved in elite gymnastics', *Sports Orthopaedics and Traumatology*, 32: 375–379 (2016).

Rumsby, B., 'Fewer Englishman than ever on show in the Premier League', *Daily Telegraph*, 18 May 2016.

Serdula, M.K., et al., 'Do obese children become obese adults? A review of the literature', *Prev Med*, 1993; 22(2): 167–177.

Syed, M., *Bounce* (London: Fourth Estate, 2010).

Taylor, E.D., et al., 'Orthopedic complications of overweight in children and adolescents', *Pediatrics* 2006; 117(6): 2167–2174.

Teasdale, N., et al., 'Obesity alters balance and movement control', *Current Obesity Research*, 2013; 2: 235–240.

Timm, N.L., et al., 'Chronic ankle morbidity in obese children following an acute ankle injury', *Arch Pediatr Adolesc Med*, 2005; 159(1):33–36.

Vanlint, S., 'Vitamin D and obesity', *Nutrients*, 2013; 5: 949–56.

Vasagar, J., Mansell, W., 'School sports fields in danger as government relaxes rules', *The Guardian*, 14 August 2012.

Vaughan, R., 'Surge in number of school playing fields sold off', Inews.co.uk, 3 January 2017.

Walden, M., et al., 'Anterior cruciate ligament injury in elite football: a prospective three-cohort study', *Knee Surg Sports Traumatol Arthrosc*, 19(1): 11–19 (2011).

Waterlow, L., 'Changing shape of modern man: average British male is now two inches taller and a stone heavier than six decades ago', *Daily Mail Online*, 3 December 2014.

www.cyclinguk.org, Cycling UK's Cycling Statistics, 15 February 2018.

Zhao, L.-J., et al., 'Relationship of obesity with osteoporosis', *J Clinical Endo Metabolism*, 2017; 92(5): 1640–1646.

See all articles by this author **Search Google Scholar** *for this author* **David Z. Hambrick** *2Michigan State University*

See all articles by this author **Search Google Scholar** *for this author* Perspect Psycholo Sci, 11(3): 333–350 (2016).

Chapter 8

Anton, B., et al., 'Can we delay aging? The biology and science of aging', *Ann N Y Acad Sci*, 2005; 1057: 525–535.

Cadbury, R. MP, co-chairwoman, all-party parliamentary cycling group, 'Cycleways not headgear', *Sunday Times*, 2 September 2018.

Cooper, R., et al., 'Physical capability in mid-life and survival over 13 years of follow-up: British birth cohort study', *BMJ*, 348: g2219 (2014).

Da Costa, J.P., et al., 'A synopsis on aging – theories, mechanisms and future prospects', *Ageing Res Rev*, 29: 90–112 (2016).

Fixx, J., The Long Distance Runner: A Definitive Study (London: Random House, 1977).

Holden, L., 'How fast will you jog at 80? Take the running-age test to find out', *The Times*, 16 October 2018.

Li, Y., et al., 'Healthy lifestyle and life expectancy free of cancer, cardiovascular disease, and type 2 diabetes', *BMJ*, 17 (11 January 2020).

McNally, S., 'Regular physical exercise: the "miracle cure to ageing",' *BMJ*, 359: 108–110 (21 October 2017).

NICE Guidelines 2017 'Osteoporosis: assessing the risk of fragility fracture'.

Streppel, M.T., et al., 'Mortality and life expectancy in relation to long-term cigarette, cigar and pipe smoking: the Zutphen Study', *Tob Control* 16(2): 107–13 (April 2007).

Torjesen, I., 'Rates of gout continue to rise in UK, but GP care has not improved', *BMJ*, 348: g239 (2014).

www.cyclinguk.org, Cycling UK's Cycling Statistics, 15 February 2018.

Chapter 9

Baiju, D.S.R., James, L.A., 'Parachuting: A sport of chance and expense', *Injury* 34: 25–217 (2013).

Greenberg, M.R., et al., 'Unique obstacle race injuries at an extreme sports event: a case series', *Annals of Emergency Medicine*, 63: 361–66 (2014).

Hawley, A., et al., 'Obstacle course runs: review of acquired injuries and illnesses at a series of Canadian events (RACE). *Canadian Journal of Emergency Medicine,* 18(S1): S37 (2016).

Lee, C.T., Williams, P., Hadden, W.A., 'Parachuting for charity: is it worth the money? A 5-year audit of parachute injuries in Tayside and the cost to the NHS. *Injury,* 30(4): 283–87 (1999).

Momaya, A., et al., 'When celebrations go wrong: a case series of celebrating in sports', *J Sports Medicine and Physical Fitness*, 57(3): 267–271 (2017).

www.bbc.co.uk/news, 'World's "first" bungee jump in Bristol captured on film', 10 December 2014.

Chapter 10

Mays, K., 'Bruno comeback gathers momentum', *Daily Telegraph*, 23 April 1992.

Pitt, N., 'Boxing returns to the Albert Hall', *Sunday Times*, 3 March 2019.

Pitt, N., 'Ingle kids get chance to win fight of their lives', *Sunday Times*, 4 May 2014.

Prynn, J., 'Thomas A Becket pub: buy Sir 'Enry's gym for a knockout price', *Evening Standard*, 10 June 2015.

www.bbc.co.uk/sport, 'Scott Westgarth: British boxer dies after winning fight in Doncaster', 26 February 2018.

Chapter 11

Anderson, C. and Sally, D., *The Numbers Game* (London: Penguin Books, 2014).

Critchley, M., 'Police dispute Mourinho's "escort" complaint', *The Independent*, 4 October 2018.

Daniels, R., *Blackpool Football: The Official Club History* (London: Robert Hale, 1972).

Dickinson, M., 'Check-ups for managers as stress takes huge toll', *The Times*, 23 May 2019.

Finkelstein, D., 'Nine top managers won't last season', *The Times*, 22 September 2018.

Gheerbrant, J., 'Players should be selfish. They, not the clubs, know if they are fit to play', *The Times*, 4 January 2020.

Heffernan, C., 'The story of Frank Buckley and monkey glands at Wolves', thesefootballtimes.co, 5 August 2015.

Hirst, P., 'Mellow Jose Mourinho has put in hours to shed moody image', *The Times*, 21 November 2019.

Hirst, P. and Jones, P., 'United anger at Southgate over Jones. FA gave him six injections, reveals Mourinho', *The Times*, 18 November 2017.

Hughes, M., 'Exclusive: Jose Mourinho has hurt game, says Graeme Le Saux', *The Times*, 15 October 2015.

Hughes, M. and Hirst, P., 'Mourinho orders United injury probe', *The Times*, 9 November 2016.

Kay, O., 'Chelsea v Swansea match report', *The Times*, 15 August 2015.

Kuper, S. and Szymanski S., *Soccernomics* (London: Harper Collins, 2018).

Lewis, D., 'Jose Mourinho hits back at Sergio Ramos after dig over Fabregas and Costa's Spain absence', *Daily Mirror*, 23 November 2014.

McCarra, K., 'Mourinho accused of getting facts wrong', *The Guardian*, 19 October 2006.

Samuel, M., 'Jose Mourinho, stop needling Chelsea and come clean,' *Daily Mail Online*, 16 March 2010.

Smith, R., 'FA silence on Chelsea doctor "disappointing", says QC', *The Times*, 9 September 2015.

The Guardian, 'United doctor quits following Ferguson bust-up', 24 May 2006.

The Independent, 'Football: Mourinho shows doctor the door after Robben dispute', 9 February 2005.

Todd, O., 'Jose Mourinho and his rows over medical staff: Eva Carneiro is not the first to face criticism from the Chelsea manager', *Daily Mail Online*, 12 August 2015.

Wallace, S., 'Eva Carneiro: video emerges showing full extent of Jose Mourinho's tirade against Chelsea doctor and physio Jon Fearn', *The Independent*, 13 August 2015.

www.bbc.co.uk/sport, 'British and Irish Lions: Stuart Hogg to have cheek injury assessed', 11 June 2017.

Chapter 13

Bird, J., 'It was very painful: Diego Costa confirms he had massage using horse placenta and electroshocks in bid to be fit for 2014 Champions League final … and it was administered by doctors smoking two cigarettes', *Daily Mail Online*, 27 April 2020.

Bonham, S., 'Arsenal's Robin van Persie to soothe ankle pains with placenta massage', *The Guardian*, 16 November 2009.

Collins, P., 'Diego Costa forced off after nine minutes of Champions League final with hamstring injury (and he could be out of World Cup)', *Daily Mail Online*, 24 May 2014.

Daily India, 'Van Persie, Johnson's placenta therapist under investigation', 20 November 2009.

Daily Mail Online, 'Robin van Persie set for five-month injury absence as Arsenal striker undergoes ankle surgery', 28 November 2009.

Daily Mirror, 'Robin van Persie set for lengthy spell on the sidelines after suffering "bad ankle injury"', 14 November 2009.

Daily Telegraph, 'Champions League Final 2014: Atletico Madrid's Diego Costa undergoes controversial muscle treatment', 21 May 2014.

Jones, S., 'Rafa Benitez pulls a Christmas quacker. Liverpool want to sign Belgrade placenta doctor, Marijana Kovacevic', *Daily Mail Online*, 24 December 2009.

McNulty, P., Match report of Champions League Final. Real Madrid 4-1 Atlético Madrid, www.bbc.co.uk/sport, 25 May 2014.

Metro online, 'Serbian horse-placenta football clinic is illegal', 25 November 2009.

Richardson, A., 'Cristiano Ronaldo will have his Euro 2016 final injury treated by famous "placenta doctor"', *The Sun*, 13 July 2016.

Smith, G., 'Robin van Persie's treatment the embryo of a brilliant idea', *The Times*, 21 November 2009.

Sydney Morning Herald, 'Serbs quack down on miracle Marijana', 24 November 2009.

Triggle, N., 'A new miracle cure for injuries', www.bbc.co.uk/news, 17 November 2009.

www.eurosport.co.uk, 'Cristiano Ronaldo to have knee treated by famous "placenta doctor"', 13 July 2016.

www.talkingpaws.com, 'Diego Costa heads to Belgrade for horse placenta injection in bid to cure hamstring injury', 21 May 2014.

Chapter 14

Gallagher, J., et al., 'Oral health-related behaviours reported by elite and professional athletes', *British Dental Journal,* 2019; 227; 276–280.

Needleman, I., et al., 'Oral Health and elite sports performance', *Br J Sports Med,* 2015; 49(1): 3–6.

Redknapp, J., 'Jamie Redknapp on the life of an injured footballer: I was like a walking episode of Casualty and tried every cure', *Daily Mail,* 18 November 2009.

Sergei Vikharev Obituary, *The Times*, 27 June 2017.

Sunday Times, 'Dutch left with less bite', 15 June 2014.

Turner, N., 'Arsenal's van Persie reveals dental trouble', www.goal.com, 31 May 2009.

Van Burm, F., Goedhardt, A., 'Preliminary evidence for the efficacy of cranial osteopathy in footballers.', *BJSM*, 2017; 51: 284.

Whipple, T., 'Don't look a gifted athlete in the mouth – it won't be pretty', *The Times*, 26 August 2019.

Whitwell, L., 'Louis van Gaal slammed by Dutch fitness coach after Robin van Persie suffers groin strain', *Daily Mail*, 5 June 2014.

www.bbc.co.uk/sport, 'Redknapp injury woe', 21 July 2000.

www.sport.co.uk, 'Van Persie follows Gerrard and Malouda wisdom in dental stakes', 1 June 2009.

www.skysports.com, 'Van Persie's teeth trouble', 31 May 2009.

Chapter 15

Allen-Mills, T., 'Mo Farah's former coach Alberto Salazar is run to ground at last', *The Times*, 6 October 2019.

Bates, D., 'The Monday Overview: to rest or not to rest?' *The Times*, 3 December 2018.

BBC TV, *Only Fools and Horses*, Heroes and Villains episode, 1996.

Brand, G., 'How Bosman rule changed football – 20 years on', www.skysports.com, 15 December 2015.

Conn, D., 'Portsmouth save their money for millionaires while paupers go unpaid', *The Guardian*, 22 April 2010.

Davis, M., 'Premier League festive fixtures lead to an increase in injuries, says analyst', www.bbc.co.uk/sport, 4 January 2018.

Dickinson, M., 'Winter break will not turn England into world-beaters', *The Times*, 2 March 2018.

Eirale, C. and Ekstrand, J., 'Targeted Topic: Sports medicine in football. Epidemiology of injury in football', *Aspetar Sports Medicine Journal*, 2013; 2: 144–149.

Ekstrand, J. and Spreko, A., Released on Twitter, 1 March 2018.

Ekstrand, J. et al., 'Communication quality between the medical team and the head/coach manager is associated with injury burden and player availability in elite football clubs', *BJSM*, 2019; 53(5): 304–308.

Gheerbrandt, J., 'Players should be selfish. They, not the clubs, know if they are fit to play', *The Times*, 4 January 2020.

Hirst, P., 'Solskjaer hits back at "medieval" Van Persie', *The Times*, 4 January 2020.

Hynes, R., 'Stephen Ward reveals extent of alleged Roy Keane and Harry Arter bust-up in Irish training', *Irish Mirror*, 11 September 2018.

Jones, S., 'Eddie Jones should take a leaf out of Fiji's playbook', *Sunday Times*, 3 June 2018.

Joyce, P., 'How World Cup has caused an injury epidemic in the Premier League', *The Times*, 20 November 2018.

Kuper, S. and Szymanski S., *Soccernomics* (London: Harper Collins, 2018).

Lowe, A., 'Eddie Jones hits back at Bath owner and says: don't tell me what to do', *The Times*, 31 May 2018.

Lowe, A., 'England misled us on Cokanasiga injury, say Bath', *The Times*, 25 November 2019.

Lowe, A., 'Premiership and RFU struck deal over injuries', *The Times*, 5 December 2018.

Robertson, G., 'Historic clubs being driven into the dirt – yet game does nothing', *The Times*, 27 July 2019.

Sheen, T., 'Team GB funding cuts are killing British basketball', *The Independent*, 20 February 2016.

Slot, O., 'Call for action on bad injuries', *The Times*, 10 January 2019.

Slot, O., 'Five-week South Africa tour will increase fears for Lions', *The Times*, 5 June 2018.

Slot, O., 'Rugby World Cup: Billy Vunipola is irreplaceable – so why risk him against the US?', *The Times*, 24 September 2019.

Stone, M., 'Football medicine in England: A personal perspective on protocols, standards, and moving the field forward', *BJSM* blog, 13 September 2014.

Syed, M., 'Few people have been less suited to coaching than this vile bully Roy Keane', *The Times*, 17 September 2018.

The Times, 'Former England star Richards retires at 31 because of injury', 27 July 2019.

The Times, 'Varnish appeals against ruling', 15 March 2019.

'twohundredpercent.net, 'The Maximum Wage and Retain and Transfer: A Match Made in Hell, for Players', 26 January 2011.

Walsh, D., 'Justice has finally caught up with Alberto Salazar – but who will he take down with him?', *Sunday Times*, 6 October 2019.

www.bbc.co.uk/sport, 'Premier League fixture congestion "absurd" as teams count Christmas cost,' 3 January 2020.

www.bbc.co.uk/sport, 'Winter break in England: Premier League, FA and EFL discuss February break', 27 February 2018.

www.mondaq.com, Allsop, M., 'Anti-deprivation rule did not prevent "Football Creditors" of a football club being paid in full before other unsecured creditors', 10 July 2012.

Ziegler, M., 'Ban coaches from giving orders to team doctors, report urges', *The Times*, 23 April 2017.

Ziegler, M., 'City anger over fixture pile up', *The Times*, 18 October 2019.

Ziegler, M., 'Jess Varnish loses employment tribunal legal case against British Cycling', *The Times*, 17 January 2019.

Ziegler, M., 'Jess Varnish tells employment tribunal that British Cycling had "extreme control" over her', *The Times*, 11 December 2018.

Ziegler, M., 'Little gifts from Premier League giants would have big benefits for those in lower leagues', *The Times*, 28 March 2020.

Ziegler, M., 'More injuries in teams where managers ignore doctors', *The Times*, 24 August 2018.

Ziegler, M., 'Premier League winter break will go ahead in 2020', *The Times*, 9 June 2018.

Ziegler, M., 'Sky doctor Richard Freeman pulls out of Jess Varnish tribunal hearing', *The Times*, 12 December 2018.

Ziegler, M., 'Winter break would alleviate injury problems', *The Times*, 21 November 2018.

Chapter 16

Ackford, P., 'Another Casualty of Hard-Knock Life', *The Times*, 17 May, 2014.

Barnes, S., 'Obsession with size has created monster', *The Times*, 4 May 2018.

Bates, D., 'Revealed the shocking truth about rugby's drug problem,' *The Times*, 3 May 2018.

De Menzies, J., 'Sam Warburton retirement a "red flag" for rugby union, admits World Rugby chief Agustin Pichot amid injury crisis', *The Independent*, 22 July 2018.

Dickinson, M., 'Sam Warburton interview: "I did not enjoy 80% of my career but I'd do it all over again"', *The Times*, 7 September 2019.

England Professional Rugby Injury Surveillance Project Steering Group, 2017–2018 RFU PRISP report.

English, T., 'Will the Six Nations bring less brutality and more beauty?', www.bbc.co.uk/sport, 1 February 2019.

Hill, N.E., et al., 'Changes in northern hemisphere male international rugby union players' body mass and height between 1955 and 2015', *BMJ Open Sport and Exercise Medicine Journal*, 2018; 4: e000459.

James, S., 'My knees were so sore – my body just couldn't cope any more', *The Times*, 25 August 2018.

Jenkins, V., 'Story-Book Finish puts paid to England', *Sunday Times*, 1 March 1970.

Jones, S., 'England take the crown', *Sunday Times*, 5 April 1988.

Jones, S., 'Victim of the sport he loves', *Sunday Times*, 22 July 2018.

Jones, S., 'We must find way to stop adding injury to insult', *Sunday Times*, 21 January 2018.

Leith, W., 'How a kick in the head created the world's best heart surgeon', *The Times Magazine*, 30 March 2019.

Lowe, A., 'Radical laws to improve rugby safety', *The Times*, 21 March 2019.

Milburn, P., 'Brute force: reducing the impact of rugby collisions', theconversation.com, 10 April 2014.

Poortmans, J.R. and Francaux, M., 'Adverse effects of creatine supplementation', *Sports Medicine*, 2000; 30(3): 155–170.

Quarrie, K.L., et al., 'Managing player load in professional rugby union: a review of current knowledge and practices', *BJSM*, 2016. 51(5), bjsports-2016-096191.

Slot, O., 'British and Irish Lions tours at risk after English rugby season is extended until late June', *The Times*, 23 October 2018.

Slot, O., 'Chalmers on sidelines after losing out in battle of bulk', *The Times*, 14 June 2014.

Slot, O., 'Clubs to monitor uber-boss Eddie Jones in fragile training deal', *The Times*, 18 September 2018.

Slot, O., 'Rugby is at last waking up to the scale of the injury crisis', *The Times*, 10 January 2019.

Slot, O., 'The Ruck podcast: teams threatened with World Cup ban in move to reduce training', *The Times*, 10 September 2018.

Stoney, E., 'Club measures how hard rugby's hits really are', *New York Times*, 18 April 2013.

Ungoed-Thomas, J. and Bowen, J., 'Injuries get worse as weight in rugby stars leaps 25%', *Sunday Times*, 20 January 2019.

Walsh, D., 'Our conveyor belt is broken and we've got to mend it quickly. Interview with Rob Andrew and Michael Lynagh', *Sunday Times*, 12 November 2017.

Walsh, D., 'Video footage of sickening injuries fills parents with dread and pushes rugby closer to crisis', *Sunday Times*, 24 March 2019.

Warburton, S., *Open Side* (Glasgow: HarperCollins, 2019).

Warburton, S., 'Against France, England should keep faith with pure physicality', *The Times*, 9 February 2019.

Ziegler, M., 'South African school rugby suffering rise in steroid use', *The Times*, 31 October 2018.

Ziegler, M., 'South Africa's efforts undone by doping stars and schoolboys', *The Times*, 16 September 2019.

Chapter 17

AFP, 'Clermont "responsible" for Jamie Cudmore's concussion-related issues – neurologist', 22 January 2019.

Bleaney, R., 'Cillian Willis to sue Sale Sharks over concussion which ended his career', *The Guardian*, 23 August 2016.

Broadbent, R., 'Eubank calls for trial of concussion gumshield', *The Times*, 24 October 2019.

Bywater, A., 'Howley: France broke the rules', *Sunday Times*, 19 March 2017.

Costello, M., 'Concussion in sport: Are safety and equality compatible in women's boxing?' www.bbc.co.uk/sport, 14 December 2017.

Covassin, T. and Elbon, R.J., 'The female athlete: The role of gender in the assessment and management of sport-related concussion', *Clin Sports Med*, 2011; 30: 125–131.

Critchley, M., 'Punch drunk syndrome: the chronic encephalopathy of boxers', *Hommage à Clovis Vincent*, 1949.

Critchley M., 'Medical aspects of boxing, particularly from a neurological point standpoint', *BMJ*, 1957; 1 5015: 357–362.

Crompton, S., 'Can lots of small blows to the head cause dementia?', *The Times*, 12 November 2019.

Cummiskey, G., 'Cillian Willis concussion case due before court next year', *The Irish Times*, 19 September 2018.

BIBLIOGRAPHY

Cummiskey, G., 'Cillian Willis to sue Sale Sharks over concussion. Case will the first time a professional rugby player has sued over head trauma', *Irish Times*, August 23, 2016.

Cummiskey, G., 'How head injuries finished the rugby career of Cillian Willis', *Irish Times*, 23 March 2019.

Daily Mail, 'The Catch-22 of concussion: Top surgeon claims team doctors fear the sack ... for trying to protect their players', 9 November 2014.

Davidson, A., 'Ryan Giggs criticised as Daniel James "fakes his concussion"', *The Times*, 15 October 2019.

England Professional Rugby Injury Surveillance Project Steering Group, 2017–2018 RFU PRISP report.

Gilmartin, S. and Ryan, J., 'A temporal comparative study of women's rugby injuries presenting to an emergency department', *Irish Medical Journal*, 112(9); 1004.

Hamilton, J., 'Where to draw the line?', *Sunday Times*, 29 July 2018.

Hughes, M., 'Vertonghen blow prompts FIFA to look at concussion substitutes', *The Times*, 2 May 2019.

Hume, P., et al., 'A comparison of cognitive function in former rugby union players compared with former non-contact-sport players and the impact of concussion history', *Sports Medicine*, 2016; 47(6): 1–12.

Jacob, G., 'Jan Vertonghen "not concussed" against Ajax', *The Times*, 3 May 2019.

Jones, C., 'Cillian Willis: Premiership coaches fear impact of legal action over concussion', www.bbc.co.uk/sport, 25 August 2016.

Jones, S., 'Rugby set to make jackal an endangered species', *Sunday Times*, 24th March 2019.

Joyce, P. and Ziegler, M., 'Hapless Lorius Karius was concussed during Champions League Final, say doctors', *The Times*, 5 June 2018.

Kay, B., 'Tough training will serve England well even if it boils over', *The Times*, 2 March 2019.

Kay, B., 'Using ex-players on panels is the only way to get fair hearing,' *The Times*, 22 September 2018.

Kerr, Z.Y., et al., 'Concussion incidence and trends in 20 high school sports', *Pediatrics*, 2019 Nov;144(5): e20192180.

Ling, H., et al., 'Mixed pathologies including chronic traumatic encephalopathy account for dementia on retired association football (soccer) players', *Acta Neuropathol*, 2017; 133: 337–352.

Lowe, A., 'Almost half of world's top players felt pressured to play while injured', *The Times*, 4 December 2018.

Lowe, A., 'Call to ban tackles above waist', *The Times*, 22 December 2018.

Lowe, A., 'Panel will review French "concussion" row', *The Times*, 6 February 2018.

Lowe, A., 'Plan to ban rugby tackles above the waist', *The Times*, 9 August 2019.

Lowe, A., 'Rugby World Cup: Concussion rate falls amid crackdown on high tackles', *The Times*, 30 October 2019.

Mackay, D.F., et al., 'Neurodegenerative disease mortality among former professional soccer players'. *N England J Med* 2019: 381: 1801–1808.

Martland, H., 'Punch drunk', *Journal of the American Medical Association*, 1928; 91(15): 1103–1107.

Meagher, G., 'Marcus Smith lands 26 points for Harlequins as Sale are shredded. Tom Curry injured in heavy defeat', *The Observer*, 1 September 2018.

Milburn, P., 'Brute force: reducing the impact of rugby collisions', theconversation.com, 10 April 2014.

Omalu, B., et al., 'Chronic traumatic encephalopathy in a National Football League player', *Neurosurgery*, 2005; 57(1): 128–134.

O'Reilly, P., 'Whistle blown on high hits', *Sunday Times*, 15 September 2019.

Peters, S., 'As Sale struggle for form, Steve Diamond continues to look out of touch with the modern game', *The Independent*, 23 September 2019.

Peters, S., 'New tackle rules won't reduce concussion' *Sunday Times*, 29 July 2018.

Peters, S., 'Rugby's concussion tests are "laughable", claims England star Corbisiero', *Daily Mail Online*, 8 March 2014.

Quinlan, A., 'Alan Quinlan: Yes, rugby matters, but so does a person's life', *Irish Independent*, 24 September 2016.

Robinson, G., 'Shocking Toulouse concussion highlights powerless governance', *Sydney Morning Herald*, 15 May 2014.

Rudd, A., 'Vertongen sparks fears by returning to pitch despite sickening blow', *The Times*, 1 May 2019.

rugbyandthelaw.com, 'The Cilllian Willis Case', 13 February 2019.

Rugby World, 'International Survey Highlights Player Concerns', January 2019.

Schaerlaeckens, L., 'U.S. Soccer makes right call in proposing youth ban on heading', sports.yahoo.com, 10 November 2015.

Schofield, D., 'Florian Fitz concussion case highlights persistent danger to players', *The Times*, 17 May 2014.

Slot, O., 'Concussion is terrifying rugby into making mistakes', *The Times*, 6 February 2018.

Slot, O., 'I applaud trial but it just won't work', *The Times*, 9 August 2019.

Slot, O., 'Lower tackle height trial for juniors', *The Times*, 26 May 2018.

Slot, O., 'Pat Lambie: After five concussions I was relieved when a broken knee ended my career', *The Times*, 4 March 2019.

Slot, O., 'The trial that fixed rugby? Not so simple', *The Times*, 8 December 2018.

Slot, O., 'Trial Law to lower rugby tackle height', *The Times*, 25 July 2018.

Slot, O., 'Will rugby look the same in ten years' time', *The Times*, 25 July 2018.

Slot, Owen, 'Rise in concussions ends low tackle trial', *The Times*, 25 January 2019.

Smith, G., 'Shearer tackles dementia with a deft touch', *The Times*, 14 November 2017.

Souster, M., 'David Denton forced to quit rugby after concussion injury', *The Times*, 16 September 2019.

Taylor, L., 'Do Schär and Ospina incidents show football has a concussion problem?', *The Guardian*, 28 March 2019.

The Times, 'Tinkering with tackling is only right', 15 January 2019.

Waldron, T., 'English Premier League Adopts New In-Game Concussion Rules', archive. thinkprogress.org, 14 August 2014.

Walsh, D., 'Concussion, dementia – rugby faces a crisis', *Sunday Times*, 19 March 2017.

Walsh, D., 'We all enjoy physicality and fearlessness in rugby games, but the death of a young player in France proves the sport has become far too violent', *Sunday Times*, 16 December 2018.

Warshaw, A., 'FIFA medical chief d'Hooghe uses Shar incident to warn of dangers of concussion', www.insideworldfootball.com, 1 April 2019.

Westerby, J., 'Abuse of Head Injury protocols is inevitable, says expert', *The Times*, 21 March 2017.

Westerby, J., 'Drop tackle height further', *The Times*, 26 July 2018.

Westerby, J., 'Extra time for spit test', *The Times*, 5 October 2017.

Westerby, J., 'Harry Ellis: I was lost after I retired. There is no quick fix for depression', *The Times*, 2 March 2019.

Winter, H., 'Hard medical facts that football can no longer ignore', *The Times*, 22 October 2019.

www.bbc.co.uk/sport, 'George North: Northampton Saints avoid sanction over head injury', 21 December 2016.

www.bbc.co.uk/sport, 'Pat Lambie: Racing 92 and South Africa fly-half retires with concussion symptoms', 20 January 2019.

www.bbc.co.uk/sport, 'Rugby Concussions: RFU head of medicine defends HIA process', 18 January 2017.

www.bbc.co.uk/sport, 'Rugby Injuries: Eight-point plan to reduce risks includes review of laws,' 26 March 2018.

www.bbc.co.uk/sport, 'Six Nations: France HIAs against Ireland under investigation', 4 February 2018.

www.bbc.co.uk/sport, 'Uini Atonio: France rebuked over Head Injury prop swap against Wales', 16 June 2017.

Ziegler, M., 'Doctor admits he made a mistake over Nordin Amrabat concussion', *The Times*, 22 June 2018.

Ziegler, M., 'Medics need instant video to assess head injuries', *The Times*, 15 October 2019.

Ziegler, M., 'Uefa calls for temporary subs in concussion cases', *The Times*, 30 May 2019.

Chapter 18

Bolton, P., 'Diamond so abrasive', *Daily Telegraph*, 7 February 2005.

Daily Mail, 'Bloodgate doctor Wendy Chapman cleared of deception over cutting rugby player's lip', 26 August 2010.

Hathaway, A., 'Despairing Saints denied at the death', *Sunday Times*, 6 February 2005.

Jacob, G., 'West Ham career over for Carroll', *The Times*, 13 March 2019.

Jones, S., 'Hill leads rout in second half', *Sunday Times*, 8 April 2001.

Moore, B., 'Bloodgate doctor Wendy Chapman must be allowed to return to work', *Daily Telegraph*, 26 August 2010.

Northcroft, J., 'Can Carroll be fit for purpose', *Sunday Times*, 25 August 2019.

Roan, D., 'British Cycling: Team Sky "gamed system" over use of therapeutic use exemptions', www.bbc.co.uk/sport, 20 November 2017.

Sharp, J.C.M., Murray, G.D., and Macleod, D.A.D., 'A unique insight into the incidence of rugby injuries using referee replacement reports', *Br J Sports Med*, 2001; 35: 34–37.

Souster, M., 'Richards: England "cheated at World Cup"', *Sunday Times*, 14 April 2019.

The Guardian, 'Newcastle's Carroll arrested over attack on woman', 21 September 2008.

Westerby, J., 'I feel sick reliving it every day', *The Times*, 11 April 2019.

www.bbc.co.uk/sport, 'Steve Diamond: Sale Sharks director of rugby defends methods after row', 1 January 2019.

www.casemine.com/judgement/uk, Brennan vs Health Professions Council, 2011.

Young, C., 'Steven Taylor's jaw broken after "bust up" with Newcastle team-mate Andy Carroll', *Daily Mail*, 23 March 2010.

Chapter 19

Active People Survey, 10 October 2015–September 2016, Sport England.

Chapter 20

Hansen, S., 'Waisake Naholo back from broken leg to make World Cup debut against Georgia', *Belfast Telegraph*, 30 September 2015.

Hooper, R., 'Bradley Wiggins out of The Jump after breaking leg', *Huffington Post*, 13 February 2017.

Jack Fingleton Obituary, *Wisden Cricketers' Almanack 1982* (London: Queen Anne Press, 1982).

Kenny, S., 'Sir Bradley Wiggins Just Became the Latest Athlete to Break a Bone on Channel 4's "The Jump"', Mpora.com, 13 February 2017.

Lowe, A., 'A witchdoctor found three lady spirits who wanted to punish me, *The Times*, 9 November 2017.

Otto, T., 'All Blacks star makes miracle recovery from broken leg thanks to witchdoctor', www.news.co.au, 8 September 2015.

Peters, S., 'Joe Marler recovered from broken leg in less than a month after drinking two pints of full fat milk a day', *Daily Mail Online*, 2 February 2017.

Price, R., 'All Black Waisake Naholo's traditional healing raises scepticism in surgeon', www.stuff.co.nz, 31 August 2015.

Radd, A., 'Northamptonshire. Gone South', *Wisden Cricketers' Almanack 2005*, (London: Queen Anne Press, 2005).

Swann, G., *The Breaks Are Off* (London: Hodder & Stoughton, 2011).

Tucker, J., 'Waisake Naholo's so-called "miracle cure" no surprise to those familiar with traditional medicine www.stuff.co.nz, October 9 , 2015.

TV New Zealand, 27 September 2015.

www.bt.com/sport, 'Joe Marler to miss start of Six Nations after suffering leg fracture', 12 January 2017.

Chapter 21

Austin, E., 'It might have looked like Ellie had it all, but she didn't feel it', *Sunday Times Magazine*, 23 September 2018.

Barnes, S., 'Ben Stokes trial: cricket's wild men know no boundaries', *Sunday Times*, 19 August 2018.

Briggs, S., 'Amiss unearths helmet that changed the world', *Daily* Telegraph, 28 April 2005.

Bruckner, P., et al., 'Traumatic cricket-related fatalities in Australia: a historical review of media reports', *Medical Journal of Australia*, 2018; 208(6): 261–264.

Carrick, M., *Between the Lines: My Autobiography* (London: Blink Publishing, 2018).

Chalabi, M., 'How many Britons have taken illegal drugs and who are they?' *The Guardian*, 25 July 2013.

Christie, C.J., Todd, A.I., King, G.A., 'The energy cost of batting during a simulated batting work out', *Science and Medicine in Sport and Exercise*, 2008; 11: 581–584.

Davis, N., 'What forced cricketer James Taylor to retire?', *The Guardian*, 16 April 2016.

Di Pietro, V., et al., 'MicroRNAs as novel biomarkers for the diagnosis and prognosis of mild and severe traumatic brain injury', *Journal of Neurotrauma*, 2017; 34:1948–1956.

Drezner, J.A., et al., 'Electrocardiographic interpretation in athletes: the "Seattle Criteria"', *British Journal of Sports Medicine*, 2013; 47: 122–124.

Finocchiaro, G., et al., 'Etiology of sudden death in sports: Insights from a United Kingdom regional registry', *J Am Coll Cardiology*, 2016; 67(18): 2108–2115.

Frith, D., *Silence of the Heart*. (Edinburgh: Mainstream Publishing, 2001).

Heitger, M., et al., 'Impaired eye movements in post-concussion syndrome indicate suboptimal brain function beyond the influence of depression, malingering or intellectual ability', *Brain*, 209; 132: 2850–2871.

Hill, A., 'Cricket stress drives players to suicide', *The Guardian*, 22 April 2001.

ICC News, 'ICC set to implement WADA-compliant code', 15 July 2010.

Jones, M.E., et al., 'Osteoarthritis and other long-term health conditions in former elite cricketers', *Journal of Science and Sports Medicine in Sport*, 2018; 21: 558–563.

Link, M.S., Estes, N.A.M. III, 'Sudden cardiac death in the athlete: bridging the gaps between evidence, policy and practice', *Circulation*, 2012; 125: 516–524.

List of Association Footballers who died while playing. Wikipedia.

Mitchell, J.H., et al., 'Task Force 8: Classification of Sports', *JACC* 2005; 45(8): 1364–1367.

National Institute on Drug Abuse. National Institutes of Health (USA). Report 2001.

Noakes, T.D., Durandt, J.J., 'Physiological requirements of cricket', *J Sports Sciences*, 2000; 18: 919–929.

Orchard, J.W., et al., 'Incidence and prevalence of elite male cricket injuries using updated consensus definitions', *Open Access Journal of Sports Medicine*, 2016: 7; 187–194.

Pelliccia, A. et al., 'Recommendations for competitive sports participation in athletes with cardiovascular disease', *European Heart Journal*, 2005; 26: 1422–1445.

Preston, N., 'Recodification of the Laws', *Wisden Cricketers' Almanac 1980* (London: Queen Anne Press, 1980).

Preston, N., 'The Ugly Helmet', *Wisden Cricketer's Almanac 1979* (London: Queen Anne Press, 1979).

Sharma, S., et al., 'Cardiac screening before participation in sports, *The New England Journal of Medicine*, 2013; 369: 21;2049–2053.

Slot, O., 'Will rugby still look the same in ten years' time?', *The Times*, 25 July 2018.

Stokes, B., *Fire Starter* (London: Headline Publishing, 2017).

Taliep, M.S., et al., 'The effect of a 12-over bowling spell on bowling accuracy and pace in cricket fast bowlers', *J Human Movement Studies*, 2003; 45: 197–217.

USA Today, 'A timeline of MLB's drug-testing rules', 28 March 2014.

Winter, H., 'World Mental Health Day: Football leading the way on breaking silence about depression', *The Times*, 10 October 2018.

Woodcock, J., 'Donning the Helmet', *Wisden Cricketers' Almanac 1981* (London: Queen Anne Press, 1981).

Woodcock, J., 'More Bouncers', *Wisden Cricketers Almanac 1982* (London: Queen Anne Press, 1982).

www.bbc.co.uk/sport, 'Ellie Soutter death: father criticises pressure on athletes', 31 July 2018.

www.bbc.co.uk/sport, 'Kate Cross: England Bowler "didn't' know her purpose" during anxiety struggles', 16 August 2018.

Chapter 22

Bowes, W.E., 'F.S. Trueman – Fiery Fred', *Wisden Cricketers' Almanack 1970* (London: Sporting Handbooks Ltd, 1970).

Brian Taylor Obituary, *The Times*, 26 June 2017

Dennis, R., et al., 'Bowling workload and the risk of injury in elite cricket fast bowlers', *J Sci and Med in Sport*, 2003; 6(3): 359–367.

Dennis, R.J., Finch, C.F., Farhart, P.J., 'Is bowling workload a risk factor for injury to Australian junior cricket fast bowlers?', *British Journal of Sports Medicine*, 2005; 39: 843–846.

Fordyce, T., 'English Cricket's Blackout', www.bbc.co.uk/sport, 22 May 2007.

Gregory, P.L., Batt, M.E., Wallace, W.A., 'Is risk of fast bowling injury in cricketers greatest in those who bowl most? A cohort of young English fast bowlers', *British Journal of Sports Medicine*, 2004; 38(2)P 125–128.

Joyce, P., 'Rooney: Watford defeat spelt end of United career', *The Times*, 11 July 2017.

Kuper, S. and Szymanski S., *Soccernomics* (London: Harper Collins, 2018).

Orchard, J.W., James, T., Portus, M., 'Fast bowlers in cricket demonstrate up to 3- to 4-week delay between high workloads and increased risk of injury', *AJSM*, 2009; 37: 1186–1192.

Paton, G., 'Only a third of schools offer cricket', *Daily Telegraph*, 20 May 2010.

Petersen, C.J., et al., 'Movement patterns in cricket vary by both position and game format', *J Sports Sci*, 2010; 28: 45–52.

Rosenwater, I., 'A History of Wicket-covering in England', *Wisden Cricketers' Almanack 1970* (London: Sporting Handbooks Ltd, 1970).

Sajad, K., 'Where are all the black English cricketers?' www.bbc.co.uk/sport, 1 August 2018.

Selvey, M., 'Frank Tyson: perhaps the fastest bowler of them all', *The Guardian* 27 September 2015.

Smith, E., 'Seventh Heaven for Jimmy as England Lord it over the Windies', *Sunday Times*, 10 September 2017.

The Economist, 'Class and cricket. A lower-order collapse', 12 March 2013.

Chapter 23

Watkins, S., *Beyond the Limit* (London: MacMillan, 2001)

Watkins, S., *Life at the Limit* (London: MacMillan, 1996)

Williams, A., 'Is this where Michael Schumacher suffered ski injury? Treacherous off-piste rocks where F1 ace is believed to have fallen are revealed', *Daily Mail Online*, 29 January 2013.

Chapter 24

Allen, N., et al., 'The effect of a comprehensive injury audit program on injury incidence in ballet: A 3-year prospective study', *Clin J Sports Med*, 2013;23(5): 373–378.

Allen N., et al., 'Musculoskeletal injuries in dance: A systematic review', *International Journal of Physical Medicine and Rehabilitation*, 2014; 3: 1.

Drinkwater, B.L., et al., 'Bone mineral density after resumption of menses in amenorrheic athletes', *JAMA*, 1986; 256: 380–382.

Evening Standard, 'Begona Cao gets right to the pointe', 20 July 2011.

Hewett, E.M., Tufano, J.J., 'Bone health in female ballet dancers: a review', *European Journal of Sport and Exercise Sciences*, 2015; 3: 2.

Hoch, A.Z., et al., 'Association between the female athlete triad and endothelial dysfunction in dancers', *Clin J Sports Med*, 2011; 21: 119–125.

John, E., 'Begona Cao. I was doing a solo and heard my foot crack', *The Guardian*, 5 September 2006.

Justin Howse Obituary, *Daily Telegraph*, 3 February 2013.

Kadel, N.J., Teitz, C.C., Kronmal, R.A., 'Stress fractures in ballet dancers', *American Journal of Sports Medicine*, 1992; 20: 445–449.

Kaufmann, B.A., et al., 'Bone density and amenorrhoea in ballet dancers are related to decreased metabolic rate and lower leptin levels', *The Journal of Clinical Endocrinology and Metabolism*, 2002; 87: 2777–2783.

Liederbach, M., 'Functional testing and evaluation of the dancer. Proceedings of the Principles of Dance Medicine Conference', *NYU Hospital for Joint Diseases*, 2007.

Luke, A.C., et al., *Determinants of injuries in young dancers*, Med Probl Perform Art, 2002; 17(3): 105–112.

Mountjoy, M., et al., 'IOC consensus statement: beyond the Female Athlete Triad – Relative Energy Deficiency in Sport (RED-S)', *BJSM*, 2014: 48; 491–497.

Raastad, R.S., Raastad, T., Sundgot-Borgen, J., 'Prevalence of the female athletic triad in the Norwegian National Ballet', selected abstracts from the 15 Annual Meeting of the International Association for Dance Medicine and Science, 2005; 9: 63.

Ribbans, W.J., 'Best foot forward: An orthopaedic odyssey through the world of dance', *J Applied Arts and Health*, 2010; 1(1): 52–60.

Roberts, K.J., Nelson, N.G., McKenzie, L., 'Dance-related injuries in children and adolescents treated in US emergency departments in 1991–2007', *J Phys Act Health*, 2013; 10(2): 143–150.

The Times, 'Dancers in Dash from Hotel to save Ballet', 17 January 1995.

www.olympic.org, IOC Consensus Statement on the Female Athlete Triad, 2005.

Yannaouklia, M., et al., 'Bone mineral density in young active females: the case of dancers', *Int J Sport and Nutrition and Exercise Metabolism*, 2004; 14: 285–297.

Chapter 25

Breithaupt, M.D., 'Zur pathologie des menschlichen fusses [To the pathology of the human foot]. *Med Zeitung*, 1855; 24: 169.

Daily Telegraph, 'Dates prove Christine Ohuruogu is no cheat', 8 November 2007.

Ennis, J., *Unbelievable* (London: Hodder & Stoughton, 2012).

Hemery, D., *Another Hurdle* (Portsmouth, New Hampshire: Heinemann, 1976).

Hullinger, C.W., 'Insufficiency fracture of the calcaneus similar to March Fracture of the metatarsal', *JBJS Am* 1944; 26(4): 751–757.

Jones, R., 'Fracture of the base of the fifth metatarsal bone by indirect violence', *Ann Surg*, 1902; 35: 697–700.

Le Vay, D., *The History of Orthopaedics* (Nashville, TN: Parthenon Publishing, 1990).

Rogers, J., et al., 'Posterior ankle impingement syndrome: A clinical review with reference to horizontal jump athletes', *Acta Orthop Belg*, 2010; 76(5): 572–579.

Rutherford, G., *Unexpected* (London: Simon & Schuster, 2016).

Sir Roger Bannister Obituary, *The Times*, 5 March 2018.

www.bbc.co.uk/sport, 'Olympic Champion Dame Kelly Holmes "cut herself daily"', 24 September 2017.

www.bbc.co.uk/sport, 'Rutherford braced for trials test', 19 July 2007.

Chapter 26

British Orthopaedic Association, 'Consultant Staffing Requirements for an Orthopaedic Service in the National Health Service', 1995.

Bysouth, A., 'Winter Olympic stats: Norway's record haul, Germany's Golden Games and more', www.bbc.co.uk/sport, 25 February 2018.

Davas, M., 'Stress fractures of the tibia in athletes or "shin soreness"', *JBJS Br,* 1958; 40(B): 227–239.

Galasko, C. and Batt, M., 'Taking the Plunge', *Surgeons' News,* September 2018.

Kuper, S. and Szymanski S., *Soccernomics* (London: Harper Collins, 2018).

Noakes, Tim., *Challenging Beliefs* (London: Zebra Press, 2012).

Royal College of Surgeons of Edinburgh, 'The Sporting Knife. Sports medicine through the ages' in *From Here Health,* the College's official quincentenary publication, 2006.

Williams, J.G.P., *Sports Medicine* (London: Edward Arnold Publishers, 1962)

Chapter 27

Arnot, C., 'Injury Time', *The Guardian,* 21 November 2000.

Black, S., *Blackie: The Steve Black Story* (Edinburgh: Mainstream Sport, 2005).

Kuper, S. and Szymanski S., *Soccernomics* (London: Harper Collins, 2018).

Chapter 28

Amin, N.H., et al., 'Performance outcomes after repair of complete Achilles tendon ruptures in national basketball association players', *Am J Sports Med,* 2013; 41(8): 1864–1868.

Andrew, J., 'Manchester City star Gabriel Jesus gives the thumbs up after he undergoes operation on broken metatarsal', *Daily Mail,* 17 February 2017.

BMJ, 'Doctors' use of Facebook, Twitter and WhatsApp leads to 28 GMC investigations', 9 September 2017.

Brennan, S., 'Manchester City player Ilkay Gundogan explains why he'll never be the same player again', *Manchester Evening News,* 12 January 2018.

Cash, P., 'Nadal must shorten points if he wants to lengthen his career', *Sunday Times,* 9 September 2018.

Ducker, J., 'Manchester City ready to sign Ilkay Gundogan despite injury after Pep Guardiola tells club to complete deal', *Daily Telegraph,* 22 May 2016.

Fraser, D., 'Sant Packing. Arsenal News: Gunners star Santi Cazorla flies out to Barcelona … to seek a cure for persistent Achilles injury', *Scottish Sun,* 20 November 2016.

General Medical Council, 'Advertising Guidance from the General Medical Council', October 1995.

Haskell, J., 'The toe pinged back like broken elastic', www.bbc.co.uk/sport, 6 September 2016.

Hirst, P., 'Courtois can leave, says Sarri', *The Times,* 6 August 2018.

Hughes, M., 'Arsenal turn to Emery', *The Times,* 22 May 2018.

Hughes, M. and Hirst, P., 'Mourinho orders United injury probe', *The Times,* 9 November 2016.

Irvine, D.H., 'The advertising of doctors' services', *Journal of Medical Ethics,* 1991; 17: 35–40.

Jackson, J., 'Vincent Kompany ruled out again as Manchester City target last 16', *The Guardian,* 22 November 2016.

Kirkley, A., et al., 'Operative versus non-operative treatment of Achilles tendon ruptures: a quantitative review', *Clin J Sports Med,* 1997; 7: 207–211.

Kuper, S. and Szymanski S., *Soccernomics* (London: Harper Collins, 2018).

Lowe, S., 'Santi Cazorla: "every time they sewed me up, it split again, more liquid"', *The Guardian*, 7 September 2018.

Morgan, S., 'From worse to worse. Santi Cazorla's injury is "worst I have known" says Arsene Wenger as he refuses to rule out midfielder never playing again', *The Sun*, 16 November 2017.

Myers, C., 'The "surgeon ego" must be excised to accelerate progress in surgical culture', *BMJ*, 24 November 2018.

Möller, M., et al., 'Acute rupture of the tendon Achilles: A prospective randomised study of comparison between surgical and non-surgical treatment', *JBJS Br*, 2001; 83: 843–848.

Parekh, S.G., et al., 'Epidemiology and outcomes of Achilles tendon ruptures in the National Football League', presented at the American Academy of Orthopaedic Surgeons 73rd Annual Meeting, Chicago, March 2006.

Robson, J., 'Man City midfielder De Bruyne is in the hands of the doctor Guardiola trusts most in bid to make Barcelona clash', *Manchester Evening Telegraph*, 5 October 2016.

Scott, C., 'It doesn't feel like a battle now, says Murray as he plots return', *The Times*, 7 March 2019.

Scott, C., 'Wimbledon is unlikely, says Murray', *The Times*, 7 March 2019.

Sokout, O., 'Santi Cazorla ends 636-day injury nightmare to play for Villarreal', *Marca*, 17 July 2018.

Stuart F., 'Murray eyes return after secret surgery', *The Times*, 9 January 2018.

Sweet, G., 'Jesus under knife. Gabriel Jesus has surgery in Barcelona to repair fractured metatarsal and faces eight weeks out', *The Sun*, 17 February 2017.

The Times, 'Bale in race to be fit for Wales's Ireland Qualifier', 25 November 2016.

The Times, 'Hudson-Odoi to miss Chelsea pre-season after surgery', 25 April 2019.

The Times, 'Rüdiger ruled out of Chelsea's run-in after knee surgery', 1 May 2019.

The Times Magazine, 'Meet my surgeon', 16 June 2018.

Wikipedia, List of Premier League Managers. Accessed 6 January 2019.

www.bbc.co.uk/sport, 'Santi Carzola: Villareal midfielder on Arsenal, gangrene and magic tricks', 20 September 2018.

www.skysports.com, 'Average tenure of managers in England just 1.23 years', 5 June 2015.

Ziegler, M., *The Times*, 18 January 2018.

Chapter 29
Ashton, N., 'Doc's Crock Shock. Sunderland sue doctor for £13 million over flop Ricky Alvarez in a lawsuit that could change transfers forever', *The Sun*, 13 September 2019.

Faculty of Occupational Medicine, 'Ethics Guidance for occupational health practice 2012'.

Faculty of Sport and Exercise Medicine, 'Code of Conduct, Clause 8.3', 2010.

Gaughan, J., 'Manchester United to spend more than £15m paying up Wayne Rooney contract as star agrees 50 per cent wage cut to rejoin Everton', *Daily Mail*, 7 July 2017.

General Medical Council, 'Good Medical Practice', 2013.

Keegan, M., 'Tottenham youngster who was left severely brain damaged after collapsing wins £7m in damages for club doctors' decision to let him play with known heart problem', *Daily Mail Online*, 4 October 2016.

Majendie, M., 'Rob Chakraverty: England football team doctor's job not in doubt despite injection controversy', *Evening Standard*, 5 March 2018.

NHS Litigation Authority. Report 2015–2016.

NHS Resolution. Annual Report and Accounts, 2018–2019.

Redelmeier, D.A. and Greenwald, J.A., 'Competing risks of mortality with marathons: retrospective analysis', *BMJ*, 2007; 335: 1275–1277.

Redman, N., 'Personal Risk Mitigation – Is your Indemnity fit for purpose?', BASEM Reports. Spring 2017.

Roan, D., 'British Cycling: Team Sky "gamed system" over use of therapeutic use exemptions', www.bbc.co.uk/sport, 20 November 2017.
Smyth, C., 'Health Service faces £77bn negligence claim', *The Times*, July 14 2018.
The Independent, 'Jack Collison: The story of one footballer's broken Premier League dreams', 7 November 2015.
The Times, 'Team Sky timeline: history of success and controversy', 12 December 2018.
www.bbc.co.uk/sport, 'Neymar: Paris St-Germain sign Barcelona forward for world record 222m euros', 3 August 2017.
Ziegler, M., 'Wiggins "Jiffy Bag" investigation may have been compromised', *The Times*, 13 January 2018.

Chapter 30
Anderson, L., 'Bloodgate: were the punishments fair?', *Br J Sports Med,* 2011; 45(12); doi:10.1136/*BJSM*. 2011.083881.
Chartered Society of Physiotherapists, 'Core Standards of Practice (Standard 3.4)', 2005.
Collins, D., 'Doctors "spied on" ailing Sir Alex Ferguson in Salford Royal hospital', *Sunday Times*, 2 December 2018.
Daily Telegraph, 'Briton dies in Tour de France', 14 July 1967.
Daly, M. and Morris, J., 'Sir Bradley Wiggins: Former team doctor "surprised" at drug prescription', BBC News, 23 September 2016.
Devitt, B.M. and McCarthy, C., '"I am in blood Stepp'd in so far...": ethical dilemmas and the sorts team doctor', *Br J Sports Med,* 2010; 44: 175–178.
Doyle, G., 'Ireland's Conor Murray hits out at "mad injury rumours"', *The Times*, 24 October 2018.
Football League/Premier League Contract (Form 13A). Clause 6.2.2. 2010–2011.
Fraser, S., 'Andy Murray: My hip is killing me. I can't go through that anymore', *The Times*, 12 January 2018.
Fraser, S., 'Andy Murray interview: I can get back to the top – but third child comes first', *The Times*, 11 October 2019.
Fraser, S., 'Andy's punishing regime worried me, says mother', *The Times*, 16 January 2019.
Fraser, S., 'Emotional Murray wins first title since operation', *The Times*, 21 October 2019.
Fraser, S., 'I don't know how long I'll last, says emotional Andy Murray after beating James Duckworth at Brisbane International', *The Times*, 1 January 2019.
Fraser, S., 'If I can play with a metal hip then so can Murray', *The Times*, 17 January 2019.
Fraser, S., 'I'd like to play until my eldest daughter is able to watch me', *The Times*, 9 January 2018.
Fraser, S., 'Murray eyes return after hip surgery', *The Times*, 9 January 2018.
Fraser, S., 'Murray hope fading.', *The Times*, 14 January 2019.
Fraser, S., 'Murray playing through the pain', *The Times*, 31 December 2018.
General Medical Council, 'Guidelines: Confidentiality. Clause 34', 2009.
Green, M., *Nobody Hurt in Small Earthquake* (Portsmouth, New Hampshire: Heinemann,1990).
Hirst, P., 'United staff member taken to hospital,' *The Times*, 13 July 2019.
Holm, S. and McNamee, M., 'Ethics in sports medicine', *BMJ*, 2009;339.
Jacob, G., 'Jack Wilshere ruled out for six weeks as West Ham United sweat on Marko Arnautovic fitness', *The Times*, 18 September 2018.
John Orchard Retweeted: David J. Chao, MD @ProFootballDoc saying '"Surgery is success" now, is like "Excellent pick" right after draft. Time will tell. Hope it's true'.
Jordan, D., 'Andy Murray "battered and bruised" but hopeful after hip resurfacing', *The Times*, 29 January 2019.
Malone, R., 'England may be without Greaves', *Daily Telegraph*, 22 July 1966.
Medical Defence Union, 'Factsheet for Consultants: Sport and Exercise Medicine', 2009.
Orchard, J., 'Who owns the information?', *Br J Sports Med,* 2002; 36: 16–18.

Ribbans, W.J., et al., 'Sports medicine, confidentiality and the press', *BJSM*, 2013; 47(1): 40–43.

Roan, D., 'Patient confidentiality applies, unless you are a footballer', *The Cobbler*, Northampton Town match programme, 14 October 2018.

Scott, C., 'It doesn't feel like a battle now, says Murray as he plots return', *The Times*, 7 March 2019.

~~Scott, C., 'Wimbledon is unlikely, says Murray', *The Times*, 7 March 2019.~~

Slot, O., 'Murray to stay at Munster until 2022', *The Times*, 11 October 2018.

Tavares, S., 'Andy Murray injury: what is the Birmingham Hip Resurfacing System?', *The Times*, 12 January 2019.

www.bbc.co.uk/sport, 'Andy Murray: Former British number one has resurfacing surgery on hip', 29 January 2019.

www.whufc.com, 'Wilshere undergoes successful surgery', 17 September 2018.

Ziegler, M., 'Semenya hits IAAF with breach claim', *The Times*, 19 February 2019.

Chapter 31

Kujala, U.M., Sarna, S., Kaprio, J., 'Cumulative incidence of Achilles tendon rupture and tendinopathy in male former elite athletes', *Clin J Sport Med*, 2005; 15(3): 133.

Myklebust, G., Skolberg, A., Bahr, R., 'ACL injury incidence in handball; 10 years after the Norwegian ACL prevention study: important lessons learned', *BJSM*, 2013;47(8); 476–479.

Rutherford, A., *A Brief History of Everyone Who Ever Lived. The Stories in Our Genes* (London: Weidenfeld & Nicolson, 2017).

Smith, O., 'Mapped: The world's tallest (and shortest) countries', *Daily Telegraph*, 7 October 2017.

van Middelkoop, M., Erasmus, M.C., 'Prevalence and incidence of lower extremity injuries in male marathon runners', *Scand J Med Sci Sports*, 2008; 18: 140–4.

Chapter 32

Conn, D., '"I thought it was appalling": anger over Atletico fans attending Anfield', *The Guardian*, 22 March 2020.

Corsin, A., et al., 'Football cannot restart soon during the COVID-19 emergency! A critical perspective from the Italian experience and a call for action'. *BJSM*, March 2020. doi:10.1136/bjsports-2020-102306

Ferguson, N.M., et al., 'Report 9: Impact of non-pharmaceutical interventions (NPIs) to reduce COVID-19 mortality and healthcare demand', Imperial College COVID-19 Response Team, 16 March 2020. DOI: https://doi.org/10.25561/77482

Mortimer, H., 'Coronavirus: Cheltenham Festival "may have accelerated" virus', www.bbc.co.uk/sport, 30 April 2020.

Myer, G.D., et al., 'Does the NFL lockout expose the Achilles Heel of competitive sport?' *J Orthop Sports Phys Ther*, 2011;41(10): 702–705.

Rees, P., 'Wales v Scotland Six Nations match called off 24 hours before kick-off', *The Guardian*, 13 March 2020.

Sabbagh, D., Morris, S., Cook, C., 'Experts call for inquiry into local death toll after Cheltenham Festival', *The Guardian*, 21 April 2020.

The Cricketer, 'County cricketers agree to extend support package to protect first-class game. Players from all 18 first-class counties have agreed to continue to be furloughed if requested, while wage deductions have been capped at 20 per cent', 1 June 2020.

The Independent, 'Premier League's restart hamstrung by injury fears', 11 June 2020.

Thorpe, L., 'Liverpool coronavirus deaths soared after Athletic Madrid match, 3 June 2020.

www.bbc.co.uk/sport, 'Coronavirus: Calls for inquiry on Cheltenham Festival go-ahead', 23 April 2020.

www.bbc.co.uk/sport, 'Premier League begins fixture planning for 2022 World Cup season', 24 October 2019.

BIBLIOGRAPHY

www.bbc.co.uk/sport, 'RFU says grassroots playing return in England approved by DCMS', 8 August 2020.

Chapter 33

Ardern, C.L., et al., 'Fifty-five per cent return to competitive sport following anterior cruciate ligament reconstruction surgery: an updated systematic review and meta-analysis including aspects of physical functioning and contextual factors', *Br J Sports Med*, 2014; 48(21): 1543–1552.

British Orthopaedic Association. Evidence submitted (WP 60) to Parliamentary Select Committee (WP60). 15 March 2006.

Chambers, S., et al., 'The accuracy of magnetic resonance imaging (MRI) in detecting meniscal pathology', *J R Nav Med Serv*, 2014; 100(2): 157–160.

Lowe, A., 'Miracle and magic sponge ease fitness worries for Jones', *The Times*, 31 January 2018.

McCutchan, J.D.S., Bewley, B., Redden, J.F., 'Does knee ligament disruption spell the end of a professional footballer's career? A study of outcome following reconstruction', *JBJS Br*, 1994.76-B: Suppl 1: 48.

Peters, S., 'George North: "It's amazing, I'm covering more ground – but taking more big hits"', *Sunday Times*, 28 October 2018.

Song, Y.D., et al., 'Is knee magnetic resonance imaging overutilized in current practice?', *Knee Surgery and Related Research*, 2015; 27(2): 95–100.

INDEX

van Persie, Robin 143–144, 146, 149
van Velze, Gerrit-Jan (GJ) 201
Vancouver 41
Varnish, Jess 161
Varsity Match 24
Vaughan, Michael 220
Verheijen, Raymond 149, 358
Vertongen, Jan 190
Vikharev, Sergei 150
Villa Park 21, 342
Vilsack, Tom 86
Voce, Bill 227, 245
von Ribbentrop, Joachim 56
Voronoff, Serge 133

Walcott, Theo 17
Wales 26, 56, 65, 136, 153, 178, 182, 193, 286, 292, 294, 343, 362
Walker, Kyle 345
Walker, Max 238
Waller, Max 230
Walsh, Stella (Stanisława Walasiewicz) 74
Walters, Dougie 213
Warburton, Sam 182
Ward, Stephen 163
Warne, Shane 233
Warner, Plum 213
Warren, Gavin 26, 347
Warrington Wolves 42
Warwick 337
Warwickshire 214, 237, 357
The Washington Post 61
Wasps RFC 11, 55, 161, 172, 195, 199–200
Waterloo 83
Waterville Valley 116
Watford 301, 346, 351, 360
Watkins, Sid, Professor 251–252
Watson, Anthony 183
Watson, Michael 120, 123–125
Watt, Steve 125
Webb, Jonathan 56

Webb, Neil 306
Webb, Sarah 72
Webster, Mike 188
Weitz, Greta 68
Wellington, Duke of 83
Welsh Institute for Sport 294
Wembley 21, 60, 120, 123, 137, 218, 246
Wenger, Arsène 146, 303
West Bromwich Albion 129, 188
West, Bryan 170
West Ham United 206, 301, 321
West Indies 218, 355
West Middlesex Hospital 175
Westaby, Stephen 183
Westgarth, Scott 126
Wexham Park 283
What'sApp 299
Whitby, Dennis 269
White, Cameron 34, 215
White Hart Lane 137, 225, 313
White Lodge, Richmond 258
Whitlock, Max 87
Wigan Borough 137
Wiggins, Bradley, Sir 165, 205, 211, 312, 322
Wilde, Oscar 195
Wilkinson, Jonny 28, 175–176, 292
Willey, David 215, 219
Willey, Peter 229
Williams, JGP (John) 282–283
Williams, JPR 56, 183
Williams, Sonny Boy 183–184
Williams, Tom 203
Willis, Cillian 199–200
Willis, Nigel 210
Wilshere, Jack 321
Wilson, David 252–253, 255
Wimbledon 16, 42, 58, 73
Windsor 58
Winehouse, Amy 50, 234
Winstone, Howard 125
Winter break 159, 359

Also available at all good book stores

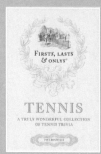

9781785316364

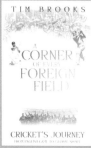

9781785316395

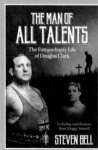

9781785316821

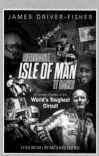

9781785315497

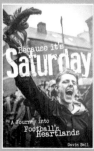

9781785316463

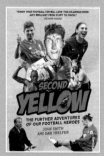

9781785316791

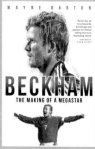

9781785316760

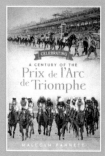

9781785317248

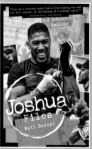

9781785313912

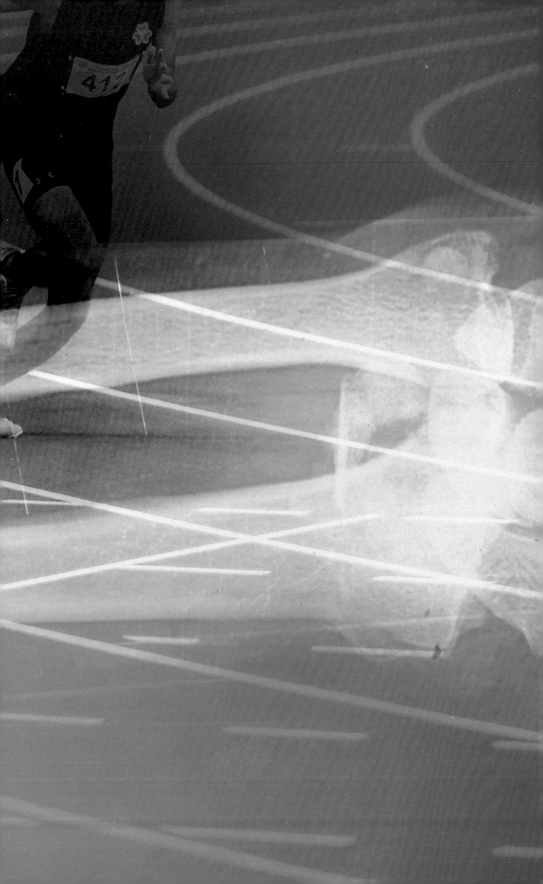